T0226984

Heart Failure in Adult Congenital Heart Disease

Editors

ALEXANDER R. OPOTOWSKY
MICHAEL J. LANDZBERG

HEART FAILURE CLINICS

www.heartfailure.theclinics.com

Consulting Editors
MANDEEP R. MEHRA
JAVED BUTLER

Founding Editor
JAGAT NARULA

January 2014 • Volume 10 • Number 1

ELSEVIER

1600 John F. Kennedy Boulevard • Suite 1800 • Philadelphia, Pennsylvania, 19103-2899

http://www.theclinics.com

HEART FAILURE CLINICS Volume 10, Number 1
January 2014 ISSN 1551-7136, ISBN-13: 978-0-323-26392-4

Editor: Barbara Cohen-Kligerman
Developmental Editor: Susan Showalter

© 2014 Elsevier Inc. All rights reserved.

This periodical and the individual contributions contained in it are protected under copyright by Elsevier, and the following terms and conditions apply to their use:

Photocopying
Single photocopies of single articles may be made for personal use as allowed by national copyright laws. Permission of the Publisher and payment of a fee is required for all other photocopying, including multiple or systematic copying, copying for advertising or promotional purposes, resale, and all forms of document delivery. Special rates are available for educational institutions that wish to make photocopies for non-profit educational classroom use. For information on how to seek permission visit www.elsevier.com/permissions or call: (+44) 1865 843830 (UK)/(+1) 215 239 3804 (USA).

Derivative Works
Subscribers may reproduce tables of contents or prepare lists of articles including abstracts for internal circulation within their institutions. Permission of the Publisher is required for resale or distribution outside the institution. Permission of the Publisher is required for all other derivative works, including compilations and translations (please consult www.elsevier.com/permissions).

Electronic Storage or Usage
Permission of the Publisher is required to store or use electronically any material contained in this periodical, including any article or part of an article (please consult www.elsevier.com/permissions). Except as outlined above, no part of this publication may be reproduced, stored in a retrieval system or transmitted in any form or by any means, electronic, mechanical, photocopying, recording or otherwise, without prior written permission of the Publisher.

Notice
No responsibility is assumed by the Publisher for any injury and/or damage to persons or property as a matter of products liability, negligence or otherwise, or from any use or operation of any methods, products, instructions or ideas contained in the material herein. Because of rapid advances in the medical sciences, in particular, independent verification of diagnoses and drug dosages should be made.

Although all advertising material is expected to conform to ethical (medical) standards, inclusion in this publication does not constitute a guarantee or endorsement of the quality or value of such product or of the claims made of it by its manufacturer.

Heart Failure Clinics (ISSN 1551-7136) is published quarterly by Elsevier Inc., 360 Park Avenue South, New York, NY 10010-1710. Months of publication are January, April, July, and October. Business and editorial offices: 1600 John F. Kennedy Boulevard, Suite 1800, Philadelphia, PA 19103-2899. Periodicals postage paid at New York, NY, and additional mailing offices. Subscription prices are USD 235.00 per year for US individuals, USD 382.00 per year for US institutions, USD 80.00 per year for US students and residents, USD 280.00 per year for Canadian individuals, USD 442.00 per year for Canadian institutions, USD 300.00 per year for international individuals, USD 442.00 per year for international institutions, and USD 100.00 per year for Canadian and foreign students/residents. To receive student and resident rate, orders must be accompanied by name of affiliated institution, date of term, and the *signature* of program/residency coordinator on institution letterhead. Orders will be billed at individual rate until proof of status is received. Foreign air speed delivery is included in all *Clinics* subscription prices. All prices are subject to change without notice. **POSTMASTER:** Send address changes to *Heart Failure Clinics*, Elsevier Health Sciences Division, Subscription Customer Service, 3251 Riverport Lane, Maryland Heights, MO 63043. **Customer Service: 1-800-654-2452 (US and Canada). From outside of the US and Canada, call 314-447-8871. Fax: 314-447-8029. For print support, e-mail: JournalsCustomerService-usa@elsevier.com. For online support, e-mail: JournalsOnlineSupport-usa@elsevier.com.**

Reprints. For copies of 100 or more of articles in this publication, please contact the Commercial Reprints Department, Elsevier Inc., 360 Park Avenue South, New York, NY 10010-1710. Tel.: 212-633-3874; Fax: 212-633-3820; E-mail: reprints@elsevier.com.

Heart Failure Clinics is covered in *MEDLINE/PubMed (Index Medicus).*

Printed and bound by CPI Group (UK) Ltd, Croydon, CR0 4YY

Transferred to digital print 2013

Contributors

CONSULTING EDITORS

MANDEEP R. MEHRA, MD
Professor of Medicine, Harvard Medical
School; Co-Director, BWH Cardiovascular; and
Executive Director, Center for Advanced Heart
Disease, Brigham and Women's Hospital,
Boston, Massachusetts

JAVED BUTLER, MD, MPH
Professor of Medicine, Director, Heart
Failure Research, Emory University, Atlanta,
Georgia

EDITORS

ALEXANDER R. OPOTOWSKY, MD, MPH
Boston Adult Congenital Heart and Pulmonary
Hypertension Service, Boston Children's
Hospital; Brigham and Women's Hospital,
Harvard Medical School, Boston,
Massachusetts

MICHAEL J. LANDZBERG, MD
Boston Adult Congenital Heart and Pulmonary
Hypertension Service, Boston Children's
Hospital; Brigham and Women's Hospital,
Harvard Medical School, Boston,
Massachusetts

AUTHORS

NASER AMMASH, MD
Professor of Medicine, Mayo Clinic, Rochester,
Minnesota

MAURICE BEGHETTI, MD
Pediatric Cardiology Unit, Department of the
Child and Adolescent, Children's Hospital,
University of Geneva, Geneva, Switzerland

PIERRE-LUC BERNIER, MD, MPH, FRCSC
Assistant Attending in Clinical Surgery,
Columbia University Medical Center,
New York, New York

WENDY M. BOOK, MD
Director, Division of Cardiology, Department of
Internal Medicine, Emory Adult Congenital
Heart Center; Professor of Medicine, School of
Medicine, Emory University, Atlanta, Georgia

CRAIG S. BROBERG, MD, MCR
Director, Adult Congenital Heart Program;
Associate Professor, Cardiovascular Medicine,
Knight Cardiovascular Institute, Oregon Health
and Science University, Portland, Oregon

JONATHAN BUBER, MD
Boston Adult Congenital Heart and Pulmonary
Hypertension Service, Department of
Cardiology, Boston Children's Hospital;
Department of Medicine, Brigham and
Women's Hospital, Boston, Massachusetts

LUKE J. BURCHILL, MBBS, PhD
Advanced Cardiac Imaging Fellow, Section of
Cardiovascular Imaging, Cleveland Clinic,
Cleveland, Ohio

JACK M. COLMAN, MD, FRCPC
University of Toronto Program in Pregnancy
and Heart Disease, Obstetric Medicine
Program, Division of Cardiology, Mount Sinai
Hospital; Toronto Congenital Cardiac Centre
for Adults, Peter Munk Cardiac Centre,
University Health Network, Toronto, Canada

GERHARD-PAUL DILLER, MD, PhD, MSc
Division of Adult Congenital and Valvular Heart
Disease, Department of Cardiovascular
Medicine, University Hospital Muenster,
Münster, Germany

ANNE M. DUBIN, MD
Professor of Pediatrics, Department of
Pediatric Cardiology, Lucile Packard
Children's Hospital, Stanford University,
Palo Alto, California

AKL C. FAHED, MD
Department of Genetics, Harvard Medical
School; Department of Medicine,
Massachusetts General Hospital, Boston,
Massachusetts

SUSAN M. FERNANDES, LPD, PA-C
Adult Congenital Heart Program at Stanford,
Lucile Packard Children's Hospital, Stanford
Hospital and Clinics, Stanford University
School of Medicine, Palo Alto, California

WAYNE J. FRANKLIN, MD
Director, Texas Adult Congenital Heart
Program, Texas Children's Hospital; Assistant
Professor of Medicine and Pediatrics, Baylor
College of Medicine, Houston, Texas

MARC GEWILLIG, MD, PhD
Professor of Pediatric Cardiology, Leuven
University Hospital, Leuven, Belgium

JONATHAN GINNS, MD
Assistant Professor of Clinical Medicine,
Columbia University Medical Center,
New York, New York

DAVID J. GOLDBERG, MD
Division of Cardiology, The Children's Hospital
of Philadelphia, Philadelphia, Pennsylvania

JASMINE GREWAL, MD, FRCPC
University of British Columbia Cardiac
Obstetrics Clinic and Pacific Adult Congenital
Heart Clinic, Division of Cardiology, St. Paul's
Hospital, University of British Columbia,
Vancouver, British Columbia, Canada

PAUL KHAIRY, MD, PhD
Director, Montreal Heart Institute, Adult
Congenital Heart Center and Canada Research
Chair, Université de Montréal, Montreal,
Québec, Canada

ADRIENNE H. KOVACS, PhD, CPsych
Psychologist, Toronto Congenital Cardiac
Centre for Adults, Peter Munk Cardiac Centre,
University Health Network; Assistant
Professor, Department of Psychiatry, Faculty
of Medicine, University of Toronto, Toronto,
Ontario, Canada

ERIC V. KRIEGER, MD
Assistant Professor of Medicine, Division of
Cardiology, Seattle Adult Congenital Heart
Service, Seattle Children's Hospital, University
of Washington Medical Center, University of
Washington School of Medicine, Seattle,
Washington

NEAL K. LAKDAWALA, MD
Division of Cardiovascular Medicine, Brigham
and Women's Hospital; Division of Cardiology,
VA Boston Health Care, Harvard Medical
School, Boston, Massachusetts

MICHAEL J. LANDZBERG, MD
Boston Adult Congenital Heart and Pulmonary
Hypertension Service, Boston Children's
Hospital; Brigham and Women's Hospital,
Harvard Medical School, Boston,
Massachusetts

ARIANE J. MARELLI, MD, MPH
Professor of Medicine and Director, McGill
Adult Unit for Congenital Heart Disease
(MAUDE Unit), McGill University Health Center,
McGill University, Montreal, Quebec, Canada

GIUSEPPE MARTUCCI, MD, FRCPC
Department of Interventional Cardiology,
McGill University Health Centre, Royal Victoria
Hospital, Montréal, Québec, Canada

JOHN E. MAYER Jr, MD
Cardiovascular Surgery, Boston Children's
Hospital; Professor of Surgery, Harvard
Medical School, Boston, Massachusetts

DOFF MCELHINNEY, MD, FACC
Department of Pediatrics, Langone Medical
Center, New York University, New York,
New York

LUC MERTENS, MD, PhD
Section Head Echocardiography, and
Professor, Pediatrics, The Hospital for Sick
Children, University of Toronto, Toronto,
Ontario, Canada

SEEMA MITAL, MD
Division of Cardiology, Department of
Pediatrics, Hospital for Sick Children,
University of Toronto, Toronto, Ontario,
Canada

BLANDINE MONDÉSERT, MD
Adult Congenital Center, Montreal Heart
Institute, Université de Montréal, Montreal,
Québec, Canada

PHILIP MOONS, PhD, RN
Professor, Department of Public Health and
Primary Care, KU Leuven; Advanced Practice
Nurse, Division of Congenital and Structural
Cardiology, Department of Cardiovascular
Sciences, University Hospitals Leuven,
Leuven, Belgium; Guest Professor, The Heart
Centre, Copenhagen University Hospital,
Copenhagen, Denmark

DAVID LUÍS SIMÓN MORALES, MD
Professor of Surgery and Pediatrics, Clark-
Helmsworth Chair of Pediatric Cardiothoracic
Surgery, Chief, Pediatric Cardiothoracic
Surgery, Executive Co-Director, Cardiovascular
Surgery, Cincinnati Children's Hospital Medical
Center, Cincinnati, Ohio

KARA S. MOTONAGA, MD
Clinical Assistant Professor of Pediatrics,
Stanford University, Palo Alto, California

VENKATACHALAM MULUKUTLA, MD
Cardiology Fellow, Pediatric Cardiology,
Texas Children's Hospital, Houston, Texas

DARREN MYLOTTE, MB, MRCPI, MD
Department of Interventional Cardiology,
McGill University Health Centre, Royal Victoria
Hospital, Montréal, Québec, Canada

HIDEO OHUCHI, MD, PhD
Departments of Pediatric Cardiology and Adult
Congenital Heart Disease, National Cerebral
and Cardiovascular Center, Suita, Osaka,
Japan

ALEXANDER R. OPOTOWSKY, MD, MPH
Boston Adult Congenital Heart and Pulmonary
Hypertension Service, Boston Children's
Hospital; Brigham and Women's Hospital,
Harvard Medical School, Boston,
Massachusetts

**NICOLO PIAZZA, MD, PhD, FRCPC, FESC,
FACC**
Department of Interventional Cardiology,
McGill University Health Centre, Royal Victoria
Hospital, Montréal, Québec, Canada

JONATHAN RHODES, MD
Associate Professor of Pediatrics, Harvard
Medical School; Department of Cardiology,
Boston Children's Hospital, Boston,
Massachusetts

AMY E. ROBERTS, MD
Division of Genetics, Department of
Cardiology, Boston Children's Hospital,
Boston, Massachusetts

FRED H. RODRIGUEZ III, MD
Assistant Professor of Medicine and
Pediatrics, Section of Cardiology, Sibley Heart
Center Cardiology, Emory University, Atlanta,
Georgia

ROBERT E. SHADDY, MD
Jennifer Terker Professor of Pediatrics, Chief,
Division of Pediatric Cardiology, Vice Chair,
The Children's Hospital of Philadelphia,
Perelman School of Medicine, University of
Pennsylvania, Philadelphia, Pennsylvania

CANDICE K. SILVERSIDES, MD, FRCPC
University of Toronto Program in Pregnancy
and Heart Disease, Obstetric Medicine
Program, Division of Cardiology, Mount Sinai
Hospital; Toronto Congenital Cardiac Centre
for Adults, Peter Munk Cardiac Centre,
University Health Network, Toronto, Canada

GARRICK C. STEWART, MD
Center for Advanced Heart Disease, Division of
Cardiovascular Medicine, Brigham and
Women's Hospital; Instructor in Medicine,
Harvard Medical School, Boston,
Massachusetts

CHET R. VILLA, MD
Cardiology Fellow, Cincinnati Children's
Hospital Medical Center, Cincinnati, Ohio

Contents

> The impact of lifelong exposure to myocardial dysfunction in populations with congenital heart disease (CHD) is becoming increasingly recognized. Most children born with CHD now reach adulthood and the long-term sequelae of treatment are contributing to substantial comorbidity. The combination of structural changes present at birth with changes resulting from cardiac surgery can result in heart failure. This article reports on the current state of knowledge on the epidemiology of heart failure in this patient population.

> Although heart failure is a diagnosis made on clinical grounds, cardiac imaging remains essential for quantifying ventricular remodeling and function, and for identifying potentially reversible causes of heart failure. Various nongeometric methods for the assessment of ventricular function have been developed, and 3-dimensional imaging is also gaining ground in its clinical applications. This review focuses on the application of noninvasive imaging strategies in the assessment of heart failure in congenital heart disease, specifically echocardiography, cardiac magnetic resonance imaging, and computed tomography. Both traditional and emerging techniques are discussed, and their potential applications and limitations are explored.

> As the longevity of patients with congenital heart disease improves, the number surviving to adulthood will continue to rise. Consequently, practicing physicians can expect to encounter an increasing number of adult patients with various congenital cardiac conditions. Impaired exercise tolerance in this patient population is exceptionally common; adult patients with congenital heart disease have reduced exercise capacity compared with healthy, age-matched counterparts. The different methods of evaluating exercise capacity, the characteristic physiologic abnormalities encountered in patients with various congenital cardiac conditions, the pathophysiologic mechanisms that may account for these abnormalities, and the clinical implications of these findings are discussed.

> Complex congenital heart disease (CHD) is a chronic medical condition to which patients are expected to adapt throughout their lives. Many patients are at risk of

developing heart failure in adulthood and their comprehensive care requires an inter-disciplinary approach. North American studies indicate that adults with CHD are at increased risk of psychosocial difficulties. Research suggests that adults with heart failure caused by acquired heart disease are also likely to experience impaired psychosocial functioning and quality of life (QOL). Thus, adults with CHD who develop heart failure are a particularly vulnerable group with regard to psychosocial functioning and QOL.

Most adults with congenital heart disease show high levels of natriuretic peptide (NP) when compared with normal controls. Levels of norepinephrine and NP were strongly related to outcome in studies that included many symptomatic patients, especially those with unrepaired congenital heart disease, Eisenmenger syndrome, and pulmonary hypertension. Limited data are available regarding serial assessment of biomarkers; such information could provide additional important information to help identify patients at risk, as demonstrated during patient follow-up and pregnancy.

As patients with congenital heart disease age with increasingly complex lesions, heart failure and arrhythmias have emerged as leading sources of morbidity and mortality. The two are intertwined, as one may herald, beget, or aggravate the other. Moreover, arrhythmias in adults with congenital heart disease and heart failure can be poorly tolerated or life threatening. There is, therefore, much interest in promptly and accurately diagnosing arrhythmias and identifying risk factors for sudden death. This article appraises current knowledge regarding diagnostic tools for arrhythmias in adults with congenital heart disease and heart failure and comments on their prognostic value where relevant.

Arrhythmias have long been recognized as a major cause of morbidity and mortality in the adult with congenital heart disease. It is important for the clinician to accurately diagnose these disturbances and be cognizant of the full array of antiarrhythmic agents and devices available to treat these conditions. This review discusses the most common arrhythmias encountered in this population and the therapeutic options available. Specific issues unique to this population are also addressed.

Dramatic advances in the diagnosis and treatment of congenital heart disease (CHD), the most common inborn defect, have resulted in a growing population of adults with CHD. Eisenmenger syndrome (ES) represents the extreme form of pulmonary arterial hypertension associated with CHD, characterized by markedly increased pulmonary vascular resistance with consequently reversed or bidirectional shunting. While ES is a direct consequence of a heart defect, it is a fundamentally multisystem syndrome with wide-ranging clinical manifestations. The introduction of targeted pulmonary hypertension therapies has subtly shifted clinical focus from preventing iatrogenic and other adverse events toward cautious therapeutic activism.

The essence of a Fontan circuit is the creation of the Fontan "neoportal system," which allows for oxygenation at near normal levels, but at the cost of a chronic state of systemic venous congestion and decreased cardiac output. The heart, while still the engine of the circuit, cannot compensate for this major flow restriction: the ventricle has lost control of the output and venous congestion. Systolic and diastolic ventricular dysfunction may aggravate the hemodynamic burden. The abnormal hemodynamics affect organs outside the heart and may lead to liver cirrhosis/malignancy, protein-losing enteropathy, or plastic bronchitis. The chronic low flow state causes an increase of pulmonary (and systemic) vascular resistance and ventricular filling pressures, causing failure of the Fontan to be progressive with increasing functional impairment.

Heart disease, present in 0.5% to 3% of pregnant women, is an important cause of morbidity and the leading cause of death among pregnant women in the developed world. Certain heart conditions are associated with an increased risk of heart failure during pregnancy or the postpartum period; for these conditions, management during pregnancy benefits from multidisciplinary care at a center with expertise in pregnancy and heart disease. This article focuses on cardiac risks and management strategies for women with acquired and congenital heart disease who are at increased risk of heart failure during pregnancy.

 Videos of valve repair accompany this article

The tricuspid valve is frequently affected in adults with congenital heart disease but is also frequently overlooked. Disease of this valve can occur primarily or develop secondary to changes in the right ventricle caused by other disease states. The embryology and anatomy of the tricuspid valve are important to understanding pathogenesis of valve dysfunction in congenital heart disease. Clinical findings can be subtle. Multimodality imaging may be necessary to fully assess the cause and impact of tricuspid valve lesions. More research is needed in pathophysiology, imaging, and treatment in this area.

There are diverse mechanisms by which congenital left-sided cardiac lesions can precipitate heart failure. Left heart outflow obstruction can impose abnormal pressure load on the left ventricle, inducing adverse remodeling, hypertrophy, and diastolic and systolic dysfunction. Abnormalities in left ventricular inflow can increase pulmonary venous pressure, predisposing to pulmonary edema. In addition, inborn abnormalities in left ventricular myocardial structure and function can impair both systolic and diastolic function and manifest as heart failure later in life. In this article, the different mechanisms, outcomes, and treatments of heart failure in patients with congenital left-sided lesions are discussed.

Heart failure is a common late complication in adults with congenital heart defects, both repaired and unrepaired. The onset of clinical heart failure is associated with increased morbidity and mortality. Some patients with congenital heart disease may benefit from medications shown to improve survival in the population with acquired heart failure, but these same therapies may be of no benefit to other patients. Further studies are needed to better guide the choice of medical therapies.

In the context of congenital heart disease (CHD), the complex biochemical and physiologic response to the pressure- or volume-loaded ventricle can be induced by stenotic and shunt/regurgitant lesions, respectively. A range of transcatheter therapies have recently emerged to expand the therapeutic potential of the more traditional surgical and medical interventions for heart failure in patients with CHD. Together, these complementary interventions aim to treat the growing patient population with adult CHD (ACHD). In this article, the most commonly used transcatheter interventions for heart failure in patients with ACHD are reviewed.

Individuals with adult congenital heart disease (ACHD) are at a great risk for heart failure, and the underlying anatomic features are important predictors of heart failure. As the ACHD population grows older, multiple events—including years of an altered physiology, the neurohormonal cascade, and many still unknown—culminate in ventricular failure. Surgical device therapy is an effective method in supporting patients with heart failure. Ventricular assist devices have been used with success in bridging ACHD patients to heart transplantation or destination therapy.

Heart transplantation has become an increasingly common and effective therapy for adults with end-stage congenital heart disease (CHD) because of advances in patient selection and surgical technique. Indications for transplantation in CHD are similar to those in other forms of heart failure. Pretransplant assessment of CHD patients emphasizes evaluation of cardiac anatomy, pulmonary vascular disease, allosensitization, hepatic dysfunction, and neuropsychiatric status. CHD patients experience longer waitlist times and higher waitlist mortality than other transplant candidates. Adult CHD patients undergoing transplantation carry an early hazard for mortality compared with non-CHD recipients, but by 10 years posttransplant, CHD patients have a slight actuarial survival advantage.

Heart Failure in Congenital Heart Disease: A Confluence of Acquired and Congenital   219

Akl C. Fahed, Amy E. Roberts, Seema Mital, and Neal K. Lakdawala

Heart failure (HF) is a common cause of morbidity and mortality in congenital heart disease (CHD), with increasing prevalence because of improved treatment options and outcomes. Genetic factors and acquired postnatal factors in CHD might play a major role in the progression to HF. This article proposes 3 routes that lead to HF in CHD: rare monogenic entities that cause both CHD and HF; severe CHD lesions in which acquired hemodynamic effects of CHD or surgery result in HF; and, most commonly, a combined effect of complex genetics in overlapping pathways and acquired stressors caused by the primary lesion.

HEART FAILURE CLINICS

DOWNLOAD
Free App!

Review Articles
THE CLINICS

NOW AVAILABLE FOR YOUR iPhone and iPad

Foreword

Adults with Congenital Heart Disease: Growing Pains

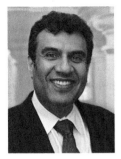 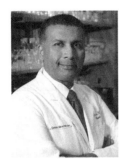

Mandeep R. Mehra, MD   Javed Butler, MD, MPH

Consulting Editors

Adults with congenital heart disease now outnumber children with an estimated prevalence of 3 per 1000. Terrific advances in surgical correction of anatomic defects, widespread recognition of avoiding teratogenicity, improved rates of maternal vaccination, prevention of illnesses during pregnancy, and improvements in more accurate clinical recognition of congenital heart defects are some principal reasons for this growing but welcome imbalance. Indeed, this group of patients exhibits a unique complexity coupled with the layering of manifestations of more traditional risk-marker-driven and metabolically sustained cardiac perturbations such as hypertension, hyperlipidemia, obesity, coronary heart disease, and unique arrhythmias. This has led to the resurgence of a specialty in its own right, one that requires a skill set that spans pediatric and adult medicine, singular experience in disease identification, appreciation of altered anatomical-physiological interactions, and knowledge of therapeutics often found only in select teams based at large academically oriented institutions.

The adult with congenital heart disease may represent a daunting task to the general clinician but epitomizes a versatile opportunity for mechanistic understanding of disease guided by incisive appreciation for unique therapeutic challenges. Take the right ventricle in congenital heart disease, for example. This chamber can be anatomically a systemic ventricle or a single ventricle, or it can be subject to uniquely abnormal loads or electrical stimulation. These facets all allow the physiologist and clinician to learn more about the pathophysiology of the ventricle, allowing for possible evolution of therapeutic stances in areas where the right heart is diseased due to noncongenital cause. The Fontan circulation, which represents a hemodynamic compromise, is interesting to observe in its natural history. As it fails with age and loses hemodynamic efficiency, a model of right heart failure emerges that challenges the clinician critically to find ways to support the circulation despite the absence of a contractile right-sided pump. An arrhythmia, which may be well tolerated in structurally normal hearts, can be hemodynamically devastating and prognostic. Such rhythms may challenge the clinician to develop and employ advanced techniques in catheter ablation or robotic magnetic navigation to treat the substrate. More recently, the subcutaneous defibrillator has become available in selected patients with congenital heart disease in whom transvenous lead implantation is unachievable or contraindicated. Finally, the development of pulmonary arterial hypertension is a common complication of congenital heart disease and at extremes can manifest as the Eisenmenger syndrome. Observations in the natural history of survival of Eisenmenger syndrome compared with common varieties of pulmonary arterial hypertension have taught us that prognosis is vastly determined by the expression of right heart

Heart Failure Clin 10 (2014) xiii–xiv
http://dx.doi.org/10.1016/j.hfc.2013.11.001
1551-7136/14/$ – see front matter © 2014 Elsevier Inc. All rights reserved.

heartfailure.theclinics.com

failure and right ventricular adaptation rather than the hemodynamic load itself.

In this issue of *Heart Failure Clinics*, we see an extraordinary constellation of well-constructed topics that include the breadth and depth of knowledge in adults with congenital heart disease. These articles take us on an extensive journey ranging from the pathophysiology, to the epidemiology and the anatomic, physiological, and electrical aberrations that signal progressive disease. Furthermore, the state of the art in surgical and interventional techniques is discussed, including the role of end-stage therapy as with mechanical circulatory support and transplantation. Yet, the editors do not ignore the importance of psychological and sociodynamic factors that can influence adherence and access to as well as outcomes from treatment in this unique subset of patients.

All in all, this is a masterful compendium on heart failure in the setting of adults with congenital heart disease.

Mandeep R. Mehra, MD
BWH Heart and Vascular Center
Brigham and Women's Hospital
75 Francis Street
A Building, 3rd Floor, Room AB324
Boston, MA 02115, USA

Javed Butler, MD, MPH
Emory Clinical Cardiovascular Research Institute
1462 Clifton Road NE, Suite 504
Atlanta, GA 30322, USA

E-mail addresses:
MMEHRA@partners.org (M.R. Mehra)
javed.butler@emory.edu (J. Butler)

Preface

Evolving Perspectives on Heart Failure in Adults with Congenital Heart Disease

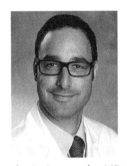 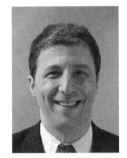

Alexander R. Opotowsky, MD, MPH   Michael J. Landzberg, MD

Editors

It may be argued that a sizable subset, even the majority, of adults living with congenital heart disease (CHD) have heart failure as defined by Zipes and Braunwald, "the pathophysiologic state in which the heart is unable to pump blood at a rate commensurate with the requirements of the metabolizing tissues or can do so only from an elevated filling pressure."[1] A proposed alternative definition, "heart failure is the label for a cardiovascular syndrome that is lacking uniform criteria for definition," would perhaps best align with heart failure among adults with CHD.[2]

This topic is of increasing interest and importance, as reflected in the number of publications relating to both CHD and heart failure published annually (**Fig. 1**), and not only because adults with CHD comprise a growing aging population with more clinically apparent heart failure.[3,4] As importantly, heart failure syndromes in adults with CHD are vastly heterogeneous, are often sustained or in flux over a lifetime, and highlight the frequently overlooked role of multisystem dysfunction and complex systems biology integral to understanding clinical presentation. Research may require identifying physiologically consistent subsets from the diverse universe of CHD, resulting in small populations to study. As a result,

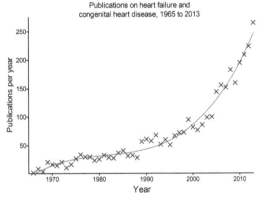

Fig. 1. Number of publications listed on PubMed (www.pubmed.org) using MESH terms for both "heart failure" and "congenital heart disease," 1965 to 2013. Data for 2013 extrapolated from publications listed through August 2013.

systematic scientific investigation can be challenging. The presence of unique, some might say unnatural, arrangements, however, provides opportunities for rich exploration.

This issue of *Heart Failure Clinics* includes articles on a broad range of topics related to the syndrome of heart failure in adults with

Heart Failure Clin 10 (2014) xv–xvi
http://dx.doi.org/10.1016/j.hfc.2013.10.005
1551-7136/14/$ – see front matter © 2014 Published by Elsevier Inc.

heartfailure.theclinics.com

CHD. How is it that patients with no subpulmonary ventricle,[5] or with a morphologic right ventricle ejecting into the systemic circulation, or with systemic pulmonary artery pressures and chronic cyanosis may live seemingly normal lives without subjective limitation well into adulthood?[6] How do these patients successfully adapt to intrinsic cardiovascular dysfunction and associated psychosocial stress and strain?[7] As more women with previously fatal forms of CHD survive to adulthood, pregnancy has become increasingly common[8–10]; how do the hemodynamic and neurohormonal changes of pregnancy interact with underlying CHD?[11] Can we extrapolate the prognostic value of specific biomarkers or standard imaging assessment or effectiveness of medical therapies for the systemic left ventricle to the systemic right ventricle, or to patients with a single ventricle?[12–14] This issue of *Heart Failure Clinics* reflects the efforts of clinicians and investigators across the globe with a shared goal to answer these and other questions to improve the lives of patients with CHD and better understand how what superficially appears to be physiologically applicable only to a few patients may help us understand the wider syndrome of heart failure, however defined, in the general population.

Alexander R. Opotowsky, MD, MPH
Boston Adult Congenital Heart and Pulmonary
Hypertension Service
Boston Children's Hospital
Brigham and Women's Hospital
300 Longwood Avenue, Bader 209
Boston, MA 02115, USA

Michael J. Landzberg, MD
Boston Adult Congenital Heart and Pulmonary
Hypertension Service
Boston Children's Hospital
Brigham and Women's Hospital
300 Longwood Avenue, Bader 209
Boston, MA 02115, USA

E-mail addresses:
alexander.opotowsky@childrens.harvard.edu
(A.R. Opotowsky)
mike.landzberg@cardio.chboston.org
(M.J. Landzberg)

REFERENCES

1. Zipes DP, Braunwald E. Braunwald's heart disease: a textbook of cardiovascular medicine. Philadelphia: W.B. Saunders; 2005.
2. Coronel R, de Groot JR, van Lieshout JJ. Defining heart failure. Cardiovasc Res 2001;50:419–22.
3. Rodriguez FH 3rd, Moodie DS, Parekh DR, et al. Outcomes of heart failure-related hospitalization in adults with congenital heart disease in the United States. Congenit Heart Dis 2012.
4. Rodriguez FH, Marelli AJ. The Epidemiology of heart failure in adults with congenital heart disease. Heart Fail Clin 2013;10(1):1–7.
5. Gewillig M, Goldberg DJ. Failure of the Fontan circulation. Heart Fail Clin 2013;10(1):105–16.
6. Opotowsky AR, Landzberg MJ, Beghetti M. The exceptional and far-flung manifestations of heart failure in Eisenmenger syndrome. Heart Fail Clin 2013; 10(1):91–104.
7. Kovacs AH, Moons P. Psychosocial functioning and quality of life in adults with congenital heart disease and heart failure. Heart Fail Clin 2013;10(1):35–42.
8. Opotowsky AR, Siddiqi OK, D'Souza B, et al. Maternal cardiovascular events during childbirth among women with congenital heart disease. Heart 2012;98:145–51.
9. Tobler D, Fernandes SM, Wald RM, et al. Pregnancy outcomes in women with transposition of the great arteries and arterial switch operation. Am J Cardiol 2010;106:417–20.
10. Said SM, Dearani JA, Silversides CK, et al. Longer-term issues for young adults with hypoplastic left heart syndrome: contraception, pregnancy, transition, transfer, counselling, and re-operation. Cardiol Young 2011;21(Suppl 2):93–100.
11. Grewal J, Silversides CK, Colman JM. Pregnancy in women with heart disease: risk assessment and management of heart failure. Heart Fail Clin 2013; 10(1):117–30.
12. Ohuchi H, Diller GP. Biomarkers in adult congenital heart disease heart failure. Heart Fail Clin 2013; 10(1):43–56.
13. Burchill LJ, Mertens L, Broberg CS. Imaging for the assessment of heart failure in congenital heart disease: ventricular function and beyond. Heart Fail Clin 2013;10(1):9–22.
14. Book WM, Shaddy RE. Medical therapy in adults with congenital heart disease. Heart Fail Clin 2013; 10(1):167–78.

The Epidemiology of Heart Failure in Adults with Congenital Heart Disease

Fred H. Rodriguez III, MD[a],*, Ariane J. Marelli, MD, MPH[b]

KEYWORDS

- Congenital heart disease • Myocardial dysfunction • Heart failure • Epidemiology

KEY POINTS

- There are more adults than children with congenital heart disease and this population is rapidly growing.
- Lifelong exposure to myocardial dysfunction results from repeated surgical interventions and chronically abnormal biventricular loading conditions.
- Heart failure in adults with congenital heart disease can result from systolic and diastolic dysfunction and is most common in patients with tetralogy of Fallot, transposition of the great arteries, and single ventricle physiology.
- The presence of heart failure in this population adversely affects mortality and morbidity and data are needed to quantify and prevent this complication.
- Hospitalizations because of heart failure in adults with congenital heart disease in the United States increased substantially from 1998 to 2005, making this problem an important public health issue.

INTRODUCTION

The impact of lifelong exposure to myocardial dysfunction in populations with congenital heart disease (CHD) is becoming increasingly recognized. Most children born with CHD now reach adulthood and the long-term sequelae of treatment are contributing to substantial comorbidity.[1,2] Improved survival is achieved at a cost of repeated interventions. The combination of structural changes present at birth with changes resulting from cardiac surgery can result in heart failure.[3,4] Thus, the effect of chronic myocardial dysfunction is amplified and increasing survivorship is resulting in longer time windows to express heart failure. Heart failure has been cited as the leading cause of cardiovascular death in adults with CHD.[5] Although guidelines for the management of chronic heart failure in acquired cardiovascular conditions exist,[6] there are no directives on preventing complications or improving outcomes from chronic heart failure in the CHD population. To date, there are few data to substantiate the incidence and prevalence of heart failure in adults with CHD. This article reports on the current state of knowledge on the epidemiology of heart failure in this patient population and the current data sources that may enable better characterization of this complex condition in adults with CHD.

ADULTS WITH CONGENITAL HEART DISEASE: HOW FAST ARE THE NUMBERS GROWING?

The reported prevalence of CHD at birth is approximately 8/1000 live births, although reports vary between 4/1000 and 50/1000.[7,8] In the United

[a] Section of Cardiology, Sibley Heart Center Cardiology, Emory University, 2835 Brandywine Road, Suite 300, Atlanta, GA 30341, USA; [b] McGill Adult Unit for Congenital Heart Disease (MAUDE Unit), McGill University Health Center, McGill University, 687 Pine Avenue West, Montreal, QC H3A 1A1, Canada
* Corresponding author.
E-mail address: fred.rodriguez@emory.edu

Heart Failure Clin 10 (2014) 1–7
http://dx.doi.org/10.1016/j.hfc.2013.09.008
1551-7136/14/$ – see front matter © 2014 Elsevier Inc. All rights reserved.

States, the Centers for Disease Control (CDC) has reported birth prevalence rates between 8 and 10/1000 live births.[9] Continental variations in birth prevalence have been reported, from 6.9/1000 births in Europe to 9.3/1000 in Asia.[10] In 26,598 live births between 2000 and 2005 in Europe, the prevalence at birth of CHD was reported to be up to 13/1000 live births.[11] Advances in medical and surgical therapy have led to an increase in the survival of patients with CHD and therefore an increased prevalence in the general population. There has been an increase in the median age at death in those with severe CHD by more than 20 years since 1987.[12] The prevalence of CHD increased by 22% in children and 85% in adults with severe CHD from 1985 to 2000 such that in 2000, the prevalence of CHD in Quebec was 4/1000 adults and 12/1000 children.[2] The median age of those alive with severe CHD has also increased from 11 to 17 years as observed from 1985 to 2000 and is expected to further increase between 2000 and 2020.[2]

The mortality rates of patients born with CHD have declined in recent decades.[13] From 1979 to 1997, age-adjusted population death rates from all defects declined 39% in the United States from 2.5 to 1.5/100,000 or 1.9% per year.[14] During the same observation period, mortality declined for both simple and complex lesions such as transposition of the great arteries (TGA), tetralogy of Fallot (TOF), atrioventricular septal defect, and aortic coarctation (COA).[14] Despite such progress, CHD remains the most common cause of infant death associated with birth defects.[13] As more children with moderate to severe defects are reaching adult age, there has been a shift in mortality.[12] In a population-based cohort in Quebec, a total of 8561 deaths occurred in 71,686 patients with CHD (11.9%) followed for 982,363 patient-years from 1987 to 2005.[12] However, long-term survival after surgical repair of complex defects remains compromised, with survival rates decreasing from the third and fourth decade onward.[15]

Anatomic severity of CHD is 1 of several important contributors to disease burden. The proportion of patients with adult CHD (ACHD) with complex or severe lesions has been estimated and measured, and varies from 10% to 15% on a population level[1,2,7,16] but is as high as 30% in select tertiary care centers.[1,2,8,16] Using estimates of survival by cohort and the Bethesda disease severity classification, approximately 15% of adults are expected to have lesions of great complexity; those with moderate lesions were estimated to account for approximately one-third of patients.

HEART FAILURE DEFINITIONS AND POPULATIONS: WHO IS AT RISK?
Scope of the Problem

Heart failure has been defined as a "complex clinical syndrome that can result from any structural or functional cardiac disorder that impairs the ability of the ventricle to fill with or eject blood."[6] Heart failure is 1 of the most common causes for hospitalization in acquired heart disease and is associated with significant morbidity and mortality. Mortality during heart failure–related hospitalization has been reported to be between 3% and 13%.[17,18]

Heart failure in patients with ACHD can be complex, with symptoms of right heart failure, left heart failure, or even inadequate end-organ perfusion, which is seen in patients with portal hypertension and end-stage liver failure who have decreased systemic vascular resistance in the setting of a normal ejection fraction. Systolic dysfunction occurs in patients but is often not caused by the ischemic changes seen in the general adult population. Coronary arteries may be compromised during cardiac surgery during operations such as an arterial switch, Ross procedure, Nikaidoh procedure, or Bentall procedure when coronary arteries are translocated and resewn into an aortic or neoaortic root. Left-sided obstructive lesions such as aortic valve stenosis, subaortic stenosis, and coarctation of the aorta may lead to left ventricular hypertrophy in patients, resulting in impaired ventricular relaxation. Left ventricular noncompaction may result in a steady and progressive decline in function either early or late in life. Patients who develop bundle branch blocks may have dyssynchrony and an eventual decline in systolic function. Patients who require a pacemaker may have a pacer-dependent decrease in cardiac function over time. The prevalence of heart failure is highest in patients with single ventricle physiology, TOF, and TGA (**Fig. 1**).[19]

Diastolic dysfunction is being increasingly recognized in both left-sided and right-sided CHD. Impaired relaxation and diastolic dysfunction in the left ventricle may occur many years after an initial operation and can cause left atrial hypertension and symptoms of dyspnea and exercise intolerance.[20] Measuring function of the right ventricle (RV) remains a challenge compounded by the fact that the RV in CHD can be in the subaortic or subpulmonary position. The geometrically challenging crescent-shaped RV exhibits a wide range of physiologic responses to pressure and volume overload resulting in systolic and diastolic dysfunction.[21] Impaired relaxation of the RV may precede systolic dysfunction and be a sensitive marker of myocardial dysfunction.[22]

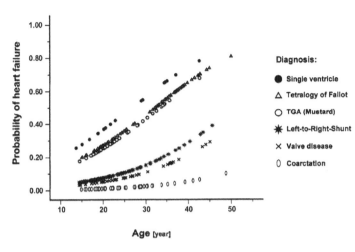

Diagnosis:

● Single ventricle

△ Tetralogy of Fallot

○ TGA (Mustard)

✳ Left-to-Right-Shunt

✕ Valve disease

◯ Coarctation

Fig. 1. The probability of heart failure versus age and type of heart defect. (*From* Norozi K, Wessel A, Alpers V, et al. Incidence and risk distribution of heart failure in adolescents and adults with congenital heart disease after cardiac surgery. Am J Cardiol 2006;97(8):1241; with permission.)

Patients with TOF now have more than a 90% chance of survival to adulthood, although many of these patients have evidence of pulmonary insufficiency, right ventricular enlargement, and impaired exercise capacity. Many others experience arrhythmias, either atrial or ventricular, caused by hemodynamic stressors as well as surgical changes. Many patients with repaired TOF experience right heart failure signs and symptoms such as hepatic congestion, peripheral edema, increased filling pressures, and peripheral edema. There is also a subset of patients with repaired tetralogy who have reduced left ventricular systolic function and experience symptoms of left ventricular failure such as pulmonary edema and orthopnea. These patients with left ventricular dysfunction are at increased risk for sudden cardiac death.[23] They may also have diastolic dysfunction of the left ventricle, particularly those who were repaired late.[24,25]

The prevalence of TGA in the United States is 4.73/10,000 live births, and more than 90% are now surviving to adulthood. From the late 1960s to the late 1980s/early 1990s, many of these patients underwent the Mustard or Senning operations. As surgical trends changed, patients usually undergo the Jatene arterial switch operation in the contemporary period, and many centers demonstrate low surgical mortality. However, the numerous atrial suture lines and burden of arrhythmias in Mustard/Senning patients, as well as the long-standing effects of a systemic RV lead to symptoms of heart failure in many patients. Many patients require a pacemaker and numerous others have depressed right ventricular systolic function and tricuspid regurgitation.

Patients born with single ventricle physiology often are palliated with the Fontan procedure, separating deoxygenated blood, which directly enters the lungs and systemic oxygenated blood flow. Compared with those with a repaired simple left to right shunt, those adolescents and adults who underwent Fontan palliation for single ventricle physiology have an odds ratio of more than 7 for developing heart failure.[19] Symptoms of heart failure develop because of systolic dysfunction, diastolic dysfunction, or sometimes because of decreased systemic vascular resistance seen in portal hypertension and cirrhosis. Hepatic congestion and portal hypertension occur in patients after the Fontan operation, and cardiac cirrhosis can develop. Patients with a failing Fontan have been described as those with a deterioration in exercise tolerance, persistent arrhythmias, worsening peripheral edema, and protein-losing enteropathy, all of which may be classified as evidence of heart failure. There is a decrease in survival of more than 15 years after the Fontan operation. Actuarial freedom from death or transplantation has been reported as 87%, 83%, and 70% at 15, 20, and 25 years after surgery, respectively.[26] Death in this group is related to heart failure in 7%.[26]

Pulmonary hypertension may develop in patients with CHD, regardless of whether they have been palliated/repaired or not.[27] Long-standing left to right shunting in patients with CHD may lead to irreversible pulmonary hypertension. Muscularization of the pulmonary vascular bed is demonstrated by increased pulmonary arterial pressures and right ventricular strain, which may result in symptoms of dyspnea and heart failure.

THE NUMBERS: WHAT DO WE KNOW?
Obtaining Data

In the United States there are an increasing number of data sources available to identify patients with ACHD and their cross-sectional outcomes.

The Nationwide Inpatient Sample (NIS) is the largest all-payer inpatient care database in the United States, containing data from approximately 8 million hospital stays each year. This estimates data for more than 39 million hospitalizations. It is the only US national hospital database containing charge information on all patients, regardless of payer, including persons covered by Medicare, Medicaid, private insurance, and the uninsured. Studies using this database have assessed trends in hospitalizations for patients with ACHD in the United States.[28] The inpatient National Claims History files from the Centers for Medicare & Medicaid Services (CMS) identifies information on patient demographics (age, sex, race), admission and discharge dates, and principal and secondary diagnosis codes (as coded by the *International Classification of Diseases, Ninth Revision, Clinical Modification*). The Healthcare Cost & Utilization Project (HCUP) Kids' Inpatient Database (KID) is drawn from the State Inpatient Discharge (SID) database, which captures 90% of all US discharges each year. The KID subset captures a random sample of 2 to 3 million discharges per year in more than 3700 hospitals in 38 states, making it the largest database on hospital care of newborns, infants, children, and adolescents (age <21 years) in the United States. It was designed by the Agency for Healthcare Research and Quality to document variables pertinent to health care delivery in children. Data include up to 15 diagnostic codes and procedural codes that use the *International Classification of Disease, 9th Revision* (ICD-9) classification. Studies using the KID database have investigated factors associated with increased resource utilization for CHD,[29] mortality after CHD surgery,[30] as well as the prevalence, morbidity, and mortality of heart failure–related hospitalizations in CHD in children.[31]

There are some population-based registries with long-term follow-up. The Québec Congenital Heart Disease Database was created by fusing outpatient, inpatient, and death registry data and applying validated algorithms. It contains 28 years of longitudinal data from 1983 to 2010 on more than 100,000 patients with CHD across the life span. Diagnoses conform to ICD-9, which has 24 codes to designate CHD anomalies.[2] Studies from the Québec CHD database have characterized epidemiologic changes in survival, death, and surgery in ACHD as well as disease burden from medical complications and health services utilization.[2,12] The Dutch CONgenital CORvitia (CONCOR) national registry has been developed to facilitate research into the etiology of CHD, as well as its outcome.[32] Clinical data such as demographics, diagnosis, clinical events, and

procedures as well as patient and family history are obtained from medical records. Currently more than 100 Dutch hospitals are participating, including all 8 tertiary referral centers from which 70% of patients originate. Studies have aimed to assess mortality and causes of death, and to determine which cardiovascular complications predict mortality in adults with CHD as well as assess surgery in adults with CHD.[5,33]

The CDC in the United States funds the National Birth Defects Prevention Study (NBDPS), which is the largest population-based study in the United States looking at risk factors for and potential causes of birth defects. The CDC collects data with researchers from other study sites, collectively called the Centers for Birth Defects Research and Prevention (CBDRP). Data from the CDC have been used to assess the prevalence of CHD in neonates[9] and investigate temporal trends in survival of infants with critical and noncritical CHD.[34]

Reporting Data

Some studies have used these data sources to assess the prevalence of outcomes in ACHD, including heart failure admissions.[28,35] Currently, 5.7 million Americans are estimated to have heart failure, and up to 30% of people who have heart failure die within 1 year of diagnosis.[13,36] Patients with CHD contribute a minority subset of these patients, but the number of patients with heart failure–related hospitalization in the United States has been steadily increasing.[13,28] In addition, patients with complex ACHD with heart failure often have multiple comorbidities that complicate their medical care.

From 1998 to 2005, the number of hospitalizations of patients with ACHD in the United States increased 102%, and heart failure–related hospitalizations increased by 82% (**Fig. 2**)[28] Of approximately 84,000 hospitalizations of adults with CHD in the United States in 2007, 17,000 had a diagnosis of heart failure.[35] The overall prevalence of heart failure among hospitalized patients with ACHD was noted to be significantly greater than that reported for hospitalizations in the general adult population. The overall mortality of patients with ACHD with heart failure was 4.1%, which was significantly greater than patients with ACHD without heart failure, even after controlling for age and comorbidities (**Fig. 3**).[35]

In an assessment of patients with ACHD in Europe from 1998 to 2003, New York Heart Association (NYHA) functional class worsened in 6%.[37] For cyanotic defects and Fontan circulation, heart failure class increased in 21% and 17%,

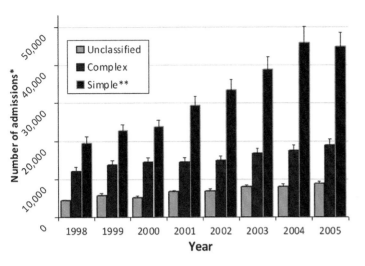

Fig. 2. Annual number of ACHD admissions in the United States categorized by level of defect complexity. * Data represent hospital admissions for adults 18 years of age. The analysis used sampling weights to produce nationally representative estimates and accounted for the complex survey design. Error bars represent the standard error. ** Classifications are based on the 32nd Bethesda Conference document and other published reports. Simple diagnoses with coexisting complex diagnoses or pulmonary hypertension were classified as complex. ACHD adults with congenital heart disease. (*From* Opotowsky AR, Siddiqi OK, Webb GD. Trends in hospitalizations for adults with congenital heart disease in the U.S. J Am Coll Cardiol 2009;54(5):462; with permission.)

respectively. In only 1% of patients with coarctation did functional class worsen. Among patients with atrial septal defects, the NYHA class improved more often than it worsened.

With regard to particular lesions, it has been demonstrated that at least 14% of patients with repaired TOF have NYHA class 2 or greater symptoms.[23] Given that TOF represents 10% of all CHD, 90% of tetralogy patients reach adult age, and recent studies have demonstrated that at least 14% experience heart failure symptoms, there is a large and increasing cohort of adults with tetralogy who require vigilant monitoring for worsening heart failure. The risk for heart failure in adolescents and adults with repaired TOF is significantly greater than in those with repaired simple left to right shunts (odds ratio 4.65).[19]

In an analysis of pulmonary hypertension in ACHD in Quebec, of 38,430 adults alive with

CHD in 2005, 2212 had a diagnosis of pulmonary hypertension (~6%, prevalence 58/1000).[27] Shunts were the most common lesion in this population. Heart failure occurred at least once in 31% with CHD-related pulmonary hypertension during follow-up. Although the median age of these adults was in the sixth decade of life, pulmonary hypertension was associated with a more than doubling of all-cause mortality and tripling of morbid complications, which were reflected in a more than 3-fold increase in hospitalization days, especially to coronary and intensive care units. Also in Quebec in a cohort of geriatric patients with ACHD age 65 years or greater,[38] heart failure was detected in 21% of the population ranging between 20% and 27% of those with severe CHD, shunt lesions and valvular disease. The modest rate of heart failure suggests that many of the older adults with severe lesions in this study had balanced or minor variants allowing them to survive to an advanced age, or had operated lesions with favorable results. However, as more adults with moderate to severe CHD have undergone palliation, the prevalence of CHD in the geriatric population will increase.

A recently reported study demonstrated gaps in time when patients with ACHD are not receiving medical care.[39] Forty-two percent of all patients with ACHD surveyed reported a gap in cardiology care. This suggests that ACHD with heart failure may not be accounted for when epidemiologic studies take place. Within the ACHD population, 36% had mild CHD, 50% had moderate CHD, and 14% had severe CHD. Eight percent of patients had at least 1 gap in care lasting more than 10 years. The first gap in care occurred during

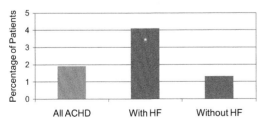

* Odds ratio 3.3, 95% CI 2.6-4.1

Fig. 3. Mortality of hospitalized adult patients with CHD with and without heart failure (HF). (*From* Rodriguez FH, third, Moodie DS, Parekh DR, et al Outcomes of heart failure-related hospitalization in adults with congenital heart disease in the United States. Congenit Heart Dis 2012 Nov 16; doi:10.1111/chd.12019 [E-pub ahead of print]; with permission.)

the transitional period of young adulthood (mean, 19.9 years; median, 19 years). The complexity of CHD was associated with gaps in care: 59% of patients with mild CHD, 42% with moderate CHD, and 26% with severe disease reported care gaps ($P<.0001$).

THE FUTURE: HOW DO WE GET THERE?

Ongoing projects to better track patients with ACHD with and without heart failure are ongoing. International collaborations and registries have demonstrated longitudinal follow-up of these complex patients for the assessment of comorbidities, and will continue to become more sophisticated in their evaluation of medical issues specific to the ACHD population. The advent of mandated electronic medical records in the United States may help to better track patients and their symptoms and allow for longitudinal follow-up. A method of linking inpatient and outpatient records may help to assess the success (or failure) of current therapies and allow for the improved care of patients. Many quality improvement initiative projects are ongoing to follow patients with ACHD.

In the United States, the Congenital Heart Futures Act of the Affordable Care Act authorized the CDC to "enhance and expand infrastructure to track the epidemiology of congenital heart disease and organize such information into a nationally-representative, population-based surveillance system." This would facilitate "further research into the types of health services patients use and to identify possible areas for educational outreach and prevention." This project is to develop robust, population-based estimates of the prevalence of CHD focusing on adolescents and adults to better understand survival, health care utilization, and long-term outcomes and improve diagnosis, treatment, and prevention.

SUMMARY

The complex nature of CHD and the wide variety of medical treatments and surgical repairs have resulted in a growing population of adults with CHD. Heart failure is becoming increasingly recognized as an important comorbidity resulting from prolonged survival. Assessing the lifelong impact of myocardial dysfunction and heart failure in this population can be challenging. This is related at least in part to data collection procedures and variations in measurement of heart failure both clinically and noninvasively. Existing data indicate that a significant proportion of adults with CHD experience symptoms of heart failure, particularly those with moderate to complex anatomy, and that this complication affects health services utilization. As more data become available, improved monitoring, longitudinal follow-up, and risk stratification of heart failure will help to improve the quality of care for the adult population with CHD.

REFERENCES

1. Warnes CA, Liberthson R, Danielson GK, et al. Task force 1: the changing profile of congenital heart disease in adult life. J Am Coll Cardiol 2001;37(5):1170-5.
2. Marelli AJ, Mackie AS, Ionescu-Ittu R, et al. Congenital heart disease in the general population: changing prevalence and age distribution. Circulation 2007;115(2):163-72.
3. Bolger AP, Coats AJ, Gatzoulis MA. Congenital heart disease: the original heart failure syndrome. Eur Heart J 2003;24(10):970-6.
4. Book WM. Heart failure in the adult patient with congenital heart disease. J Card Fail 2005;11(4):306-12.
5. Verheugt CL, Uiterwaal CS, van der Velde ET, et al. Mortality in adult congenital heart disease. Eur Heart J 2010;31(10):1220-9.
6. Hunt SA, Abraham WT, Chin MH, et al. ACC/AHA 2005 guideline update for the diagnosis and management of chronic heart failure in the adult: a report of the American College of Cardiology/American Heart Association Task Force on Practice Guidelines (Writing Committee to Update the 2001 Guidelines for the Evaluation and Management of Heart Failure): developed in collaboration with the American College of Chest Physicians and the International Society for Heart and Lung Transplantation: endorsed by the Heart Rhythm Society. Circulation 2005;112(12):e154-235.
7. Marelli A. The future of ACHD care symposium: changing demographics of congenital heart disease. Prog Pediatr Cardiol 2012;34(2):85-90.
8. Hoffman JI, Kaplan S. The incidence of congenital heart disease. J Am Coll Cardiol 2002;39(12):1890-900.
9. Reller MD, Strickland MJ, Riehle-Colarusso T, et al. Prevalence of congenital heart defects in metropolitan Atlanta, 1998-2005. J Pediatr 2008;153(6):807-13.
10. van der Linde D, Konings EE, Slager MA, et al. Birth prevalence of congenital heart disease worldwide: a systematic review and meta-analysis. J Am Coll Cardiol 2011;58(21):2241-7.
11. Dolk H, Loane M, Garne E, European Surveillance of Congenital Anomalies Working G. Congenital heart defects in Europe: prevalence and perinatal mortality, 2000 to 2005. Circulation 2011;123(8):841-9.

12. Khairy P, Ionescu-Ittu R, Mackie AS, et al. Changing mortality in congenital heart disease. J Am Coll Cardiol 2010;56(14):1149–57.

13. Go AS, Mozaffarian D, Roger VL, et al. Heart disease and stroke statistics–2013 update: a report from the American Heart Association. Circulation 2013;127(1):e6–245.

14. Boneva RS, Botto LD, Moore CA, et al. Mortality associated with congenital heart defects in the United States: trends and racial disparities, 1979-1997. Circulation 2001;103(19):2376–81.

15. Nieminen HP, Jokinen EV, Sairanen HI. Late results of pediatric cardiac surgery in Finland: a population-based study with 96% follow-up. Circulation 2001; 104(5):570–5.

16. Hoffman JI, Kaplan S, Liberthson RR. Prevalence of congenital heart disease. Am Heart J 2004;147(3): 425–39.

17. Fang J, Mensah GA, Croft JB, et al. Heart failure-related hospitalization in the U.S., 1979 to 2004. J Am Coll Cardiol 2008;52(6):428–34.

18. Abraham WT, Fonarow GC, Albert NM, et al. Predictors of in-hospital mortality in patients hospitalized for heart failure: insights from the Organized Program to Initiate Lifesaving Treatment in Hospitalized Patients with Heart Failure (OPTIMIZE-HF). J Am Coll Cardiol 2008;52(5):347–56.

19. Norozi K, Wessel A, Alpers V, et al. Incidence and risk distribution of heart failure in adolescents and adults with congenital heart disease after cardiac surgery. Am J Cardiol 2006;97(8):1238–43.

20. Tede NH, Child JS. Diastolic dysfunction in patients with congenital heart disease. Cardiol Clin 2000; 18(3):491–9.

21. Mertens LL, Friedberg MK. Imaging the right ventricle–current state of the art. Nat Rev Cardiol 2010;7(10):551–63.

22. Addetia K, Sebag IA, Marelli A, et al. Right ventricular end-diastolic wall stress: does it impact on right atrial size, and does it differ in right ventricular pressure vs volume loading conditions? Can J Cardiol 2013;29(7):858–65.

23. Ghai A, Silversides C, Harris L, et al. Left ventricular dysfunction is a risk factor for sudden cardiac death in adults late after repair of tetralogy of Fallot. J Am Coll Cardiol 2002;40(9):1675–80.

24. Borow KM, Green LH, Castaneda AR, et al. Left ventricular function after repair of tetralogy of fallot and its relationship to age at surgery. Circulation 1980; 61(6):1150–8.

25. Aboulhosn JA, Lluri G, Gurvitz MZ, et al. Left and right ventricular diastolic function in adults with surgically repaired tetralogy of Fallot: a multi-institutional study. Can J Cardiol 2013;29(7):866–72.

26. Khairy P, Fernandes SM, Mayer JE Jr, et al. Long-term survival, modes of death, and predictors of mortality in patients with Fontan surgery. Circulation 2008;117(1):85–92.

27. Lowe BS, Therrien J, Ionescu-Ittu R, et al. Diagnosis of pulmonary hypertension in the congenital heart disease adult population impact on outcomes. J Am Coll Cardiol 2011;58(5):538–46.

28. Opotowsky AR, Siddiqi OK, Webb GD. Trends in hospitalizations for adults with congenital heart disease in the U.S. J Am Coll Cardiol 2009;54(5): 460–7.

29. Connor JA, Gauvreau K, Jenkins KJ. Factors associated with increased resource utilization for congenital heart disease. Pediatrics 2005;116(3):689–95.

30. Marelli A, Gauvreau K, Landzberg M, et al. Sex differences in mortality in children undergoing congenital heart disease surgery: a United States population-based study. Circulation 2010;122(Suppl 11):S234–40.

31. Rossano JW, Kim JJ, Decker JA, et al. Prevalence, morbidity, and mortality of heart failure-related hospitalizations in children in the United States: a population-based study. J Card Fail 2012;18(6): 459–70.

32. van der Velde ET, Vriend JW, Mannens MM, et al. CONCOR, an initiative towards a national registry and DNA-bank of patients with congenital heart disease in the Netherlands: rationale, design, and first results. Eur J Epidemiol 2005;20(6):549–57.

33. Zomer AC, Verheugt CL, Vaartjes I, et al. Surgery in adults with congenital heart disease. Circulation 2011;124(20):2195–201.

34. Oster ME, Lee KA, Honein MA, et al. Temporal trends in survival among infants with critical congenital heart defects. Pediatrics 2013;131(5):e1502–8.

35. Rodriguez FH 3rd, Moodie DS, Parekh DR, et al. Outcomes of heart failure-related hospitalization in adults with congenital heart disease in the United States. Congenit Heart Dis 2012. http://dx.doi.org/10.1111/chd.12019.

36. Chen J, Normand SL, Wang Y, et al. National and regional trends in heart failure hospitalization and mortality rates for Medicare beneficiaries, 1998-2008. JAMA 2011;306(15):1669–78.

37. Engelfriet P, Boersma E, Oechslin E, et al. The spectrum of adult congenital heart disease in Europe: morbidity and mortality in a 5 year follow-up period. The Euro Heart Survey on adult congenital heart disease. Eur Heart J 2005;26(21):2325–33.

38. Afilalo J, Therrien J, Pilote L, et al. Geriatric congenital heart disease: burden of disease and predictors of mortality. J Am Coll Cardiol 2011; 58(14):1509–15.

39. Gurvitz M, Valente AM, Broberg C, et al. Prevalence and predictors of gaps in care among adult congenital heart disease patients: HEART-ACHD (The Health, Education, and Access Research Trial). J Am Coll Cardiol 2013;61(21):2180–4.

Imaging for the Assessment of Heart Failure in Congenital Heart Disease
Ventricular Function and Beyond

Luke J. Burchill, MBBS, PhD[a], Luc Mertens, MD, PhD[b],
Craig S. Broberg, MD, MCR[c],*

KEYWORDS

- Heart defect • Congenital • Echocardiography • Cardiac magnetic resonance • Heart failure
- Clinical assessment

KEY POINTS

- Assessment of heart failure often relies on accurate cardiac imaging.
- Current noninvasive imaging modalities include many nongeometric methods for ventricular function that are ideally suited for the unique challenges of congenital heart disease.
- Research is still needed to aid in understanding how imaging parameters may guide management.

INTRODUCTION

Heart failure (HF) is a clinical syndrome with multiple causes. Patients with adult congenital heart disease (ACHD) typically have more than 1 substrate for developing HF, including prolonged cyanosis, myocardial damage related to multiple surgical and interventional procedures, chronic pressure/volume loading related to residual lesions, intrinsic myocardial disease, and HF secondary to arrhythmia. Clinical HF assessment is generally based on symptoms (exertional dyspnea, orthopnea, paroxysmal nocturnal dyspnea), physical findings related fluid retention (distended neck veins, edema, ascites), and insufficient cardiac output (reduced peripheral perfusion with colder extremities, orthostasis, circulatory shock). While not universal in patients with HF and a structurally normal heart, these findings tend to be even more unreliable among adults with congenital

heart disease (CHD). Use of additional more objective measures of HF such as biomarkers, measured exercise capacity, and ventricular performance is particularly helpful for this patient population. This article focuses on the use of echocardiography, cardiac magnetic resonance imaging (CMR), and cardiac computed tomography (CT) techniques, and their use in the management of ACHD patients with HF. These imaging modalities are increasingly being used to replace cardiac catheterization, which still is the gold standard for measuring ventricular pressures, cardiac output, and vascular resistance. Each modality offers unique information and has specific limitations; given the heterogeneity of CHD vulnerable to HF, all have a role and are considered here (**Table 1**). Despite an expanding array of imaging options, a major challenge in HF management is to integrate the findings with other clinical data to

Disclosures: None.
[a] Section of Cardiovascular Imaging, Cleveland Clinic, Cleveland, OH, USA; [b] Pediatrics, The Hospital for Sick Children, University of Toronto, Toronto, Ontario, Canada; [c] Adult Congenital Heart Program, Cardiovascular Medicine, Knight Cardiovascular Institute, Oregon Health and Science University, UHN 62, 3181 Southwest Sam Jackson Park Road, Portland, OR 97239, USA
* Corresponding author.
E-mail address: brobergc@ohsu.edu

Heart Failure Clin 10 (2014) 9–22
http://dx.doi.org/10.1016/j.hfc.2013.09.013
1551-7136/14/$ – see front matter © 2014 Elsevier Inc. All rights reserved.

Table 1
Strengths and limitations of imaging modalities

Imaging Modality	Factors Influencing Choice of Modality	Strengths	Limitations
Echocardiography	Imaging capabilities	Ventricular volumes/ mass/global function (2D and 3D) Diastolic function Regional ventricular function and myocardial contractility (TDI, strain, myocardial performance index) Valvular regurgitation severity and mechanism	Volumetric methods assume uniform ventricular geometry often not present in ACHD patients Variable reproducibility Underestimation of ventricular volumes by 3D echo Limited extracardiac evaluation Retrosternal position of right ventricle may limit echocardiographic evaluation
	Technical considerations	Safe Portable Inexpensive	Poor acoustic windows Beam alignment (TDI)
CMR	Imaging capabilities	Ventricular volumes/ mass/global function Dedicated software for right ventricular functional assessment Flow measurements (valvular regurgitation) Ventricular mechanics Myocardial fibrosis and scar Extracardiac evaluation	Susceptibility metal artifact/ field distortion (coils and stents) Contraindicated in patients with pacemakers/ defibrillators and those with severe renal dysfunction Inferior to CT for coronary imaging
	Technical considerations	No ionizing radiation Enables longitudinal review without cumulative radiation exposure	Limited availability and/or expertise Long imaging times Long breath holds Claustrophobia Expense
CT	Imaging capabilities	Ventricular volumes/ mass/global function (2D and 3D) Vascular abnormalities including coronary artery disease, collaterals, and AV malformations Hybrid CT/PET for localization of regional myocardial ischemia Extracardiac evaluation	Overestimation of ventricular volumes No flow measurements
	Technical considerations	Short imaging times High resolution Higher reproducibility vs MR and echo	Ionizing radiation (7–12 mSv) Less suitable for longitudinal review owing to radiation exposure and cancer risk Iodinated contrast (nephrotoxicity, anaphylaxis) Tachycardia and arrhythmias reduce image quality Expense

Abbreviations: 2D, 2-dimensional; 3D, 3-dimensional; ACHD, adult congenital heart disease; AV, atrioventricular; CMR, cardiac magnetic resonance imaging; CT, computed tomography; MR, magnetic resonance; PET, positron emission tomography; TDI, tissue Doppler imaging.

guide medical management. Imaging should be used to obtain information that can alter treatment strategies in a meaningful way, particularly in the current era of heightened cost consciousness in health care.

VENTRICULAR FUNCTION AND CLINICAL OUTCOMES IN ACHD

A subset of ACHD patients is diagnosed with HF after presenting with symptoms and signs that coincide with advanced ventricular dysfunction[1] only after extensive compensatory hemodynamic and neurohormonal mechanisms have been exhausted. Late presentation with symptomatic HF is associated with a poor prognosis: ACHD patients with a recent HF admission have a 5-fold higher mortality rate than those without recent HF admission.[2] HF mortality is highest in those with complex CHD and accounts for at least 25% of deaths in adulthood.[3,4] In patients with ACHD, imaging techniques are essential for (1) confirming the clinical diagnosis of HF through assessment of ventricular systolic and diastolic function and cardiac output; (2) defining the underlying cause (residual lesions including residual shunts, valvular heart disease, associated coronary artery disease, underlying cardiomyopathy); (3) describing severity and guiding prognostication; and (4) assisting in evaluating the effect of treatments. When combined with other objective parameters, cardiac imaging can help to differentiate the clinical syndrome of HF from other conditions presenting with similar symptoms[5] including arrhythmia, valve dysfunction, residual shunts, anemia, pulmonary disorders, and renal and liver disease.[6–10]

The risk of HF in ACHD increases with age, defect complexity, and the number of prior surgeries,[11] and is therefore most prevalent in patients with a univentricular circulation (after the Fontan operation), a systemic right ventricle (RV) (transposition of the great arteries [TGA] after atrial switch surgery and congenitally corrected TGA), repaired tetralogy of Fallot (TOF) with severe pulmonary regurgitation, and repaired or unrepaired atrioventricular septal defect.[1,2,11] A unifying definition of HF for these ACHD subtypes is challenging because of the significant clinical, anatomic, and surgical heterogeneity. Reflecting this, most research has explored whether traditional HF parameters used in acquired heart disease also confirm the presence of HF in ACHD. Regardless of defect complexity or systemic ventricular morphology, the extent of ventricular dysfunction has been associated with a stepwise increase in New York Heart Association (NYHA)

functional class and neurohormonal upregulation, reinforcing the notion of myocardial dysfunction being a common final pathway in HF patients regardless of etiology.[12] However, this relationship is more complicated in patients with ACHD. A patient with right HF or Fontan failure is significantly different from a patient with HF resulting from acquired heart disease. More factors influence HF symptoms, rather than ventricular function only, in ACHD. This fact probably explains the weaker association between ventricular dysfunction and neurohormonal brain natriuretic peptide (BNP) upregulation, which also varies according to CHD subtype. In adults with a failing systemic RV, BNP is strongly associated with RV dysfunction, whereas this relationship is more variable in those with repaired TOF.[13] In patients with univentricular physiology the relationship between clinical symptoms, ventricular function, and biomarkers is even more complicated (as reviewed in a 2012 meta-analysis of BNP in CHD[13]), likely reflecting the unique hemodynamic characteristics of the Fontan circulation. In this patient population symptoms and signs of HF can be present, despite normal ventricular systolic function. This situation is related to the unusual circulatory system whereby the venous flow in the pulmonary circulation becomes an important regulatory factor, limiting ventricular filling and, thus, cardiac output.[14] This scenario differs significantly from HF in a patient with a biventricular circulation, which probably explains why whereas even modestly impaired peak oxygen consumption and NYHA functional class are associated with death and hospitalization in ACHD patients, ventricular dysfunction has not been shown to yield prognostic information until it becomes severe.[15] Nevertheless, HF mortality is significantly higher in ACHD patients with severe ventricular dysfunction, including those with TOF, systemic RV failure, and adults with failing Fontan physiology.[1,11,16] The additional prognostic value of confirming severe ventricular dysfunction in such patients, however, is questionable because many of these patients present with NYHA class III/IV symptoms and other unfavorable prognostic markers of advanced HF (eg, hyponatremia or renal dysfunction).

For the diagnosis of HF and follow-up of treatment, clinicians rely heavily on ejection fraction (EF) as a metric of systolic ventricular function, as measured by echocardiographic techniques. Left ventricular (LV) EF can generally reliably be obtained in a geometrically normal LV, but is more difficult to measure if the LV shape is abnormal, and is more difficult to measure in the more complex RV and even more so in any type of single ventricle. For these ventricles, functional assessment often is limited to a qualitative assessment of ventricular function. For quantitative assessment of RV and single function, cardiac magnetic resonance imaging (CMR) is considered the clinical reference technique, but its limited accessibility makes it difficult to use in the clinical follow-up in ACHD HF patients. Newer echocardiographic techniques based on nongeometric indices of ventricular function have gained more popularity, such as the myocardial performance index (MPI), and new techniques including tissue Doppler imaging and myocardial strain imaging.[17,18] Nongeometric indices may provide a more reliable measure of ventricular function than EF, and are emerging as important techniques that provide important information on the severity of dysfunction. Apart from direct functional assessment, evaluation of ventricular size (dimensions and volumes), wall thickness (degree of hypertrophy), and shape (thickness/dimension ratio) provide important information about myocardial remodeling. Unfavorable remodeling often results in myocardial fibrosis, which is linked to adverse clinical outcomes.[19–22] Tissue-characterization techniques are potentially very powerful predictive techniques, as the degree of myocardial fibrosis is likely related to poor long-term outcomes. Cardiac imaging techniques that evaluate the ventricular response to exercise also yield important prognostic information, with an abnormal ventricular response to stress in patients with a systemic RV being associated with an increased risk of HF hospitalization and death.[23]

ECHOCARDIOGRAPHY

Echocardiography is the first-line imaging modality for the evaluation of ventricular size and function in ACHD patients. Echocardiography provides invaluable insights into HF mechanisms (eg, significant valvular dysfunction), complications (eg, pulmonary hypertension), treatment response (eg, improved EF, improved diastolic function parameters), and prognosis. Guidelines for the assessment of LV and RV size and function have been published for acquired adult heart disease,[24,25] and more recently also for pediatric heart disease.[26] However, no specific echocardiographic guidelines for ACHD patients are available. The pediatric guidelines are limited by the standard adult 2-dimensional (2D) linear and volumetric methods, the need to adjust measurements for body surface area in younger patients, and the lack of validated Doppler techniques for grading valvular dysfunction in CHD. There is a need for more specific echocardiographic guidelines focusing on ACHD. This population is even more challenging than the pediatric CHD population, owing to the more limited echocardiographic windows and the association of acquired heart disease. The authors propose a systematic approach to the assessment of this population that includes the different available techniques.

Geometric Versus Nongeometric Assessment of Ventricular Function

The range of techniques being used to assess the global performance of the heart and its function at the level of the myocyte highlight the inherent challenges of quantifying ventricular function. The existing techniques can be broadly classified into 2 categories: geometric techniques that rely on an assumption of consistent ventricular size geometry, and nongeometric techniques such as Doppler that are not influenced by ventricular shape. Most methods are potentially load dependent.

Every assessment of myocardial function should start with assessing ventricular dimensions and dimensional changes. Progressive ventricular systolic dysfunction is generally associated with progressive ventricular dilatation and more spherical reconfiguration of the overall ventricular shape. The different quantification guidelines include specific recommendations for standardization of measuring LV and RV dimensions.[24–26] In ACHD patients, serial follow-up of these dimensions provide important information on ventricular remodeling or reverse remodeling on treatment. Dimensional changes can be used to assess global pump function. For the LV, the recommended measurement is EF calculation based on the biplane Simpson or area-length method; however, both methods assume an ellipsoid LV shape. There is no robust 2D technique available to estimate RV EF. The monoplane or biplane Simpson method is inaccurate because of the geometric assumptions made. For the RV, fractional area change (FAC) as measured from the apical 4-chamber view has been proposed as a good clinical alternative, as FAC correlates highly with RV EF as measured by CMR in most conditions affecting RV function. A similar approach could probably be used for a univentricular heart, but has not been well validated. More recently, 3-dimensional (3D) echocardiography has been proposed for more reliable assessment of LV and RV volumes and EF. For the LV, largely automated segmentation programs allow a rapid analysis of LV volumes and EF, but these programs are also based on normally shaped LVs. For the RV only semiautomated methods are available, which are more labor intensive and require significant manual postprocessing, limiting their application in routine clinical practice. Studies comparing 3D echocardiographic volumes with CMR as the gold standard[27–31] have confirmed a tendency for 3D imaging to underestimate volumes relative to CMR, and this should be taken into account when comparing study values. It can be difficult to obtain high-quality 3D echocardiographic images of the RV in patients with ACHD, especially when enlarged, such as in TOF or in patients with a systemic RV; this limits the application of 3D techniques. In patients with structurally normal hearts, the predominant contraction pattern is longitudinal. Tricuspid annular planar excursion is a simple measurement that provides a reasonably accurate measure of RV longitudinal contractile function in the lateral wall of the RV. However, it is a regional parameter that does not always correlate with global RV function in patients with abnormal segmental RV motion, and is also influenced by tricuspid regurgitation.

Because of the limitations of geometric techniques in patients with ACHD, nongeometric methods are potentially good alternative or, at least, complementary methods for assessing ventricular function. These techniques include measurements based on Doppler intervals such as dP/dt and the MPI, tissue Doppler imaging (TDI) measuring myocardial velocities, and myocardial deformation methods measuring myocardial strain and strain rate.

Despite being widely researched, the first category of methods based on Doppler intervals has not found widespread clinical application, mainly because of the limited reproducibility of the time intervals.[32] Other problems include the heart rate and load sensitivity of these measurements, resulting in a less intuitive interpretation and an absence of published normative values for young adults with CHD of varying types. More recently, attention has shifted to the clinical applications of TDI, strain, and strain rate in ACHD and HF.

TDI uses high-amplitude/low-frequency signals from the myocardium itself to measure displacement velocity relative to the imaging probe. Measured velocity is relatively independent of ventricular geometry and less dependent on 2D image quality; however, as for any Doppler technique, alignment with the direction of myocardial motion is important. When the ultrasound beam is not aligned with the direction of ventricular motion, myocardial velocities are less accurate; this is a potential limitation in ACHD, particularly in patients with significant ventricular enlargement. Nevertheless, such limitations can generally be overcome by adjusting the probe position, and

TDI has now been validated against CMR as a reliable measure of ventricular function across a range of CHD subtypes.[33] TDI is generally used for assessing longitudinal ventricular function by obtaining measurements in the different annuli of the atrioventricular valves. In patients with CHD, the tissue Doppler velocities are typically lower than in healthy controls, this being associated with atrial arrhythmia and other clinical findings.[16,34–36] Measurement of tissue Doppler velocities should become a routine echocardiographic technique. Measurements can be used for serial follow-up even in more complex defects. Disadvantages are the load sensitivity and the fact that basal tissue Doppler velocities are regional functional parameters influenced by different factors such as regional dysfunction and atrioventricular valve regurgitation. Interpretation of changes taking these factors into account is, thus, mandatory. Although TDI can be used to calculate strain and strain rate, which have been demonstrated to be more sensitive and earlier indicators of regional dysfunction than many other techniques, speckle-tracking methods of quantifying strain are now generally more commonplace.

Speckle-Tracking Echocardiography

Speckle tracking overcomes some of the limitations of TDI through its ability to track changes in tissue velocity independent of probe position (angle independent). Using this technique, tissue movement is tracked by following "speckles" in the myocardium, which are based on the unique ultrasound signature given by a specific myocardial area. Algorithms can be applied to calculate displacement, velocity, and strain, specifically the percentage of change of length compared with the original length and strain rate, the derivative of strain over time.

Using this method, both regional (segmental) and global ventricular myocardial deformation can be assessed, as in the example shown with congenitally corrected TGA (**Fig. 1**). Many emerging studies now apply this technology for the assessment of CHD.[37–40] Not surprisingly, measurements in CHD patients differ from those in healthy controls; however, the clinical and prognostic significance of these differences are still unknown. In addition, intrinsically these methods are influenced by changes in loading conditions and also by ventricular remodeling. Strain rate seems less load-dependent but is more difficult to measure, as generally strain-rate curves are noisier and the lower frame rates of speckle-tracking echocardiography limit accurate assessment of peak strain rates. Therefore, for most

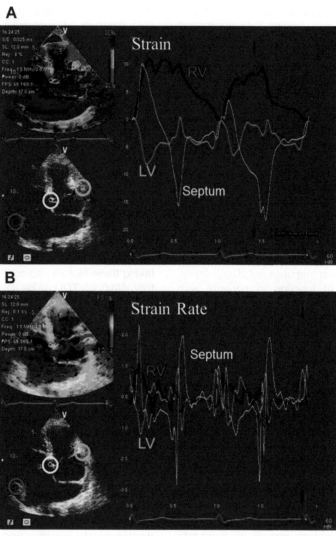

Fig. 1. Speckle-tracking strain imaging in a patient with congenitally corrected transposition of the great arteries. Regions of interest are defined in basal regions of the right and left ventricular myocardium (shown in *red, yellow*, and *green*). Algorithms track the movement of the speckle pattern within these regions, and quantitate strain (*A*) and strain rate (*B*) for each region throughout the cardiac cycle. Separately, by using a border detection algorithm, similar speckle patterns are followed for each segment from base to apex, to map strain (*C*) and to quantify global strain (*D*) for the entire heart. The example shown includes the patient with transposition with mild to moderately reduced absolute value of global strain (*D, left*), and, by comparison, a different patient with an acquired cardiomyopathy with severely reduced absolute value of global strain (*D, right*). LV, left ventricle; RV, right ventricle.

congenital heart defects it is not yet certain how these newer metrics of function can guide decisions related to patient care in adults with CHD. An exception is in patients with a systemic RV, for whom 2 studies now show an association between strain findings and clinical events in patients with TGA.[41,42] Another study showed differences between restrictive and nonrestrictive RV physiology after TOF repair.[43] Nevertheless, how the strain data influence clinical HF management is as yet unclear. One area where speckle tracking may be useful is in evaluating timing of surgery and likelihood of myocardial recovery in ACHD patients with valvular disease, or in sophisticated studies of regional dyssynchrony when cardiac resynchronization therapy is being considered. Though conceptually appealing, it is unclear both in patients with structurally normal hearts and in those with CHD whether logical inference based on imaging assessment of dyssynchrony corresponds robustly with extent of clinical response.

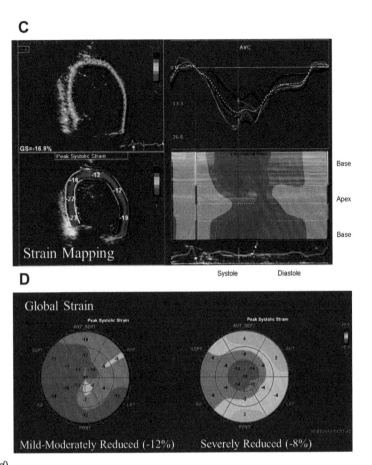

Fig. 1. (continued)

Diastolic Function

In acquired heart disease, pulsed-wave Doppler is frequently used to assess diastolic inflow across the mitral valve and LV myocardial velocities (tissue Doppler).[44] A hierarchy of diastolic dysfunction has been described, beginning with delayed relaxation and progressing to "restrictive" disease implying end-stage elevations in ventricular filling pressures. Diastolic assessment in ACHD remains controversial because of the significant variation in factors that influence transmitral pressure gradients, including, but not limited to, atrial anatomy and dimensions, atrioventricular connections, ventricular morphology, valvular regurgitation, ventricular-vascular interactions, and transpulmonary flow. The prognostic and clinical significance of diastolic dysfunction varies according to ACHD subtype. In Mustard patients, systemic RV diastolic function using standard criteria developed for the systemic LV bears no relationship to clinical status,[45] whereas an association has been reported between RV diastolic dysfunction and ventricular tachycardia in adults with TOF.[46] When

standard algorithms for grading LV diastolic dysfunction are applied to single-ventricle children after the Fontan procedure, restrictive diastolic dysfunction is said to be present in an alarming 18% to 26% of children,[47] although it is likely that the rapid early diastolic filling in these patients reflects exaggerated ventricular relaxation in the younger heart rather than true restrictive physiology. Because the ratio of E/E' compares mitral inflow against myocardial relaxation, it may be a more sensitive measure of diastolic dysfunction in Fontan patients. The finding that an E/E' of 12 correlates with a ventricular end-diastolic pressure of greater than 10 mm Hg suggests that E/E' may be a useful noninvasive parameter for tracking fluid status in patients with a failing Fontan circulation.[48]

Until parameters of diastolic dysfunction are better defined in specific ACHD groups, the authors caution against the application of standard diastolic echocardiographic algorithms in these patients. In instances where diastolic dysfunction is thought to be contributing to HF in ACHD patients, additional objective measures of HF should be sought, including direct assessment of ventricular filling pressures.

CARDIAC MAGNETIC RESONANCE IMAGING

CMR lends itself well to the evaluation of CHD by offering the potential for comprehensive imaging of the entire thorax, irrespective of anatomic variation, with a variety of options for tissue characterization. It is not surprising, then, that CMR plays an important role in clinical CHD management,[5] and in many CMR laboratories CHD indications make up to one-third of all CMR studies performed. Importantly for the purpose of HF assessment, the strengths of CMR include dynamic imaging of the moving heart combined with full visibility throughout the chest.

The mainstay of CMR is accurate measurement of blood flow, ventricular volumes, and, consequently, EF. Although EF is a 1-dimensional, load-dependent, chamber-level, gross metric of ventricular systolic function as discussed earlier, it is conceptually simple and easy to measure, and has thus become universally relied on as the standard indicator of ventricular function. Quantification of EF by CMR has been well established as being accurate and reproducible even in a structurally abnormal heart.[49] Because the method does not require assumptions about RV geometry

or position, it has become the standard for RV quantification, especially in conditions such as TOF, pulmonary atresia, Ebstein anomaly, TGA with a systemic RV, double-chambered RV, Eisenmenger syndrome, or hypoplastic left heart syndrome (**Fig. 2**). Ventricular output can be confirmed with phase-contrast velocity flow mapping, which is also useful in the assessment of valve regurgitation and stenosis, particularly the semilunar valves. Nevertheless, there remain some challenges in accurately quantifying this factor in CHD, including the RV.

Ventricular volume measurement is made from a stack of parallel short-axis images obtained and contoured in diastole and systole. Quantification requires informed contouring of the area of both ventricles in each plane, with judgment about the inclusion of imaging planes of the base that change from ventricle to atria during the cardiac cycle. The sum of areas multiplied by their thickness gives the volume (**Fig. 3A**). For the RV in particular, there is debate as to whether the trabeculations should be included as part of the ventricular mass or blood pool, and strong arguments can be made for either technique. Whereas in most RVs the trabeculations are somewhat trivial, in a severely hypertrophied ventricle, most notably a systemic RV, there is a labyrinth of trabeculations in each slice, making reproducible contouring difficult (see **Fig. 3B**). In diastole, the border of compacted myocardium

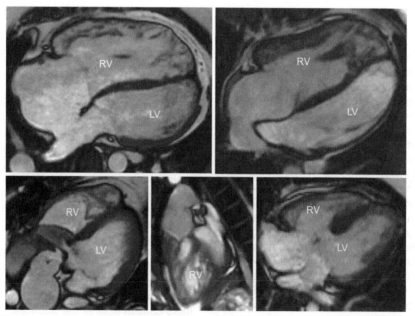

Fig. 2. Examples of magnetic resonance imaging of the right ventricle in several congenital defects such as (*clockwise from upper left*) tetralogy of Fallot, D-transposition with atrial switch palliation, unrepaired atrioventricular septal defect with Eisenmenger syndrome, double-chamber right ventricle, and double-outlet right ventricle after a Rastelli repair. LV, left ventricle; RV, right ventricle.

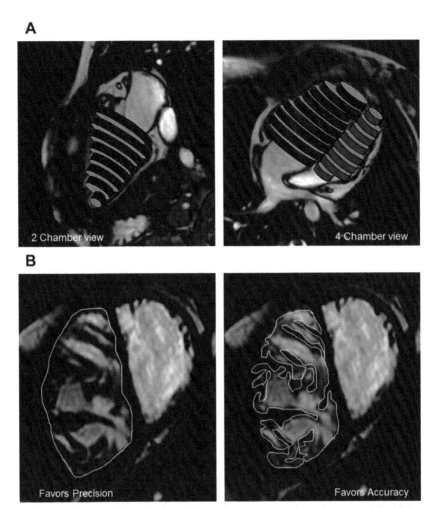

Fig. 3. Method of quantification of ventricular volumes shown as a stack of short-axis disks (*A*) in a patient with D-transposition after atrial switch palliation. Unlike echocardiography, these disks are manually contoured areas of each short-axis image (*B*). However, there is variation between laboratories regarding the techniques used to contour these areas, given the extensive trabeculations found in many patients. Some favor including the trabeculations and papillary muscles in the ventricular area (*left*), which improves precision and reproducibility. Others favor excluding these trabeculations from the ventricular area (*right*), which improves accuracy of the estimate of ventricular blood volume. It is important that serial studies use similar methodology to allow comparison.

can be traced as an alternative, yet this border becomes more indistinct in systole. There may be a small but clinically important overall impact of different techniques on volume quantification and ejection fraction,[50] but no universal method has been agreed upon. Also, some have suggested that the images be acquired in an axial plane rather than in short axis, to more easily account for the longitudinal motion of the valve plane. One comparative study found no clinically meaningful differences between the 2 methods.[51]

Myocardial Deformation Analysis

Sophisticated HF assessment beyond EF with any imaging modality depends on temporal resolution.

Newer scanners allow for faster gradients and improved temporal resolution, facilitating an emerging potential for CMR quantification of multiplanar strain, rotation, and torsion as well as some assessment of diastolic function. Although they are still mainly research tools, several of these methods to assess ventricular mechanics are attractive in CHD because of the ability to apply them 3-dimensionally across the whole heart.

One of the simplest and most established methods is the use of myocardial "tagging."[52] Images throughout a cardiac cycle are acquired after the application of an initial "prepulse" to darken the signal within defined parallel lines or grids, known as tags. Once applied, these dark lines persist on the myocardium through systole and diastole. The displacement of the lines can be tracked to quantify strain, strain rate, and rotation. The lines can be prescribed in any cardiac plane or orientation, unlike the dependence on transducer position in echocardiography. However, the number of frames acquired per cardiac cycle is usually 10 to 20, which is fewer than with echocardiography, meaning that strain calculations are not comparable between modalities.

Tag sequences have been used to demonstrate functional differences of the RV in volume loading (TOF) and pressure loading (atrial septal defect with pulmonary arterial hypertension) states, despite equivalent EF.[53] The disadvantages of tagging are the time required for acquisition (1 breath hold per slice), the fact that it is generally limited to deformation in a predefined plane (2D), and the labor intensive postacquisition analysis using various proprietary software packages. As such, to date tagging has not found widespread application outside of research.

More recently, a new method for tracking myocardial motion and deformation, known as displacement encoding with stimulated echoes (DENSE), has been developed.[54,55] The method encodes positional information into the phase of each pixel, through a process similar to phase-encoded velocity mapping, but on a tissue level similar to tissue Doppler by echocardiography. DENSE quantifies movement in 3 dimensions, with an exceptional spatial resolution that even allows differentiation of epicardium from endocardium. Higher resolution requires longer scan times and is limited by the patient's ability to hold breath. As with tagging, postimaging analysis can be onerous and time consuming, which limits the clinical applicability of DENSE, although its use in CHD is slowly emerging.

Fibrosis Detection

In addition to mechanics, tissue characterization is increasingly important and is a strong feature of CMR. Late gadolinium enhancement takes advantage of dense extracellular space to demonstrate myocardial fibrosis (**Fig. 4**). In CHD, the method has been used in TOF,[20] TGA,[19] and Fontan palliation.[22] Collectively these studies and others showed that the presence of late gadolinium enhancement correlates with increased ventricular volume, decreased EF, poorer functional class, decreased exercise capacity, and arrhythmia. Despite these associations and the universal acceptance of the technique, it detects large areas of replacement fibrosis or scar, not diffuse fibrosis that may be more of a feature of ACHD. Furthermore, the known presence of late enhancement

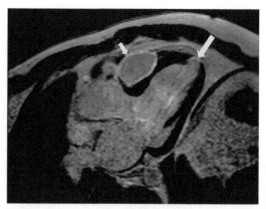

Fig. 4. Late gadolinium enhancement in a patient with tetralogy of Fallot. Normal myocardium is dark. Areas of enhanced signal are seen at the left ventricular apex (*long arrow*), likely the site of prior apical vent placement during cardiopulmonary bypass surgery, and at the right ventricular outflow tract (*short arrow*).

may not add significant prognostic information to readily available basic clinical data, or provide actionable therapeutic guidance.

Newer techniques are based on quantification of T1 and calculation of the extracellular volume fraction, an indicator of more diffuse microscopic fibrosis. In ACHD, this has been used to show more diffuse fibrosis than that seen using late gadolinium enhancement alone.[21] As these techniques emerge it will be useful, for example, to determine the clinical value of fibrosis quantification in directing pharmacotherapy. Whether the methods will be sensitive enough to show changes in an individual with tailored therapy is unknown.

COMPUTED TOMOGRAPHY

Because of the commonplace use of pacemaker/defibrillator insertion, many CHD patients will have contraindications to CMR. When echocardiography is also of insufficient quality, cardiac CT is a useful alternative for assessing ventricular volumes and function. Electrocardiographic gating of a slow heart rate allows for multiphase reformatting of short-axis cine images, providing 3D reconstruction and multiplanar measurements without the use of the geometric assumptions that limit 2D echocardiography. Low temporal resolution is a major limitation to cardiac CT; usually this is limited to 10 phases per cardiac cycle, significantly fewer than in echocardiography or CMR. Quantitative cardiac imaging analysis software is available from several vendors, and uses semiautomated techniques for endocardial border tracing and calculation of end-systolic and end-diastolic volumes, permitting derivation of stroke volume and EF. In adult patients with TOF and TGA, CT is comparable with CMR in assessing RV size and function.[56] Despite the potential to overestimate RV volumes (partly because images are acquired immediately after a contrast bolus of ~ 100 mL), CT provides superior spatial resolution and, therefore, greater precision and higher reproducibility than CMR and echocardiography.[57] It is also superior for the assessment of small structures such as more distal coronary arteries. Compared with CMR, CT image-acquisition time is shorter, an important consideration for HF patients with orthopnea and an inability to lie flat for extended periods of time.

Although temporal resolution is limited, the excellent spatial resolution of CT can be a strong advantage for specific indications. Dual-source CT is a recent innovation of particular relevance to ACHD and HF patients, as it facilitates assessment of cardiac structure, volume, and mass, even in the presence of arrhythmia and tachycardia.[58,59] With adequate visualization, wall-motion analysis is feasible with CT, and in patients suspected of having coronary artery disease or anomalies, CT is the noninvasive imaging modality of choice.[60] Similarly, CT is superior to CMR and echocardiography for evaluating collaterals and arteriovenous malformations, all of which may contribute to HF pathophysiology in ACHD patients.[60] CT may also be helpful for evaluating baffle stenosis or leaks, pulmonary vein stenosis, and in diagnosing intracardiac thrombus, recently reported in almost 2% of Fontan patients undergoing CT[61]; the potential for streaming artifact attributable to less robust prepulmonary mixing with Fontan physiology requires care when assessing for potential pulmonary thrombus or embolism.[62] Furthermore, CT can aid in the evaluation of extracardiac manifestations of ACHD and HF, including pulmonary (atrioventricular malformations), hepatic (cirrhosis, neoplasms), and neurologic (cerebral aneurysms, stroke) disease. As the number of ACHD patients with coronary artery disease increases, hybrid CT/positron emission tomography imaging may become more important for accurately localizing regional myocardial ischemia.

The primary limitations for CT in ACHD HF patients are exposure to ionizing radiation and the risk of contrast-induced nephropathy (CIN) following administration of iodinated contrast material. CIN occurs in 6% of cases after contrast-enhanced CT, and the risk is highest in patients with chronic kidney disease and diabetes.[63] Unlike CMR and echocardiography, CT does not provide quantification of dynamic blood flow (ie, regurgitant lesions) or ventricular filling pressures.

SUMMARY

HF is a clinical diagnosis made after incorporating parameters of symptoms, physical findings, laboratory tests, and exercise capacity as well as ventricular dysfunction. More sensitive indices of regional function and intrinsic myocardial contractility are increasingly being used to understand and identify subclinical dysfunction that precedes reductions in global ventricular performance. For example, abnormalities in RV strain, annular tissue velocity, and MPI in the setting of asymptomatic TOF patients with preserved RV EF indicate early subclinical RV dysfunction.[17,64,65] Emerging imaging techniques have revealed distinct and important differences in ventricular mechanics of patients with congenital heart defects. Imaging is best applied within a comprehensive clinical context and in situations where it can help guide clinical care in a meaningful way. With the development of novel techniques for myocardial assessment comes the challenge of integrating the results into clinical practice.

REFERENCES

1. Piran S, Veldtman G, Siu S, et al. Heart failure and ventricular dysfunction in patients with single or systemic right ventricles. Circulation 2002;105: 1189–94.
2. Zomer AC, Vaartjes I, van der Velde ET, et al. Heart failure admissions in adults with congenital heart disease; risk factors and prognosis. Int J Cardiol 2013. [Epub ahead of print].
3. Verheugt CL, Uiterwaal CS, van der Velde ET, et al. Mortality in adult congenital heart disease. Eur Heart J 2010;31:1220–9.
4. Oechslin EN, Harrison DA, Connelly MS, et al. Mode of death in adults with congenital heart disease. Am J Cardiol 2000;86:1111–6.
5. Warnes CA, Williams RG, Bashore TM, et al. ACC/ AHA 2008 guidelines for the management of adults with congenital heart disease: a report of the American College of Cardiology/American Heart Association Task Force on Practice Guidelines (writing committee to develop guidelines on the management of adults with congenital heart disease). Circulation 2008;118:e714–833.
6. Dimopoulos K, Okonko DO, Diller GP, et al. Abnormal ventilatory response to exercise in adults with congenital heart disease relates to cyanosis and predicts survival. Circulation 2006;113:2796–802.
7. Dimopoulos K, Diller GP, Piepoli MF, et al. Exercise intolerance in adults with congenital heart disease. Cardiol Clin 2006;24:641–60, vii.
8. Dimopoulos K, Diller GP, Petraco R, et al. Hyponatraemia: a strong predictor of mortality in adults

with congenital heart disease. Eur Heart J 2010;31: 595–601.

9. Dimopoulos K, Diller GP, Koltsida E, et al. Prevalence, predictors, and prognostic value of renal dysfunction in adults with congenital heart disease. Circulation 2008;117:2320–8.

10. Dimopoulos K, Diller GP, Giannakoulas G, et al. Anemia in adults with congenital heart disease relates to adverse outcome. J Am Coll Cardiol 2009;54:2093–100.

11. Norozi K, Wessel A, Alpers V, et al. Incidence and risk distribution of heart failure in adolescents and adults with congenital heart disease after cardiac surgery. Am J Cardiol 2006;97:1238–43.

12. Bolger AP, Sharma R, Li W, et al. Neurohormonal activation and the chronic heart failure syndrome in adults with congenital heart disease. Circulation 2002;106:92–9.

13. Eindhoven JA, van den Bosch AE, Jansen PR, et al. The usefulness of brain natriuretic peptide in complex congenital heart disease: a systematic review. J Am Coll Cardiol 2012;60:2140–9.

14. Gewillig M. The Fontan circulation. Heart 2005;91: 839–46.

15. Diller GP, Dimopoulos K, Okonko D, et al. Exercise intolerance in adult congenital heart disease: comparative severity, correlates, and prognostic implication. Circulation 2005;112:828–35.

16. Roos-Hesselink JW, Meijboom FJ, Spitaels SE, et al. Decline in ventricular function and clinical condition after Mustard repair for transposition of the great arteries (a prospective study of 22-29 years). Eur Heart J 2004;25:1264–70.

17. Norozi K, Buchhorn R, Alpers V, et al. Relation of systemic ventricular function quantified by myocardial performance index (Tei) to cardiopulmonary exercise capacity in adults after Mustard procedure for transposition of the great arteries. Am J Cardiol 2005;96:1721–5.

18. Schwerzmann M, Samman AM, Salehian O, et al. Comparison of echocardiographic and cardiac magnetic resonance imaging for assessing right ventricular function in adults with repaired tetralogy of Fallot. Am J Cardiol 2007;99:1593–7.

19. Babu-Narayan SV, Goktekin O, Moon JC, et al. Late gadolinium enhancement cardiovascular magnetic resonance of the systemic right ventricle in adults with previous atrial redirection surgery for transposition of the great arteries. Circulation 2005;111: 2091–8.

20. Babu-Narayan SV, Kilner PJ, Li W, et al. Ventricular fibrosis suggested by cardiovascular magnetic resonance in adults with repaired tetralogy of Fallot and its relationship to adverse markers of clinical outcome. Circulation 2006;113:405–13.

21. Broberg CS, Chugh SS, Conklin C, et al. Quantification of diffuse myocardial fibrosis and its association with myocardial dysfunction in congenital heart disease. Circ Cardiovasc Imaging 2010;3: 727–34.

22. Rathod RH, Prakash A, Powell AJ, et al. Myocardial fibrosis identified by cardiac magnetic resonance late gadolinium enhancement is associated with adverse ventricular mechanics and ventricular tachycardia late after Fontan operation. J Am Coll Cardiol 2010;55:1721–8.

23. Winter MM, Scherptong RW, Kumar S, et al. Ventricular response to stress predicts outcome in adult patients with a systemic right ventricle. Am Heart J 2010;160:870–6.

24. Lang RM, Bierig M, Devereux RB, et al. Recommendations for chamber quantification: a report from the American Society of Echocardiography's Guidelines and Standards Committee and the Chamber Quantification Writing Group, developed in conjunction with the European Association of Echocardiography, a branch of the European Society of Cardiology. J Am Soc Echocardiogr 2005;18: 1440–63.

25. Rudski LG, Lai WW, Afilalo J, et al. Guidelines for the echocardiographic assessment of the right heart in adults: a report from the American Society of Echocardiography endorsed by the European Association of Echocardiography, a registered branch of the European Society of Cardiology, and the Canadian Society of Echocardiography. J Am Soc Echocardiogr 2010;23:685–713 [quiz: 786–8].

26. Lopez L, Colan SD, Frommelt PC, et al. Recommendations for quantification methods during the performance of a pediatric echocardiogram: a report from the Pediatric Measurements Writing Group of the American Society of Echocardiography Pediatric and Congenital Heart Disease Council. J Am Soc Echocardiogr 2010;23:465–95 [quiz: 576–7].

27. Friedberg MK, Su X, Tworetzky W, et al. Validation of 3D echocardiographic assessment of left ventricular volumes, mass, and ejection fraction in neonates and infants with congenital heart disease: a comparison study with cardiac MRI. Circ Cardiovasc Imaging 2010;3:735–42.

28. Grewal J, Majdalany D, Syed I, et al. Three-dimensional echocardiographic assessment of right ventricular volume and function in adult patients with congenital heart disease: comparison with magnetic resonance imaging. J Am Soc Echocardiogr 2010;23:127–33.

29. Kutty S, Smallhorn JF. Evaluation of atrioventricular septal defects by three-dimensional echocardiography: benefits of navigating the third dimension. J Am Soc Echocardiogr 2012;25:932–44.

30. Takahashi K, Mackie AS, Rebeyka IM, et al. Two-dimensional versus transthoracic real-time 3-dimensional echocardiography in the evaluation

of the mechanisms and sites of atrioventricular valve regurgitation in a congenital heart disease population. J Am Soc Echocardiogr 2010;23: 726–34.

31. van der Zwaan HB, Helbing WA, Boersma E, et al. Usefulness of real-time three-dimensional echocardiography to identify right ventricular dysfunction in patients with congenital heart disease. Am J Cardiol 2010;106:843–50.

32. Colan SD, Shirali G, Margossian R, et al. The ventricular volume variability study of the Pediatric Heart Network: study design and impact of beat averaging and variable type on the reproducibility of echocardiographic measurements in children with chronic dilated cardiomyopathy. J Am Soc Echocardiogr 2012;25:842–54.e6.

33. Friedberg MK, Mertens L. Deformation imaging in selected congenital heart disease: is it evolving to clinical use? J Am Soc Echocardiogr 2012;25: 919–31.

34. Arnold R, Gorenflo M, Bottler P, et al. Tissue Doppler derived isovolumic acceleration in patients after atrial repair for dextrotransposition of the great arteries. Echocardiography 2008;25: 732–8.

35. Ramos R, Branco L, Agapito A, et al. Usefulness of tissue Doppler imaging to predict arrhythmic events in adults with repaired tetralogy of Fallot. Rev Port Cardiol 2010;29:1145–61.

36. van der Hulst AE, Roest AA, Holman ER, et al. Relation of prolonged tissue Doppler imaging-derived atrial conduction time to atrial arrhythmia in adult patients with congenital heart disease. Am J Cardiol 2012;109:1792–6.

37. Cheung EW, Liang XC, Lam WW, et al. Impact of right ventricular dilation on left ventricular myocardial deformation in patients after surgical repair of tetralogy of Fallot. Am J Cardiol 2009; 104:1264–70.

38. Friedberg MK, Fernandes FP, Roche SL, et al. Relation of right ventricular mechanics to exercise tolerance in children after tetralogy of Fallot repair. Am Heart J 2013;165:551–7.

39. Marcus KA, de Korte CL, Feuth T, et al. Persistent reduction in left ventricular strain using two-dimensional speckle-tracking echocardiography after balloon valvuloplasty in children with congenital valvular aortic stenosis. J Am Soc Echocardiogr 2012;25:473–85.

40. Moiduddin N, Texter KM, Zaidi AN, et al. Two-dimensional speckle strain and dyssynchrony in single right ventricles versus normal right ventricles. J Am Soc Echocardiogr 2010;23:673–9.

41. Kalogeropoulos AP, Deka A, Border W, et al. Right ventricular function with standard and speckle-tracking echocardiography and clinical events in adults with D-transposition of the great arteries post atrial switch. J Am Soc Echocardiogr 2012; 25:304–12.

42. Diller GP, Radojevic J, Kempny A, et al. Systemic right ventricular longitudinal strain is reduced in adults with transposition of the great arteries, relates to subpulmonary ventricular function, and predicts adverse clinical outcome. Am Heart J 2012;163:859–66.

43. Samyn MM, Kwon EN, Gorentz JS, et al. Restrictive versus nonrestrictive physiology following repair of tetralogy of Fallot: is there a difference? J Am Soc Echocardiogr 2013;26:746–55.

44. Nagueh SF, Appleton CP, Gillebert TC, et al. Recommendations for the evaluation of left ventricular diastolic function by echocardiography. J Am Soc Echocardiogr 2009;22:107–33.

45. Schaefer A, Tallone EM, Westhoff-Bleck M, et al. Relation of diastolic and systolic function, exercise capacity and brain natriuretic peptide in adults after Mustard procedure for transposition of the great arteries. Cardiology 2010;117:112–7.

46. Aboulhosn JA, Lluri G, Gurvitz MZ, et al. Left and right ventricular diastolic function in adults with surgically repaired tetralogy of Fallot: a multi-institutional study. Can J Cardiol 2013;29:866–72.

47. Anderson PA, Sleeper LA, Mahony L, et al. Contemporary outcomes after the Fontan procedure: a Pediatric Heart Network multicenter study. J Am Coll Cardiol 2008;52:85–98.

48. Menon SC, Gray R, Tani LY. Evaluation of ventricular filling pressures and ventricular function by Doppler echocardiography in patients with functional single ventricle: correlation with simultaneous cardiac catheterization. J Am Soc Echocardiogr 2011;24:1220–5.

49. Kilner PJ, Geva T, Kaemmerer H, et al. Recommendations for cardiovascular magnetic resonance in adults with congenital heart disease from the respective working groups of the European Society of Cardiology. Eur Heart J 2010;31:794–805.

50. Winter MM, Bernink FJ, Groenink M, et al. Evaluating the systemic right ventricle by CMR: the importance of consistent and reproducible delineation of the cavity. J Cardiovasc Magn Reson 2008;10:40.

51. Clarke CJ, Gurka MJ, Norton PT, et al. Assessment of the accuracy and reproducibility of RV volume measurements by CMR in congenital heart disease. JACC Cardiovasc Imaging 2012;5:28–37.

52. Zerhouni EA, Parish DM, Rogers WJ, et al. Human heart: tagging with MR imaging—a method for noninvasive assessment of myocardial motion. Radiology 1988;169:59–63.

53. Chen SS, Keegan J, Dowsey AW, et al. Cardiovascular magnetic resonance tagging of the right ventricular free wall for the assessment of long axis myocardial function in congenital heart disease. J Cardiovasc Magn Reson 2011;13:80.

54. Aletras AH, Tilak GS, Natanzon A, et al. Retrospective determination of the area at risk for reperfused acute myocardial infarction with T2-weighted cardiac magnetic resonance imaging: histopathological and displacement encoding with stimulated echoes (DENSE) functional validations. Circulation 2006;113:1865–70.

55. Spottiswoode BS, Zhong X, Lorenz CH, et al. Motion-guided segmentation for cine DENSE MRI. Med Image Anal 2009;13:105–15.

56. Raman SV, Shah M, McCarthy B, et al. Multi-detector row cardiac computed tomography accurately quantifies right and left ventricular size and function compared with cardiac magnetic resonance. Am Heart J 2006;151:736–44.

57. Sugeng L, Mor-Avi V, Weinert L, et al. Multimodality comparison of quantitative volumetric analysis of the right ventricle. JACC Cardiovasc Imaging 2010;3:10–8.

58. Stolzmann P, Scheffel H, Trindade PT, et al. Left ventricular and left atrial dimensions and volumes: comparison between dual-source CT and echocardiography. Invest Radiol 2008;43:284–9.

59. Takx RA, Moscariello A, Schoepf UJ, et al. Quantification of left and right ventricular function and myocardial mass: comparison of low-radiation dose 2nd generation dual-source CT and cardiac MRI. Eur J Radiol 2012;81:e598–604.

60. Orwat S, Diller GP, Baumgartner H. Imaging of congenital heart disease in adults: choice of modalities. Eur Heart J Cardiovasc Imaging 2013. [Epub ahead of print].

61. Lee SY, Baek JS, Kim GB, et al. Clinical significance of thrombosis in an intracardiac blind pouch after a Fontan operation. Pediatr Cardiol 2012;33: 42–8.

62. Prabhu SP, Mahmood S, Sena L, et al. MDCT evaluation of pulmonary embolism in children and young adults following a lateral tunnel Fontan procedure: optimizing contrast-enhancement techniques. Pediatr Radiol 2009;39:938–44.

63. Kooiman J, Pasha SM, Zondag W, et al. Meta-analysis: serum creatinine changes following contrast enhanced CT imaging. Eur J Radiol 2012;81: 2554–61.

64. Abd El Rahman MY, Hui W, Yigitbasi M, et al. Detection of left ventricular asynchrony in patients with right bundle branch block after repair of tetralogy of Fallot using tissue-Doppler imaging-derived strain. J Am Coll Cardiol 2005;45: 915–21.

65. Sun AM, Al Habshan F, Cheung M, et al. Delayed onset of tricuspid valve flow in repaired tetralogy of Fallot: an additional mechanism of diastolic dysfunction and interventricular dyssynchrony. J Cardiovasc Magn Reson 2011;13:43.

Exercise Physiology and Testing in Adult Patients with Congenital Heart Disease

Jonathan Buber, MD[a,b], Jonathan Rhodes, MD[c,*]

KEYWORDS

- Exercise physiology • Adults • Congenital heart diseases • Exercise testing • Exercise training

KEY POINTS

- Adult patients with congenital heart diseases comprise a heterogeneous patient population whose altered cardiovascular, pulmonary, and skeletal muscle physiology may contribute to their overall reduced exercise capacity.
- Formal exercise testing provides an important and excellent objective evaluation of patient physiology and exercise capacity.
- Specific congenital cardiac conditions and types of repair are associated with somewhat characteristic alterations of exercise physiology and the treating physician should be familiar with these distinctive patterns.
- In many conditions the degree of exercise intolerance can have significant prognostic implications.
- The role of exercise training to improve the exercise capacity and the overall survival of ACHD patients is an area of interest to many and may be part of the brighter future that awaits this patient population.

The outstanding improvement in the long-term survival of patients with congenital heart disease (CHD) is perhaps one of modern medicine's greatest triumphs. Many individuals with congenital cardiac conditions that were considered nontreatable merely 4 or 5 decades ago are now adults. As the number of individuals with CHD who survive into adulthood increases, the interest in their unique cardiovascular physiology and long-term outcomes grows and promotes vast research.

One of the early observations made by investigators of this field was that despite improvements in survival for adult patients with congenital heart disease (ACHD), these patients commonly had impaired exercise capacity. Many factors have been identified to explain this phenomenon, including residual cardiovascular defects, deconditioning, repeated surgical interventions, cardiac device implantations, multidrug therapy, and alterations in the anatomy and physiology of organ systems other than the cardiovascular system, such as the pulmonary and the musculoskeletal systems.

Regardless of the underlying mechanisms, exercise intolerance is perhaps the single most important factor responsible for the impairment in the quality of life of ACHD patients. Even simple lesions that are easily addressed at surgery or via transcatheter solutions may be associated with limited exercise capacity. Interestingly, it is common for ACHD patients' self-perception of their exercise intolerance to be unrealistically optimistic. This

Disclosures: None.
[a] Boston Adult Congenital Heart and Pulmonary Hypertension Service, Department of Cardiology, Boston Children's Hospital Boston, 300 Longwood Avenue, Boston, MA 02115, USA; [b] Department of Medicine, Brigham and Women's Hospital, Boston, MA 02115, USA; [c] Department of Cardiology, Boston Children's Hospital, 300 Longwood Avenue, Boston, MA 02115, USA
* Corresponding author.
E-mail address: jonathan.rhodes@cardio.chboston.org

Heart Failure Clin 10 (2014) 23–33
http://dx.doi.org/10.1016/j.hfc.2013.09.012
1551-7136/14/$ – see front matter © 2014 Elsevier Inc. All rights reserved.

observation has been ascribed to the fact that most of them have impaired exercise tolerance that dates back to their early childhood, causing a distorted perception of what constitutes "normal" exercise capacity. Indeed, a recent study of asymptomatic young ACHD found that their exercise capacity, when assessed with formal cardiopulmonary exercise testing (CPET), was comparable to much older adults with equivalent functional class and congestive heart failure (CHF) secondary to acquired heart disease.[1] Formal exercise testing is therefore currently considered to be an important component of the routine evaluation of ACHD patients, because it can reliably and objectively assess exercise capacity and provide valuable risk stratification data.

IMPAIRED EXERCISE TOLERANCE IN ACHD: PREVALENCE AND SPECIAL CONSIDERATIONS

Effort intolerance is experienced by patients from across the CHD spectrum, ranging from simple lesions such as mild left ventricular outflow tract obstructive lesions to complex conditions such as single ventricle physiology (**Table 1**). When CPET was performed in a large cohort of ACHD patients with various conditions, on average, peak oxygen consumption (V_{O2}) was found to be reduced in all examinees regardless of the baseline disease as compared with healthy individuals of similar age.[1] As can be appreciated from **Table 1**, different degrees of exercise intolerance do exist

within the CHD spectrum, and the general rule is that there is a good correlation between the severity of the underlying cardiac defect or the completeness of its repair and the degree of exercise intolerance.[1–4] ACHD patients with Eisenmenger physiology experience the most severe form of exercise intolerance, followed by patients with univentricular physiology and cyanosis.[4]

In normal adult subjects, exercise function tends to deteriorate with age; peak V_{O2} has been found to decline ~0.5% to 0.6% per year after age 21.[5–8] Studies in various ACHD populations have found that this decline tends to progress more rapidly, although observational data suggest that engaging in frequent physical activity may favorably alter this trend.[9]

This observation may be particularly relevant to patients with a systemic right ventricle, such as patients with L-loop transposition of the great arteries (L-loop TGA) or with D-loop TGA who underwent an atrial switch operation (either the Senning or the Mustard procedures). In these patients, severe exercise intolerance often manifests itself in the third or fourth decade of life.[10,11] In fact, almost two-thirds of patients with atrial repairs of D-loop TGA who have other associated defects or prior surgical intervention experience heart failure by the age of 45. The common explanation for this delayed presentation is failure of the systemic right ventricle and progressive insufficiency of the systemic atrioventricular valve, both of which tend to progress slowly over the years.[12] Chronotropic

Table 1
Cardiopulmonary test abnormalities encountered in patients with various congenital and acquired heart diseases

Defect	↓ Peak V_{O2}	↓ Peak HR	↓ O_2 Pulse	↑ V_E/V_{CO2}	↓ VT
Repaired TOF/Truncus	+++	++	+++	+++	++
Fontan	++++	+++	++++	++++	+++
PVOD	++++	+	++++	++++	++++
Ebstein anomaly	+++	++	+++	++	++
D-TGA S/P atrial switch	+++	++	+++	++	++
Aortic valve disease	++	+	++	+	++
Coarctation	++	+	++	+	+++
DCM	++++	+	++++	++	++++
HCM	++	+	++	+	++
Isolated PR	+	+	+	+	+

Note: This table assumes that the patient is not receiving beta-blocker or other anti-arrhythmic therapy that might impair the chronotropic response to exercise.

Abbreviations: +, implies rarely present; ++, sometimes present; +++, often present; ++++, usually present; DCM, dilated cardiomyopathy; HCM, hypertrophic cardiomyopathy; peak HR, heart rate at peak exercise; Peak V_{O2}, oxygen consumption at peak exercise; PR, pulmonary regurgitation, postvalvuloplasty; PVOD, pulmonary vascular obstructive disease; TOF, tetralogy of Fallot; Truncus, Truncus arteriosus; V_E/V_{CO2}, slope of the linear portion of minute ventilation vs carbon dioxide production curve.

incompetence, permanent pacing (which is common in this specific patient population, as discussed below), and other valvular abnormalities are additional possible mechanisms.

Similar to the general population, adult male individuals with CHD perform better at CPET than their female counterparts. An exception to this rule is patients with Eisenmenger syndrome, in whom exercise intolerance was similarly depressed for men and women.[4] These observations indicate that unless patients have severe forms of cardiac defects that combine cyanosis, decreased cardiac output and decreased pulmonary blood flow (as present in Eisenmenger syndrome), the favorable effects of male gender effects on exercise performance (ie, higher muscle mass, higher hemoglobin concentration, and better physical conditioning)[4,13,14] are applicable to the ACHD population.

POTENTIAL CONTRIBUTORS TO IMPAIRED EXERCISE CAPACITY

Impaired exercise capacity in the ACHD patient population is usually the end result of a complex interplay between multiple factors. Careful analyses may be required to identify and evaluate the magnitude and significance of each one. To simplify consideration, it is useful to divide the potential contributors into those that involve the cardiac system, and those that involve other systems, or extracardiac contributors. Naturally, much overlap can exist between these 2 categories.

The important cardiac-associated contributors include ventricular systolic or diastolic dysfunction (of either the systemic or the subpulmonary ventricle, or the function of a single ventricle), valvular stenosis or regurgitation, chronotropic incompetence, conduction abnormalities, significant arrhythmic burden, multiple open heart surgeries, intracardiac shunt, and pericardial disease. The development of heart failure, a major cause of exercise intolerance by itself, can be a common final syndrome of any of these underlying mechanisms.

The important extracardiac contributors include the presence of restrictive and/or obstructive lung disease, pulmonary vascular disease, systemic vascular disease, skeletal muscle dysfunction (including deconditioning), anemia, and iron deficiency. Drug therapy of various types can also significantly affect exercise capacity in ACHD patients by affecting both the cardiac and the extracardiac pathways.

Given that the ACHD population is highly heterogeneous, comprising patients with a large variety of primary conditions addressed by numerous different procedures, it is important to understand the patterns of exercise dysfunction that may be associated with specific cardiac anomalies or types of repairs. In the following section, the methods for evaluating exercise capacity by exercise tests are discussed, along with the changes in the various parameters that may occur in some specific congenital conditions.

EXERCISE TESTING METHODS
CPET

CPET refers to exercise testing with electrocardiogram (ECG) monitoring and expiratory gas analysis. Exercise requires dramatic changes in the amount of oxygen required for muscle function and the volume of carbon dioxide produced as a result of the increase in metabolic rate and, eventually, anaerobic production of ATP. In steady state, such changes at the cellular level are exceptionally closely matched by changes in gas exchange to maintain homeostasis.[10] Important clinical parameters that can be generated from this analysis include breath-by-breath estimates of oxygen consumption (V_{O2}), carbon dioxide production (V_{CO2}), minute ventilation (V_E), end-tidal P_{O2}, and end-tidal P_{CO2}. The parameters obtained from these estimates are of particular relevance to the assessment of the ACHD patient population and are discussed in detail.

Peak V_{O2}
For most individuals, and especially for those with cardiovascular disease, peak V_{O2} is limited by the amount of O_2 that the cardiopulmonary system can deliver to the exercising muscles and this in turn is limited by the circulatory system's ability to increase cardiac output during exercise. Hence peak V_{O2} (ie, the highest rate of V_{O2} detected during a progressive exercise test) is an excellent indicator of the capabilities of a patient's cardiovascular system.

Peak V_{O2} varies with age; it tends to increase and reach a maximum during adolescence or early adulthood and decline progressively thereafter. As noted above, it also varies by gender (with men typically having greater values than women, especially after puberty), and with body size (as larger individuals consume more oxygen than smaller individuals). This relationship is complex, however, as body composition must also be taken into account. Although body mass affects resting V_{O2}, the change in V_{O2} for a given change in workload is similar between subjects. Unlike skeletal muscle, adipose tissue consumes very little oxygen during exercise. Consequently, simply normalizing peak V_{O2} for body mass (ie, V_{O2}/kg) may be misleading. Currently, normal values for peak V_{O2}

are usually calculated from prediction equations generated from a group of normal subjects and are based on age, gender, height, and body mass. Estimates of predicted peak V_{O2} are more highly dependent on height than body mass and therefore these prediction equations partially account for the distorting effects of body habitus/adipose tissue. Ideally, prediction equations should also be generated from studies that used similar exercise equipment. Peak V_{O2} tends to be 5% to 10% higher on a treadmill compared with a cycle ergometer, and this phenomenon should be taken into account. Whichever equations are chosen by a laboratory, the validity of the predictions for the population should be established by testing several normal subjects and confirming that the predicted values agree well with the results of these tests.[15]

Heart rate during exercise

During a progressive exercise test, heart rate (HR) increases linearly in proportion with V_{O2}, from baseline levels to peak HR. The normal peak HR, for treadmill exercise, may be estimated from the equation: Peak HR = 220 − age (years).[16] Peak HR during bicycle exercise tends to be 5% to 10% lower, so it is reasonable to multiply the predicted peak HR derived from this equation by 0.925 if a bicycle exercise protocol is used.[17] In patients with chronotropic incompetence, the HR versus V_{O2} relationship tends to be depressed below the expected normal curve. In contrast, patients who cannot increase forward stroke volume normally during exercise tend to compensate by increasing their HRs more rapidly than normal during exercise and the HR versus V_{O2} relationship is elevated. Patients with impairment of both the chronotropic and the stroke volume response to exercise may have "pseudonormalization" of the HR versus V_{O2} relationship, but would be unable to achieve a normal peak HR.

Chronotropic incompetence (ie, an inability to increase HR to >80% of predicted at peak exercise) is common in the ACHD patient population, with a prevalence of ~60%. Chronotropic incompetence may be due to intrinsic malfunction of the conduction system or it may be iatrogenic, secondary to surgical or catheter-based intervention with inadvertent injury to the sinus or atrioventricular nodes, to drug therapy (mainly β-blocker, nondihydropyridine calcium channel blockers, and antiarrhythmic medications), or to chronic pacing.[18–21] ACHD patients who often require pacemaker implantation on account of sinus node dysfunction include those who have had Fontan operations and those who have undergone atrial switch procedures for D-loop TGA. Conditions for which pacemaker implantation is commonly required for AV node dysfunction include L-TGA and defects whose repair requires surgery near the atrioventricular node (eg, membranous ventricular septal defects, atrioventricular canal defects, subaortic stenosis).

Exercise testing can provide information on rate control in patients with chronic atrial fibrillation and on the adequacy of rate response for those with pacemakers. Because cycle ergometry is associated with less upper body motion, however, it may not always accurately represent rate response with more common daily activities.

More recently described indices of chronotropic incompetence, such as the HR reserve (peak HR − resting HR) and the chronotropic index (100 × (HR reserve)/(predicted peak HR − resting HR)), have not been studied widely in the ACHD patient population, and their relevance remains uncertain.[19,22]

Oxygen pulse

The oxygen pulse (O_2P) at peak exercise is the product of the forward stroke volume times the O_2 extraction at peak exercise. Under most circumstances, O_2 extraction at peak exercise is expected to vary little from patient to patient and the O_2P will be proportional to forward stroke volume.[23] Normal values for O_2P at peak exercise depend on patient size, age, and gender. Normal values may be calculated by dividing the predicted peak V_{O2} by the predicted peak HR.[15]

Important limitations of the O_2P concept should be kept in mind when interpreting these data. In patients with depressed arterial O_2 content at peak exercise (eg, patients with anemia or patients with significant arterial oxygen desaturation), O_2 extraction at peak exercise is limited and the O_2P will underestimate stroke volume. Isolated polycythemia causes the opposite effect, increasing arterial O_2 content and causing the O_2P to overestimate the stroke volume, although in most cases with ACHD high hemoglobin is due to systemic arterial desaturation. It should be also appreciated that based on the Starling curve, relative bradycardia at peak exercise should engender a compensatory increase in the stroke volume and hence the O_2P at peak exercise. Consequently, in patients with low peak-exercise HRs, the absence of a compensatory increase in O_2P, above normal predicted values, is abnormal.

The O_2P tends to be depressed in patients with conditions that impair their ability to increase forward stroke volume to appropriate levels at peak exercise. Patients with depressed ventricular function,[24] severe obstructive lesions, severe valvular regurgitation,[25,26] and pulmonary or systemic vascular disease[27,28] often have a low peak-exercise O_2P.

The O_2P is often depressed in patients who have undergone a Fontan procedure, even in the absence of ventricular or valvular dysfunction.[19] In these patients, the low O_2P probably reflects the absence of a pulmonary ventricle and the limited ability of the passively perfused pulmonary vascular bed to accommodate the high rate of blood flow normally present at peak exercise (a physiologic function that greatly influences the exercise capacity of Fontan patients). Indeed, the O_2P is one of the strongest correlates of peak work rate in patients with Fontan circulations.[19]

Skeletal muscle abnormalities, which impair oxygen extraction, such as glycogen storage diseases, mitochondrial and other metabolic defects, or severe deconditioning, will also cause the O_2P to be depressed.[29] Patients with severe deconditioning also tend to have depressed O_2P because the normal augmentation of preload and stroke volume by pumping action of the exercising skeletal muscles are impaired, in addition to mild impairment of oxygen extraction.

Ventilatory anaerobic threshold

The anaerobic threshold occurs during progressive exercise when aerobic metabolism is insufficient to meet the energy requirements of the exercising muscles. The anaerobic threshold is a physiologic phenomenon that is not affected by patient effort or motivation and may be determined on a submaximal exercise test. It is thus considered an excellent index of the cardiovascular system's capacity to support the hemodynamic demands of exercise. Because anaerobic metabolism produces CO_2 but does not consume O_2, during a progressive exercise test, the ventilatory anaerobic threshold (VT) is marked by an increase in V_{CO2} out of proportion to the associated increase in V_{O2}. Although there is debate regarding nomenclature (ventilatory threshold, anaerobic threshold, lactate threshold) and whether this reflects a true threshold effect, these distinctions have little import for clinical exercise testing.

Normal values for the VT are calculated based on established equations, which are in turn based on age, size, and gender. VT is also commonly expressed as a percentage of predicted peak V_{O2}. In the absence of cardiovascular disease, VT rarely occurs before a V_{O2} less than 40% of predicted peak V_{O2}. However, VT is often depressed below this value in patients with conditions that significantly impair the ability to increase cardiac output or oxygen delivery appropriately during exercise.[10,30]

In the ACHD patient population, the VT is often depressed in a manner similar to, or slightly less than, peak V_{O2}.[19] Therefore, when peak V_{O2} data are available, VT data do not often provide significant additional information. When a patient does not expend a maximal effort, however, peak exercise parameters may not accurately reflect his/her true clinical status. Under these circumstances, VT data may provide worthwhile insights that would otherwise be unavailable on a submaximal test.

The VT tends to be disproportionately depressed in conditions that selectively impair blood flow to the exercise muscles, such as patients' significant residual or unrepaired aortic coarctation, peripheral arterial disease, or Takayasu arteritis.

V_E/V_{CO2} slope

V_E rises linearly in proportion with V_{CO2} during progressive exercise until a point above the VT, when the accumulating lactic acidosis engenders a compensatory increase in V_E out of proportion to the increase in V_{CO2}. The V_E/V_{CO2} slope is the slope of the linear portion of this curve. Alternatively, some report the slope of the entire V_E/V_{CO2} relationship through exercise. Although this approach is slightly simpler, the value for the V_E/V_{CO2} slope calculated in this manner is effort dependent and therefore, at least theoretically, less reproducible than the aforementioned methodology. Although the values (and normal range) of the V_E/V_{CO2} slope calculated by these 2 methods are slightly different, in practice both methods provide similar information.[31]

Implications in ACHD patients

The ventilatory response to the increase in CO_2 production with exercise (expressed as V_E/V_{CO2} slope) increases progressively after the second decade of life.[32] Currently, most centers consider a V_E/V_{CO2} slope greater than 29 to 30 to be abnormal in young adults. The V_E/V_{CO2} slope is often elevated in patients with acquired CHF,[33–35] tetralogy of Fallot,[36] D-TGA after atrial switch procedure,[37] and pulmonary arterial hypertension.[27,28] Although multiple factors may influence the V_E/V_{CO2} slope, pulmonary blood flow maldistribution and consequent ventilation/perfusion (V/Q) mismatch are probably the most important pathophysiologic processes that underlie these observations and associations.[38,39]

Efficient gas exchange across the alveolar/capillary membrane requires optimal V/Q matching. Patients who have undergone repair of tetralogy of Fallot often have residual branch pulmonary artery stenoses that cause maldistribution of the pulmonary blood flow, which in turn has been linked to V_E/V_{CO2} slope elevation and depressed peak

V_{O2}.[39–41] Effective relief of these stenoses has been associated with improvements in peak V_{O2} and the V_E/V_{CO2} slope (**Fig. 1**).[39]

Patients with CHF have maldistribution of the pulmonary blood flow as a consequence of the elevated pulmonary capillary wedge pressure that accompanies CHF.[39,42] As ventricular function deteriorates and the wedge pressure rises, the pulmonary blood flow maldistribution (and consequent V/Q mismatch) worsens and the V_E/V_{CO2} slope progressively rises. Similarly, for patients who have had an atrial switch procedure for TGA, elevation of the V_E/V_{CO2} slope probably reflects the progressive systemic ventricular dysfunction that often develops in these patients as they age.

In patients with pulmonary arterial hypertension, and possibly also for patients with TGA who develop pulmonary hypertension after an atrial switch procedure, pulmonary blood flow maldistribution results from pulmonary vascular obstructive

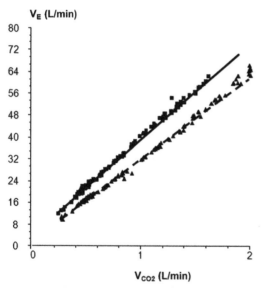

V_E (L/min)

V_{CO2} (L/min)

Fig. 1. Relationship between V_E and V_{CO2} in a patient with tetralogy of Fallot before and after successful pulmonary artery balloon angioplasty that increased left pulmonary artery blood flow from 13% to 35% of the total pulmonary blood flow. Square symbols are data points before angioplasty; triangular symbols are data points after angioplasty. The solid line represents the linear portion of the V_E/V_{CO2} relationship before angioplasty (the slope of the line is the V_E/V_{CO2} slope). The dashed line is the relationship after angioplasty. Note that, after the angioplasty, the patient's V_E was lower for any given V_{CO2}. The V_E/V_{CO2} slope decreased from 35 to 29 and was associated with an increase in the peak V_{O2} from 18.8 to 23.7 mL/kg/min and an increase in the end-tidal P_{CO2} at the anaerobic threshold from 32 to 36 mm Hg.

disease. As the vascular obstruction progresses, the maldistribution worsens; gas exchange within the lungs becomes more and more inefficient and the V_E/V_{CO2} slope rises. Hence, for these patients the V_E/V_{CO2} slope reflects the extent of disease within the pulmonary vasculature.[27,28]

The V_E/V_{CO2} slope is also commonly elevated in patients with Fontan-type circulation.[43,44] This elevation is probably also due, to a large extent, to pulmonary blood flow maldistribution (and associated V/Q mismatch) secondary to the absence of a pulmonary ventricle.[45] Right-to-left intracardiac (as seen in Eisenmenger syndrome) or intrapulmonary shunting, which is common in patients with Fontan-type circulation, will also cause elevated V_E/V_{CO2} slope. The shunting allows CO_2-rich systemic venous blood to enter the systemic arterial circulation, bypassing the pulmonary circulation. The consequent increase in arterial P_{CO2} is sensed by arterial chemoreceptors, inducing central nervous system respiratory centers to increase the patient's respiratory drive (and V_E) and causing the V_E/V_{CO2} slope to rise. The resulting alveolar hyperventilation reduces the P_{CO2} of the blood returning from the lungs and helps to normalize the patient's arterial P_{CO2}. Eliminating right-to-left shunting results in a reduction in the V_E/V_{CO2} slope (**Fig. 2**).[46]

Exercise Testing with Electrocardiographic Monitoring Without Gas Exchange

In this form of exercise testing, exercise is carried out in conjunction with continuous 12-lead ECG monitoring. The Bruce Treadmill Protocol is most commonly used, and endurance time is used as an index of exercise capacity.[47–52]

Important parameters that should be recorded during exercise testing with ECG monitoring include abnormal blood pressure responses, exercise-induced rhythm disturbances, ST changes, and arterial oxygen desaturation (either noninvasive pulse oximetry or arterial blood gas). In conjunction with myocardial perfusion imaging or stress echocardiography, it can also provide evidence of myocardial ischemia during exercise.

Implications in ACHD patients

As the concern for ischemia should always exist, especially for patients that have risk factors for atherosclerotic disease, several ACHD subpopulations are considered to be at a somewhat increased risk to develop ischemia and are routinely screened for its presence; these include patients who underwent the arterial switch operation for TGA or other procedures requiring reimplantation of the coronary arteries, patients who underwent surgical correction of anomalous

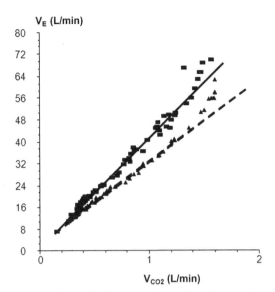

Fig. 2. Relationship between V_E and V_{CO2} in a patient with fenestrated Fontan before and after successful fenestration closure. Square symbols are data points before fenestration closure; triangular symbols are data points after closure. The solid line represents the linear portion of the V_E/V_{CO2} relationship before closure (the slope of the line is the V_E/V_{CO2} slope). The dashed line is the relationship after closure. Note that, after the fenestration closure, the patient's V_E was lower for any given V_{CO2}. The V_E/V_{CO2} slope decreased from 41 to 30 and was associated with an increase in the end-tidal PCO_2 at the anaerobic threshold from 26 to 34 mm Hg. Peak V_{O2} decreased from 34.5 to 34.4 mL/kg/min.

coronary artery origin, patients implanted with a Melody valve that was in proximity to the coronary vessels, and patients with a congenitally abnormal course of the coronary arteries that was not addressed at surgery.

The major limitation of this method of evaluation lies in the fact that endurance time is significantly influenced by factors unrelated to the cardiopulmonary system (eg, musculoskeletal system, obesity, motivation), and it thus often may not provide reliable information regarding a patient's cardiopulmonary status. Depending on the peak HR as an index of patient effort is unreliable, as many ACHD patients have sinus node dysfunction and/or are on medications that may impair the chronotropic response to exercise (see above). Hence, the ability of exercise testing with ECG monitoring to provide objective, quantitative information regarding a patient's exercise capacity is suboptimal. This testing modality also provides little information regarding the mechanisms responsible for a CHD patient's exercise limitation.

Alternative protocols or modifications of the Bruce protocol may be used if the speeds of the higher levels of the Bruce protocol are too fast for the more severely affected ACHD patients (although interpretation of endurance time then becomes even more problematic). Cycle protocols may also be used; one advantage is that there is less motion artifact with cycle testing. For these protocols, the peak work rate, rather than the endurance time, is used as an index of exercise capacity.

Many ACHD patients have baseline conduction abnormalities or otherwise grossly abnormal depolarization and repolarization patterns that impair the sensitivity and specificity of exercise-induced ST changes for the detection of myocardial ischemia. Consequently, stress echocardiography and/or myocardial perfusion imaging is often required when there is a clinical need to address this issue.

The Six-minute Walk Test

The 6-minute walk test (6MWT) is a simpler test to assess exercise capacity and is more applicable in patients who are significantly debilitated. In the 6MWT the patient is encouraged to cover as much distance walking as possible during the 6 minutes. Portable pulse oximetry may be used in the test, but the heart rhythm and electrocardiogram are not monitored.

The 6MWT has advantages. It is easy to perform, does not require sophisticated equipment, and mimics activities of daily living.[53] It has therefore commonly been used in drug trials for adults with CHF or pulmonary arterial hypertension. There are few data in ACHD.[54] However, in all but the most limited patients, it is a submaximal test. Consequently, although it correlates fairly well with V_{O2} in highly symptomatic patients, its utility and validity in patients with mild or moderate impairment are unclear.[55,56] In fact, many have advocated against using the 6MWT in such individuals, especially when the aim is to evaluate for improvement after attempted corrective intervention, due to what is known as the "ceiling effect" that can mask true clinical improvement. The test is also strongly influenced by patient motivation and other factors (such as leg length, body weight, orthopedic issues, ability to turn quickly at the ends of the course) unrelated to the cardiopulmonary system. It is difficult to control for or to quantify the influence of these variables on the outcome (distance walked) of the 6MWT. Although these issues are mitigated somewhat in drug trials that include large numbers of patients, they make the interpretation of an individual's test (or serial studies in one individual) ambiguous and difficult. On account of these considerations, the utility of the 6MWT in ACHD is limited.

THE PROGNOSTIC IMPLICATIONS OF EXERCISE TESTING IN ACHD

Several CPET parameters have been found to possess prognostic value in patients with various forms of CHD. Peak V_{O2} has been found to be an independent predictor of death and/or hospitalization for ACHD patients overall,[1] patients with repaired tetralogy of Fallot,[33] patients who have undergone atrial switch procedures for D-TGA,[57] patients with pulmonary hypertension,[27,28] and patients with CHF. Among patients with Fontan surgery, a peak V_{O2} less than 16.6 mL/kg/min was associated with a mortality risk 7.5-fold higher than patients with peak V_{O2} above this value (**Fig. 3**A). In addition, a peak HR less than 122.5 bpm was associated with a 10.6-fold increase in mortality (see **Fig. 3**B). Fontan patients who did not have any of these risk factors had an intermediate-term (4.0 ± 2.0 y) survival of 98%.[57]

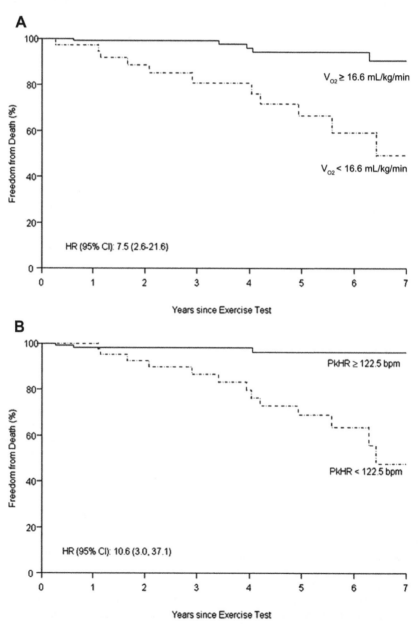

Fig. 3. Time to death for patients above and below the cutoff value for (A) weight normalized peak V_{O2} and (B) peak heart rate. CI, confidence intervals; HR, hazard ratio; PkHR, heart rate at peak exercise.

The V_E/V_{CO2} slope has also been found to possess prognostic value in patients with CHF,[35] pulmonary hypertension,[31,32] ACHD patients in general,[2] and patients with D-TGA who develop systemic (anatomic right) ventricular dysfunction following atrial switch surgery.[37] In patients with these conditions, disease progression is associated with progressive V/Q mismatch and/or impairment of gas exchange across the alveolar-capillary membrane. These pathophysiologic changes in turn cause V_E/V_{CO2} slope to become progressively elevated.

The V_E/V_{CO2} slope has also been found to carry important prognostic value in patients with repaired tetralogy of Fallot. In these patients V_E/V_{CO2} slope elevation has been linked to the presence of branch residual PA stenosis.[39,40] These stenoses can have a particularly deleterious effect on the exercise hemodynamics of the postoperative tetralogy patient. Pulmonary valve incompetency is almost always present following tetralogy repair. If the patient's pulmonary vascular bed is healthy, the tremendous decline in pulmonary vascular resistance that accompanies exercise mitigates the severity of the pulmonary regurgitation. In contrast, in patients with residual branch PA stenoses the severity of the pulmonary regurgitation is magnified during exercise and the right ventricle's pressure and volume overload are greatly exacerbated. These unfavorable hemodynamics probably account for the association between mortality and V_E/V_{CO2} slope elevation.

Although very common among Fontan patients, the degree of V_E/V_{CO2} slope elevation does not seem to be associated with increased mortality in this population.[58] This observation is probably because the V_E/V_{CO2} slope elevation encountered in these patients is to a large extent due to V/Q mismatch secondary to the absence of normal pulmonary artery pulsatility (a condition common to all Fontan patients) and, in contrast to the aforementioned conditions, is not strongly related to disease progression.

SUMMARY

Patients with ACHDs comprise a heterogeneous patient population whose altered cardiovascular, pulmonary, and skeletal muscle physiology may contribute to their overall reduced exercise capacity. As these patients are often unaware of their own exercise intolerance, formal exercise testing provides an important and excellent objective evaluation of their physiology and exercise capacity. Specific congenital cardiac conditions and types of repair are associated with somewhat characteristic alterations of exercise physiology.

The treating physician should be familiar with these distinctive patterns. In addition, in many conditions the degree of exercise intolerance can have significant prognostic implications. The role of exercise training to improve the exercise capacity and the overall survival of ACHD patients further is an area of interest to many and may be part of the brighter future that awaits this unique patient population.

REFERENCES

1. Diller GP, Dimopoulos K, Okonko D, et al. Exercise intolerance in adult congenital heart disease: comparative severity, correlates, and prognostic implication. Circulation 2005;112:828–35.
2. Dimopoulos K, Okonko DO, Diller GP, et al. Abnormal ventilatory response to exercise in adults with congenital heart disease relates to cyanosis and predicts survival. Circulation 2006;113:2796–802.
3. Fredriksen PM, Veldtman G, Hechter S, et al. Aerobic capacity in adults with various congenital heart diseases. Am J Cardiol 2001;87:310–4.
4. Kempny A, Dimopoulos K, Uebing A, et al. Reference values for exercise limitations among adults with congenital heart disease. Relation to activities of daily life–single centre experience and review of published data. Eur Heart J 2012;11: 1386–96.
5. Shephard RJ. Endurance Fitness. Toronto: University of Toronto Press; 1969.
6. Astrand P. Human physical fitness, with special reference to sex and age. Physiol Rev 1956; 36(Suppl 2):307–55.
7. Astrand I. Aerobic work capacity in men and women with special reference to age. Acta Physiol Scand 1960;49(Suppl 196):1–92.
8. Lange-Anderson K, Shephard RJ, Denolin H, et al. Fundementals of exercise testing. Geneva (Switzerland): World Health Organization; 1971.
9. Ubeda Tikkanen A, Opotowsky AR, Bhatt AB, et al. Physical activity is associated with improved aerobic exercise capacity over time in adults with congenital heart disease. Int J Cardiol 2013. [Epub ahead of print].
10. Wasserman K. The anaerobic threshold measurement to evaluate exercise performance. Am Rev Respir Dis 1984;129(2 Pt 2):S35–40.
11. Fredriksen PM, Pettersen E, Thaulow E. Declining aerobic capacity of patients with arterial and atrial switch procedures. Pediatr Cardiol 2009; 30:166–71.
12. Reybrouck T, Mertens L, Brown S, et al. Long-term assessment and serial evaluation of cardiorespiratory exercise performance and cardiac function in patients with atrial switch operation for complete transposition. Cardiol Young 2001;11:17–24.

13. Buys R, Budts W, Reybrouck T, et al. Serial exercise testing in children, adolescents and young adults with Senning repair for transposition of the great arteries. BMC Cardiovasc Disord 2012;12:88.

14. Drinkwater BL. Women and exercise: physiological aspects. Exerc Sport Sci Rev 1984;12:21–51.

15. American Thoracic Society, American College of Chest Physicians. ATS/ACCP Statement on cardiopulmonary exercise testing. Am J Respir Crit Care Med 2003;167:211–77.

16. Cooper KH, Purdy J, White S, et al. Age-fitness adjusted maximal heart rates. Med Sci Sports 1977;10:78–86.

17. Braden DS, Carroll JF. Normative cardiovascular responses to exercise in children. Pediatr Cardiol 1999;20:4–10.

18. Reybrouck T, Weymans M, Stijns H, et al. Exercise testing after correction of tetralogy of Fallot: the fallacy of a reduced heart rate response. Am Heart J 1986;112:998–1003.

19. Paridon SM, Mitchell PD, Colan SD, et al. A cross-sectional study of exercise performance during the first two decades of life following the Fontan operation. J Am Coll Cardiol 2008;52:99–107.

20. Norozi K, Wessel A, Alpers V, et al. Chronotropic incompetence in adolescents and adults with congenital heart disease after cardiac surgery. J Card Fail 2007;13:263–8.

21. Diller GP, Dimopoulos K, Okonko D, et al. Heart rate response during exercise predicts survival in adults with congenital heart disease. J Am Coll Cardiol 2006;48:1250–6.

22. McCrindle BW, Zak V, Sleeper LA, et al. Laboratory measures of exercise capacity and ventricular characteristics and function are weakly associated with functional health status after Fontan procedure. Circulation 2010;121:34–42.

23. Jones NL. Clinical exercise testing. 4th edition. Philadelphia: W.B. Saunders; 1997.

24. Mancini DM, Eisen H, Kussmaul W, et al. Value of peak exercise oxygen consumption for optimal timing of cardiac transplantation in ambulatory patients with heart failure. Circulation 1991;83:778–86.

25. Rhodes J, Fischbach PS, Patel H, et al. Factors affecting the exercise capacity of pediatric patients with aortic regurgitation. Pediatr Cardiol 2000;21:328–33.

26. Meadows J, Powell AJ, Geva T, et al. Cardiac magnetic resonance imaging correlates of exercise capacity in patients with surgically repaired tetralogy of Fallot. Am J Cardiol 2007;100:1446–50.

27. Wensel R, Opitz CF, Anker SD, et al. Assessment of survival in patients with primary pulmonary hypertension: importance of cardiopulmonary exercise testing. Circulation 2002;106:319–24.

28. Arena R, Lavie CJ, Milani RV, et al. Cardiopulmonary exercise testing in patients with pulmonary arterial hypertension: an evidence-based review. J Heart Lung Transplant 2010;29:159–73.

29. Tarnopolsky M. Exercise testing in metabolic myopathies. Phys Med Rehabil Clin N Am 2012;23:173–86.

30. Hansen JE, Sue DY, Oren A, et al. Relation of oxygen uptake to work rate in normal men and men with circulatory disorders. Am J Cardiol 1987;59:669–74.

31. Ingle L, Goode K, Carroll S, et al. Prognostic value of the VE/VCO2 slope calculated from different time intervals in patients with suspected heart failure. Int J Cardiol 2007;118:350–5.

32. Giardini A, Odendaal D, Khambadkone S, et al. Physiologic decrease of ventilatory response to exercise in the second decade of life in healthy children. Am Heart J 2011;161:1214–9.

33. Ponikowski P, Francis DP, Piepoli MF, et al. Enhanced ventilatory response to exercise in patients with chronic heart failure and preserved exercise tolerance: marker of abnormal cardiorespiratory reflex control and predictor of poor prognosis. Circulation 2001;103:967–72.

34. Chua TP, Ponikowski P, Harrington D, et al. Clinical correlates and prognostic significance of the ventilatory response to exercise in chronic heart failure. J Am Coll Cardiol 1997;29:1585–90.

35. Francis DP, Shamim W, Davies LC, et al. Cardiopulmonary exercise testing for prognosis in chronic heart failure: continuous and independent prognostic value from VE/VCO(2) slope and peak VO(2). Eur Heart J 2000;21:154–61.

36. Giardini A, Specchia S, Tacy TA, et al. Usefulness of cardiopulmonary exercise to predict long-term prognosis in adults with repaired tetralogy of Fallot. Am J Cardiol 2007;99:1462–7.

37. Giardini A, Hager A, Lammers AE, et al. Ventilatory efficiency and aerobic capacity predict event-free survival in adults with atrial repair for complete transposition of the great arteries. J Am Coll Cardiol 2009;53:1548–55.

38. Buller NP, Poole-Wilson PA. Mechanism of the increased ventilatory response to exercise in patients with chronic heart failure. Br Heart J 1990;63:281–3.

39. Sutton NJ, Peng L, Lock JE, et al. Effect of pulmonary artery angioplasty on exercise function after repair of tetralogy of Fallot. Am Heart J 2008;155:182–6.

40. Rhodes J, Dave A, Pulling MC, et al. Effect of pulmonary artery stenoses on the cardiopulmonary response to exercise following repair of tetralogy of Fallot. Am J Cardiol 1998;81:1217–9.

41. Clark AL, Gatzoulis MA, Redington AN. Ventilatory responses to exercise in adults after repair of tetralogy of Fallot. Br Heart J 1995;73:445–9.

42. Uren NG, Davies SW, Agnew JE, et al. Reduction of mismatch of global ventilation and perfusion on exercise is related to exercise capacity in chronic heart failure. Br Heart J 1993;70:241–6.

43. Grant GP, Mansell AL, Garofano RP, et al. Cardiorespiratory response to exercise after the Fontan procedure for tricuspid atresia. Pediatr Res 1988;24:1–5.

44. Troutman WB, Barstow TJ, Galindo AJ, et al. Abnormal dynamic cardiorespiratory responses to exercise in pediatric patients after Fontan procedure. J Am Coll Cardiol 1998;31:668–73.

45. Cloutier A, Ash JM, Smallhorn JF, et al. Abnormal distribution of pulmonary blood flow after the Glenn shunt or Fontan procedure: risk of development of arteriovenous fistulae. Circulation 1985;72:471–9.

46. Meadows J, Lang P, Marx G, et al. Fontan fenestration closure has no acute effect on exercise capacity but improves ventilatory response to exercise. J Am Coll Cardiol 2008;52:108–13.

47. Gibbons RJ, Balady GJ, Bricker JT, et al. ACC/AHA 2002 guideline update for exercise testing. Summary article: a report of the ACC/AHA Task Force on Practice Guidelines (Committee to Update the 1997 Exercise Testing Guidelines). J Am Coll Cardiol 2002;40:1531–40.

48. Gibbons RJ, Abrams J, Chatterjee K, et al. ACC/AHA 2002 Guideline update for the management of patients with chronic stable angina. A Report of the American College of Cardiology/American Heart Association Task Force on Practice Guidelines (Committee to Update the 1999 Guidelines for the Management of Patients with Chronic Stable Angina). J Am Coll Cardiol 2003;41:159–68.

49. Ellestad MH. Stress testing: principles and practice. 5th edition. New York: Oxford University Press; 2003.

50. Froelicher VF, Myers J. Exercise and the heart. 5th edition. Philadelphia: WB Saunders; 2006.

51. Arena R, Myers J, Williams MA, et al. Assessment of functional capacity in clinical and research settings. A Scientific Statement from the American Heart Association Committee on Exercise, Rehabilitation, and Prevention of the Council on Clinical Cardiology and the Council on Cardiovascular Nursing. Circulation 2007;116:329–43.

52. Kodama S, Saito K, Tanaka S, et al. Cardiorespiratory fitness as a quantitative predictor of all-cause mortality and cardiovascular events in healthy men and women. A meta-analysis. JAMA 2009; 301:2024–35.

53. ATS Committee on Proficiency Standards for Clinical Pulmonary Function Laboratories. ATS statement: guidelines for the six-minute walk test. Am J Respir Crit Care Med 2002;166:111–7.

54. Niedeggen A, Skobel E, Haager P, et al. Comparison of the 6-minute walk test with established parameters for assessment of cardiopulmonary capacity in adults with complex congenital cardiac disease. Cardiol Young 2005;15:385–90.

55. Olsson LG, Swedberg K, Clark AL, et al. Six minute corridor walk test as an outcome measure for the assessment of treatment in randomized, blinded intervention trials of chronic heart failure: a systematic review. Eur Heart J 2005;26:778–93.

56. Gratz A, Hess J, Hager A. Peak oxygen uptake and exercise capacity: a reliable predictor of quality of life? Eur Heart J 2009;30:1674–5.

57. Giardini A, Khambadkone S, Rizzo N, et al. Determinants of exercise capacity after arterial switch operation for transposition of the great arteries. Am J Cardiol 2009;104:1007–12.

58. Fernandes SM, Alexander ME, Graham DA, et al. Ability of exercise testing to predict morbidity and mortality in adults with Fontan surgery. Congenit Heart Dis 2011;6:294–303.

Psychosocial Functioning and Quality of Life in Adults with Congenital Heart Disease and Heart Failure

Adrienne H. Kovacs, PhD, CPsych[a,b,*],
Philip Moons, PhD, RN[c,d,e]

KEYWORDS

- Adult • Heart defects • Congenital • Quality of life • Psychosocial • Heart failure

KEY POINTS

- North American adults with congenital heart disease (CHD) are at increased risk of psychosocial difficulties, including depression and anxiety. This finding has been less consistently shown in European studies.
- Data regarding the quality of life (QOL) of adults with CHD are inconsistent, likely because of differences in study methodology.
- Adults with heart failure associated with acquired heart disease are likely to experience impaired psychosocial functioning and QOL.
- Although research is limited, it is reasonable to predict that adults with CHD who develop heart failure are vulnerable to psychosocial and QOL impairment.
- An interdisciplinary approach to clinical care and research is recommended in order to attend to the broader psychosocial and QOL implications of living with CHD and heart failure.

INTRODUCTION

Adults with congenital heart disease (CHD) represent a growing population of cardiac patients. Because patients with CHD of moderate to great complexity are not cured, CHD is considered to be a chronic medical condition to which patients are expected to adapt throughout their lives. One common adult-onset development is heart failure,[1] and approximately 1 in 4 adults with CHD die of heart failure.[2,3] An exclusive focus on medical symptoms and treatment neglects the broader psychosocial and quality-of-life (QOL) implications of living with CHD and heart failure. The 3 aims of this article are (1) to summarize what is currently known about the psychosocial functioning and QOL of adults with CHD, (2) to summarize what is known about the psychosocial functioning and QOL of adults with heart failure associated with acquired heart disease, and (3) to generate a discussion regarding the psychosocial and QOL implications of managing heart failure associated with CHD.

The authors have nothing to disclose.
[a] Toronto Congenital Cardiac Centre for Adults, Peter Munk Cardiac Centre, University Health Network, 585 University Avenue, 5-NU-523, Toronto, Ontario M5G 2N2, Canada; [b] Department of Psychiatry, Faculty of Medicine, University of Toronto, 250 College Street, 8th Floor, Toronto, Ontario M5T 1R8, Canada; [c] Department of Public Health and Primary Care, KU Leuven, Kapucijnenvoer 35 PB 7001, Leuven 3000, Belgium; [d] Division of Congenital and Structural Cardiology, Department of Cardiovascular Sciences, University Hospitals Leuven, Herestraat 49, Leuven 3000, Belgium; [e] The Heart Centre, Copenhagen University Hospital, Blegdamsvej 9, Copenhagen 2100, Denmark
* Corresponding author. Toronto Congenital Cardiac Centre for Adults, Peter Munk Cardiac Centre, University Health Network, 585 University Avenue, 5-NU-523, Toronto, Ontario M5G 2N2, Canada.
E-mail address: adrienne.kovacs@uhn.ca

Heart Failure Clin 10 (2014) 35–42
http://dx.doi.org/10.1016/j.hfc.2013.09.003
1551-7136/14/$ – see front matter © 2014 Elsevier Inc. All rights reserved.

Psychosocial functioning and QOL are interrelated, both in CHD and heart failure,[4–7] although they are distinct entities. Psychosocial functioning is an umbrella term that includes both psychological and social factors, as well as their interplay. Psychological factors include mood, anxiety, and cognitive functioning, and examples of social factors include social support and social role fulfillment (eg, employment). Psychosocial factors have been shown to affect QOL among adults with CHD.[8,9] QOL is also sometimes used as an umbrella term, in that it encompasses psychosocial functioning as well as other factors such as health symptoms and functional status, lifestyle, and life conditions.[10] It is this broadness that has hampered a solid understanding of the concept of QOL, because it has led to multiple conceptualizations and definitions, each of which is a subject for debate.[8] However, concept analyses, concept clarifications, and structural equation modeling have shown that it is most appropriate to define QOL in terms of life satisfaction.[8,11–14] As a reflection of this conceptual foundation, the following definition for QOL has been proposed: "the degree of overall life satisfaction that is positively or negatively influenced by individuals' perception of certain aspects of life important to them, including matters both related and unrelated to health."[15] Life satisfaction is being increasingly used in QOL studies of CHD, whereas heart failure studies have typically defined QOL from a functional or health status perspective. Nonetheless, health status and QOL are related, albeit distinct, concepts, and therefore should not be used interchangeably.[16]

ADULTS WITH CHD: PSYCHOSOCIAL AND QOL CONSIDERATIONS
Psychosocial Functioning of Adults with CHD

International guidelines for the care of adults with CHD underscore the importance of attending to patient psychosocial needs.[17–19] Approximately 1 in 3 North American adults with CHD experience difficulties with depression and/or anxiety,[20–23] and this includes patients considered to be well-adjusted by their cardiologists.[21] However, European data regarding psychological outcomes are less consistent. In a series of Dutch studies, the emotional functioning of adults with CHD was observed to be similar, and occasionally superior, to reference norms.[24,25] A recent Italian study similarly concluded that patient psychological well-being was comparable with reference norms.[26] German patients have been shown to be similar to reference norms in trait anxiety, although their rates of state anxiety were increased.[27] However, Portuguese adolescents and adults with CHD

have been shown to be at increased risk of psychopathology.[28]

Regardless of the presence or absence of formal psychiatric diagnoses, many adults with CHD of moderate to great complexity face typical adult stressors, such as managing careers, relationships, and finances, in addition to a unique set of stressors related to living with a chronic medical condition. It has been noted that, "psychosocial challenges are part of the everyday lives of adults with CHD, yet they are rarely addressed as part of routine medical care."[29] Intrapersonal concerns include dealing with uncertainty, balancing goals with limits, and people accepting a health condition without letting it define them; CHD has been described as the "worst part time job."[29] Interpersonal concerns include feeling different from peers, body image concerns, social isolation, overprotection from parents and teachers, and ongoing medical surveillance and interventions that disrupt lives. Although it is important to avoid generalizations because there are many high-achieving adults with CHD, as a group, they seem less likely to pursue higher education or secure employment.[25,30,31]

The impact of CHD complexity on psychosocial outcomes remains unclear. Some researchers have observed that psychosocial functioning is poorer among patients with more complex CHD,[21,28,32] whereas others have not detected this relationship.[20,23,33,34] Most likely, there are multiple factors that interact to contribute to higher or lower psychosocial functioning. The following is a list of correlates of poorer psychological functioning in adults with CHD:

- Female sex[28,32]
- Lower exercise capacity[32,35,36]
- Restrictions placed by physicians[32]
- Body image/patient perceptions of scarring[32,37]
- Perceived health status or disease severity[23,26,38]
- Poor social support/loneliness/social anxiety/poor social problem solving[23,28,39]
- Poorer academic performance[28]
- Perceived financial strain[40]

Most adults with CHD with significant depression or anxiety do not receive appropriate mental health treatment.[22,23,33] There are also no empirically evaluated psychosocial interventions for adults with CHD.[41] This is in contrast with the existence of dozens of psychological intervention trials for adults with acquired heart disease.[42] A survey of adults with CHD revealed that half report high interest in at least one area of psychological treatment, most commonly stress management and coping with heart disease.[43] Focus group research suggests that adults with CHD are interested in psychological counseling in addition to having opportunities to connect with other adults with CHD and psychoeducation (eg, wanting to understand typical psychological reactions of adults with CHD going through similar situations).[29] In addition, as a group, adults with CHD are interested in giving back to other patients; approximately one-third of patients are interested in providing peer support.[43]

QOL of Adults with CHD

In 2013, 2 systematic literature reviews on QOL in adults with CHD were published.[44,45] These 2 reviews taken together include all relevant quantitative studies published through January 2013. In general, patients have a reduced QOL if QOL is defined in terms of physical functioning.[44] However, when QOL is defined differently, QOL in patients with CHD can be similar or even better than that of healthy counterparts.[44,45] These reviews concluded that the inconsistent findings across studies could be the result of methodological limitations and differences in the definition of QOL. A major issue is whether QOL is measured in terms of functional consequences (health-related QOL) or in terms of satisfaction with life (overall QOL).

The following is a list of correlates of poorer QOL among adults with CHD:

- Lower academic performance and education[46,47]
- Lower employment rates[47]
- Fewer daily activities[48]
- Worse functional class[49]
- Lower exercise capacity[48]
- Lower social support[46,50]
- Cardiac surgery[46,50]
- Implantable cardioverter defibrillator[51]
- Physical limitations[46]
- Type D (distressed) personality[5]

Furthermore, several studies reported inconsistencies regarding the relationship between QOL and age[46,47,50,52]; sex[46,47,50]; medication[46,50]; disease severity[46,47,50]; and severity of residual lesions.[46,50] In addition, QOL seemed to be unrelated to CHD subtype,[46] cyanosis,[50] personal resources,[50] and family environment.[50]

In summary, QOL in adults with CHD reflects multiple factors and is to a limited extent determined by their heart defect. Demographic and psychosocial factors seem to play an important role in determining QOL. However, it is difficult to interpret the study findings because of inconsistencies in methods and results among these different studies.

ADULTS WITH HEART FAILURE: PSYCHOSOCIAL AND QOL CONSIDERATIONS
Psychosocial Functioning of Adults with Heart Failure

A meta-analysis of 34 publications revealed that clinically significant depression was reported in 22% of adults with heart failure, although the rate was higher in studies that used questionnaires (34%) versus studies that used diagnostic interviews (19%).[53] The relationship between depression and disease severity in heart failure is more linear than has been observed in CHD research, because this same meta-analysis concluded that depression was higher among patients with functional class IV symptoms (42%) versus class I symptoms (11%).[53]

Among adults with heart failure associated with acquired heart disease, depression is associated with higher rates of death and secondary events (risk ratio, 2.1) and there are trends toward more frequent hospitalizations and emergency department visits as well as increased health care usage.[53] Adams and colleagues[54] conducted a 12-year prospective observational study of 985 adults with heart failure (mean age, 69 years). Across the extended follow-up period, 80% of patients with increased symptoms of depression died, compared with 73% of those without increased symptoms ($P = .01$). Changes in symptoms of depression are also associated with clinical outcomes. Sherwood and colleagues[55] conducted a prospective 5-year study of 147 patients with heart failure with ejection fraction less than 40% (mean age, 57 years). After controlling for baseline depressive scores and clinical risk factors, a 1-year increase in the depression score was associated with increased risk of death or hospitalization at a mean follow-up of 5 years. In addition to depression, anxiety has also been linked with shorter event-free survival.[56]

Several psychosocial interventions for adults with heart failure have been developed and evaluated. A 2006 meta-analysis identified 6 studies in which interventions targeting depression in adults with heart failure were evaluated.[53] Despite methodological limitations, results suggested reductions in depressive symptoms.[53] Other interventions targeting psychological distress have been published after that meta-analysis. For example, a home-based disease management program resulted in reduced depression, anxiety, and heart failure hospitalization.[57] However, not all trials prove successful. A randomized, double-blind, placebo-controlled trial of sertraline revealed that this antidepressant medication was safe for patients with heart failure, although it was not superior to placebo in reducing symptoms of depression.[58]

In summary, compared with CHD research, heart failure research suggests (1) a stronger relationship between disease severity and depression, (2) the existence of a relationship between psychological factors and medical outcomes, and (3) the importance of developing and evaluating interventions focused on reducing psychological distress.

QOL of Adults with Heart Failure

Over the past decades, numerous studies on QOL in patients with heart failure have been published. QOL was assessed predominantly as part of the evaluation of specific interventions, such as pharmacologic treatments (eg, β-blockers, angiotensin-converting enzyme inhibitors, diuretics), pacing devices, exercise training and rehabilitation, or comprehensive disease management.[59,60] In these studies, QOL is mostly approached from a functional perspective. Studies in heart failure that define QOL as life satisfaction are more scant. Empirical studies showed that QOL of patients with heart failure is severely affected,[61] and is described as the lowest compared with patients with other chronic conditions, such as chronic hepatitis C infection, chronic hemodialysis, and major depression.[62]

The most important demographic determinants of QOL in patients with heart failure are gender and age. In general, QOL is more diminished in women with heart failure than in men.[61,63] Younger patients also report a poorer QOL than older patients with heart failure.[60,61] This is mainly because of higher levels of depression and anxiety, and the higher importance of loss of activities and roles for younger patients.[64] Clinical factors that are related to a lower QOL are an increasing disease severity and symptoms associated with heart failure.[61] The most commonly reported symptoms in patients with heart failure are dyspnea, fatigue, ankle edema, appetite problems, and constipation. Asymptomatic patients, or those who by treatment obtain an asymptomatic left ventricular dysfunction, have a similar QOL to individuals in the general population.[65]

THE PSYCHOSOCIAL AND QOL IMPLICATIONS OF MANAGING HEART FAILURE ASSOCIATED WITH CHD

In adults with CHD, psychosocial outcomes are inconsistent across studies and disease severity seems minimally associated with psychosocial functioning. In contrast, among adults with heart failure caused by acquired heart disease, results more clearly suggest diminished psychological functioning and there is a notable impact of disease severity. This finding leads to challenges in predicting the degree to which adults with CHD who develop heart failure experience psychosocial impairment. North American research suggests that CHD and heart failure are both associated with an increased risk of psychological distress. Risk factors for psychological distress among adults with CHD include reduced exercise capacity and lower perceived health status, both of which are common in heart failure.[23,26,32,35,36] Further, among adults with heart failure, depression is linked with various symptoms, including fatigue, sleep disturbance, and pain.[66] Thus, adults with CHD who develop heart failure may be a particularly vulnerable subset of patients at increased risk of psychological maladjustment.

There are no published studies that have been undertaken specifically to understand the impact of heart failure on the QOL of adults with CHD. However, given the detrimental effect that heart failure has on patients' QOL, particularly in younger patients, this issue should be put on the research agenda. Left ventricle ejection fraction could be used as a surrogate for heart failure. To the best of our knowledge, there is only 1 study in which the relationship between left ventricular ejection fraction and QOL has been investigated.[67] That study showed a nonsignificant correlation coefficient of these two variables of 0.1.[67] Although the New York Heart Association (NYHA) classification is sometimes used as a surrogate for heart failure severity, this approach is not advocated because data obtained in the previously mentioned study[67] showed that the correlation between left ventricular ejection fraction and NYHA class was significant ($P<.001$) but low, with $r = -0.15$ (data on file). Hence, NYHA class is not an accurate surrogate for heart failure severity.

CLINICAL RECOMMENDATIONS

Because heart failure strongly affects patients' psychosocial functioning and QOL, adults with CHD who develop heart failure should be considered an at-risk group for diminished psychosocial well-being and QOL. Clinicians managing these patients are thus encouraged to adopt a broad conceptualization of the diverse challenges faced by this patient subgroup. Although adults with CHD, with or without heart failure, comprise a heterogeneous group of individuals, **Table 1** presents a selected list of common challenges.

Table 1
Potential challenges faced by adults with CHD and heart failure

Category	Challenge
Physical	Fatigue Dyspnea Edema Restricted physical activities Medication side effects Shortened life expectancy
Behavioral	Adherence to medication regimen Adherence to a specific heart failure diet Increased frequency of medical appointments Frequent hospitalizations
Psychological	Depression Anxiety Cognitive difficulties Coping with uncertainty Coping with poor or declining health status Coping with shortened life expectancy End-of-life planning
Social	Education and/or employment restrictions Reduced social activity Overprotection (from caregivers, teachers, colleagues, friends, and so forth) Body image concerns Feeling different from others

We argue that it is not sufficient to optimize medical symptom management and that the psychosocial well-being and QOL of adults with CHD who develop heart failure should also be explicitly considered and addressed. The four As provide a heuristic for the identification and management of patient psychosocial concerns: ask, advise, assist, and arrange referral.[68] The initial step is to ask patients whether they are having difficulties with depressed mood or anxiety or have any concerns about their daily functioning. Next, it can be helpful to advise the patient regarding challenges and coping strategies often faced by patients in similar situations. Providers can also assist patients, as appropriate, with brief problem solving. Providers might also wish to arrange a consultation with a mental health professional. Adult CHD programs are thus strongly encouraged to identify suitable mental health providers, such as psychologists and psychiatrists, to whom interested patients can be referred.

Clinicians should also be aware of the possibility of diminished cognitive functioning. As a group, individuals with CHD are at greater risk of neurocognitive difficulties.[69] Further, it is known that approximately one-third to one-half of adults with heart failure experience at least some degree of cognitive impairment, particularly memory impairment and concentration difficulties.[70] Reduced cognitive functioning creates challenges for understanding health information, managing complex treatment regimens, and self-managing symptoms.[70] Thus, providers managing adults with CHD who develop heart failure should ensure that they take adequate time with patient education and should simplify care regimens as much as possible.

Given that one-quarter of adults with CHD die of heart failure,[2,3] providers must also be prepared to address issues related to advance care planning and end-of-life care. However, although most adults with CHD wish to discuss end-of-life planning and prepare advance directives, these discussions frequently do not occur.[71,72] Further, research suggests that patients do not always have documented end-of-life discussions before death and aggressive medical treatment is common.[73] Challenges with prognostication exist for adults with CHD, although these do not eliminate the need for open patient-provider communication regarding end-of-life matters.[74] In order to optimize psychosocial functioning and QOL toward the end of the lives of adults with CHD and heart failure, providers are encouraged to pay particular attention to the preparation of advance directives, understanding patients' treatment preferences, and promoting transparent end-of-life communication.[75]

FUTURE RESEARCH DIRECTIONS

There are strengths and limitations in the existing psychosocial and QOL literature pertaining to adults with CHD as well as adults with heart failure caused by acquired heart disease. The following recommendations would allow clinicians to close significant gaps in the knowledge and management of the psychosocial and QOL challenges faced by adults with CHD who develop heart failure:

- QOL research should be based on sound conceptual grounds and a common methodology.
- Multicenter research is crucial in order to better understand apparent international differences in psychosocial outcomes.
- Research specifically focused on psychosocial functioning and QOL in patients with CHD and heart failure would be valuable.

- Longitudinal research is needed in order to determine whether there are changes in psychosocial functioning and QOL over time, particularly as an adult with CHD develops heart failure.
- The impact of psychosocial functioning and QOL on medical outcomes could be elucidated.
- Interventions targeting psychosocial distress and impaired QOL should be developed and evaluated.

SUMMARY

North American studies suggest that adults with CHD are at increased risk of psychosocial difficulties. Research also suggests that heart failure caused by acquired heart disease can contribute to poorer psychosocial functioning and QOL. Although there is a paucity of research focused on adults with CHD who develop heart failure, this group of patients is more vulnerable to psychosocial and QOL impairment. Comprehensive care of these patients requires an interdisciplinary approach to optimize functioning in all domains.

REFERENCES

1. Kantor PF, Andelfinger G, Dancea A, et al. Heart failure in congenital heart disease. Can J Cardiol 2013;29(7):753–4.
2. Verheugt CL, Uiterwaal CS, van der Velde ET, et al. Mortality in adult congenital heart disease. Eur Heart J 2010;31(10):1220–9.
3. Zomer AC, Vaartjes I, Uiterwaal CS, et al. Circumstances of death in adult congenital heart disease. Int J Cardiol 2012;154(2):168–72.
4. Pike NA, Evangelista LS, Doering LV, et al. Quality of life, health status, and depression: comparison between adolescents and adults after the Fontan procedure with healthy counterparts. J Cardiovasc Nurs 2012;27(6):539–46.
5. Schoormans D, Mulder BJ, van Melle JP, et al. Patients with a congenital heart defect and type D personality feel functionally more impaired, report a poorer health status and quality of life, but use less healthcare. Eur J Cardiovasc Nurs 2012; 11(3):349–55.
6. Bunyamin V, Spaderna H, Weidner G. Health behaviors contribute to quality of life in patients with advanced heart failure independent of psychological and medical patient characteristics. Qual Life Res 2013;22(7):1603–11.
7. Mulligan K, Mehta PA, Fteropoulli T, et al. Newly diagnosed heart failure: change in quality of life, mood, and illness beliefs in the first 6 months after diagnosis. Br J Health Psychol 2012;17(3):447–62.
8. Moons P, Budts W, De Geest S. Critique on the conceptualisation of quality of life: a review and evaluation of different conceptual approaches. Int J Nurs Stud 2006;43(7):891–901.
9. Luyckx K, Missotten L, Goossens E, et al. Individual and contextual determinants of quality of life in adolescents with congenital heart disease. J Adolesc Health 2012;51(2):122–8.
10. Moons P. Why call it health-related quality of life when you mean perceived health status? Eur J Cardiovasc Nurs 2004;3(4):275–7.
11. Ferrans CE. Development of a conceptual model of quality of life. Sch Inq Nurs Pract 1996;10(3):293–304.
12. Ferrans CE. Quality of life: conceptual issues. Semin Oncol Nurs 1990;6(4):248–54.
13. Zhan L. Quality of life: conceptual and measurement issues. J Adv Nurs 1992;17(7):795–800.
14. Beckie TM, Hayduk LA. Measuring quality of life. Soc Indic Res 1997;42(1):21–39.
15. Moons P, Van Deyk K, Marquet K, et al. Individual quality of life in adults with congenital heart disease: a paradigm shift. Eur Heart J 2005;26(3):298–307.
16. Smith KW, Avis NE, Assmann SF. Distinguishing between quality of life and health status in quality of life research: a meta-analysis. Qual Life Res 1999;8(5):447–59.
17. Warnes CA, Williams RG, Bashore TM, et al. ACC/AHA 2008 guidelines for the management of adults with congenital heart disease: a report of the American College of Cardiology/American Heart Association Task Force on Practice Guidelines (Writing Committee to Develop Guidelines on the Management of Adults With Congenital Heart Disease). Developed in Collaboration With the American Society of Echocardiography, Heart Rhythm Society, International Society for Adult Congenital Heart Disease, Society for Cardiovascular Angiography and Interventions, and Society of Thoracic Surgeons. J Am Coll Cardiol 2008;52(23):e143–263.
18. Connelly MS, Webb GD, Somerville J, et al. Canadian consensus conference on adult congenital heart disease 1996. Can J Cardiol 1998;14(3):395–452.
19. Report of the British Cardiac Society Working Party. Grown-up congenital heart (GUCH) disease: current needs and provision of service for adolescents and adults with congenital heart disease in the UK. Heart 2002;88(Suppl 1):i1–14.
20. Brandhagen DJ, Feldt RH, Williams DE. Long-term psychologic implications of congenital heart disease: a 25-year follow-up. Mayo Clin Proc 1991;66(5):474–9.
21. Bromberg JI, Beasley PJ, D'Angelo EJ, et al. Depression and anxiety in adults with congenital heart disease: a pilot study. Heart Lung 2003;32(2):105–10.

22. Horner T, Liberthson R, Jellinek MS. Psychosocial profile of adults with complex congenital heart disease. Mayo Clin Proc 2000;75(1):31–6.

23. Kovacs AH, Saidi AS, Kuhl EA, et al. Depression and anxiety in adult congenital heart disease: predictors and prevalence. Int J Cardiol 2009;137(2):158–64.

24. Utens EM, Bieman HJ, Verhulst FC, et al. Psychopathology in young adults with congenital heart disease. Follow-up results. Eur Heart J 1998; 19(4):647–51.

25. van Rijen EH, Utens EM, Roos-Hesselink JW, et al. Psychosocial functioning of the adult with congenital heart disease: a 20-33 years follow-up. Eur Heart J 2003;24(7):673–83.

26. Callus E, Utens EM, Quadri E, et al. The impact of actual and perceived disease severity on preoperative psychological well-being and illness behaviour in adult congenital heart disease patients. Cardiol Young 2013;27:1–8.

27. Muller J, Hess J, Hager A. General anxiety of adolescents and adults with congenital heart disease is comparable with that in healthy controls. Int J Cardiol 2013;165(1):142–5.

28. Freitas IR, Castro M, Sarmento SL, et al. A cohort study on psychosocial adjustment and psychopathology in adolescents and young adults with congenital heart disease. BMJ Open 2013;3(1). pii:e001138.

29. Page MG, Kovacs AH, Irvine J. How do psychosocial challenges associated with living with congenital heart disease translate into treatment interests and preferences? A qualitative approach. Psychol Health 2012;27(11):1260–70.

30. Immer FF, Althaus SM, Berdat PA, et al. Quality of life and specific problems after cardiac surgery in adolescents and adults with congenital heart diseases. Eur J Cardiovasc Prev Rehabil 2005;12(2):138–43.

31. Geyer S, Norozi K, Buchhorn R, et al. Chances of employment in women and men after surgery of congenital heart disease: comparisons between patients and the general population. Congenit Heart Dis 2009;4(1):25–33.

32. van Rijen EH, Utens EM, Roos-Hesselink JW, et al. Medical predictors for psychopathology in adults with operated congenital heart disease. Eur Heart J 2004;25(18):1605–13.

33. Rietveld S, Mulder BJ, van Beest I, et al. Negative thoughts in adults with congenital heart disease. Int J Cardiol 2002;86(1):19–26.

34. Balon YE, Then KL, Rankin JA, et al. Looking beyond the biophysical realm to optimize health: results of a survey of psychological well-being in adults with congenital cardiac disease. Cardiol Young 2008;18(5):494–501.

35. Popelova J, Slavik Z, Skovranek J. Are cyanosed adults with congenital cardiac malformations depressed? Cardiol Young 2001;11(4):379–84.

36. Rose M, Kohler K, Kohler F, et al. Determinants of the quality of life of patients with congenital heart disease. Qual Life Res 2005;14(1):35–43.

37. Geyer S, Norozi K, Zoege M, et al. Psychological symptoms in patients after surgery for congenital cardiac disease. Cardiol Young 2006;16(6):540–8.

38. Norozi K, Zoege M, Buchhorn R, et al. The influence of congenital heart disease on psychological conditions in adolescents and adults after corrective surgery. Congenit Heart Dis 2006;1(6):282–8.

39. Enomoto J, Nakazawa J, Mizuno Y, et al. Psychosocial factors influencing mental health in adults with congenital heart disease. Circ J 2013;77(3):749–55.

40. Eslami B, Sundin O, Macassa G, et al. Anxiety, depressive and somatic symptoms in adults with congenital heart disease. J Psychosom Res 2013; 74(1):49–56.

41. Lane DA, Millane TA, Lip GY. Psychological interventions for depression in adolescent and adult congenital heart disease. Cochrane Database Syst Rev 2009;(1):CD004372.

42. Linden W, Phillips MJ, Leclerc J. Psychological treatment of cardiac patients: a meta-analysis. Eur Heart J 2007;28(24):2972–84.

43. Kovacs AH, Bendell KL, Colman J, et al. Adults with congenital heart disease: psychological needs and treatment preferences. Congenit Heart Dis 2009;4(3):139–46.

44. Fteropoulli T, Stygall J, Cullen S, et al. Quality of life of adult congenital heart disease patients: a systematic review of the literature. Cardiol Young 2013;23(4):473–85.

45. Apers A, Luyckx K, Moons P. Quality of life in adult congenital heart disease: what do we already know and what do we still need to know? Curr Cardiol Rep 2013;15(10):407.

46. Teixeira FM, Coelho RM, Proenca C, et al. Quality of life experienced by adolescents and young adults with congenital heart disease. Pediatr Cardiol 2011;32(8):1132–8.

47. Vigl M, Niggemeyer E, Hager A, et al. The importance of socio-demographic factors for the quality of life of adults with congenital heart disease. Qual Life Res 2011;20(2):169–77.

48. Muller J, Hess J, Hager A. Daily physical activity in adults with congenital heart disease is positively correlated with exercise capacity but not with quality of life. Clin Res Cardiol 2012;101(1):55–61.

49. Overgaard D, Schrader AM, Lisby KH, et al. Patient-reported outcomes in adult survivors with single-ventricle physiology. Cardiology 2011; 120(1):36–42.

50. Silva AM, Vaz C, Areias ME, et al. Quality of life of patients with congenital heart diseases. Cardiol Young 2011;21(6):670–6.

51. Opic P, Utens EM, Moons P, et al. Psychosocial impact of implantable cardioverter defibrillators

(ICD) in young adults with tetralogy of Fallot. Clin Res Cardiol 2012;101(7):509–19.

52. Cotts T, Malviya S, Goldberg C. Quality of life and perceived health status in adults with congenitally corrected transposition of the great arteries. J Thorac Cardiovasc Surg 2012;143(4):885–90.

53. Rutledge T, Reis VA, Linke SE, et al. Depression in heart failure a meta-analytic review of prevalence, intervention effects, and associations with clinical outcomes. J Am Coll Cardiol 2006;48(8):1527–37.

54. Adams J, Kuchibhatla M, Christopher EJ, et al. Association of depression and survival in patients with chronic heart failure over 12 years. Psychosomatics 2012;53(4):339–46.

55. Sherwood A, Blumenthal JA, Hinderliter AL, et al. Worsening depressive symptoms are associated with adverse clinical outcomes in patients with heart failure. J Am Coll Cardiol 2011;57(4):418–23.

56. De Jong MJ, Chung ML, Wu JR, et al. Linkages between anxiety and outcomes in heart failure. Heart Lung 2011;40(5):393–404.

57. Tsuchihashi-Makaya M, Matsuo H, Kakinoki S, et al. Home-based disease management program to improve psychological status in patients with heart failure in Japan. Circ J 2013;77(4):926–33.

58. O'Connor CM, Jiang W, Kuchibhatla M, et al. Safety and efficacy of sertraline for depression in patients with heart failure: results of the SADHART-CHF (Sertraline Against Depression and Heart Disease in Chronic Heart Failure) trial. J Am Coll Cardiol 2010;56(9):692–9.

59. Morgan K, McGee H, Shelley E. Quality of life assessment in heart failure interventions: a 10-year (1996-2005) review. Eur J Cardiovasc Prev Rehabil 2007;14(5):589–607.

60. Garin O, Ferrer M, Pont A, et al. Disease-specific health-related quality of life questionnaires for heart failure: a systematic review with meta-analyses. Qual Life Res 2009;18(1):71–85.

61. Jaarsma T, Johansson P, Agren S, et al. Quality of life and symptoms of depression in advanced heart failure patients and their partners. Curr Opin Support Palliat Care 2010;4(4):233–7.

62. Juenger J, Schellberg D, Kraemer S, et al. Health related quality of life in patients with congestive heart failure: comparison with other chronic diseases and relation to functional variables. Heart 2002;87(3):235–41.

63. Johansson P, Dahlstrom U, Brostrom A. Factors and interventions influencing health-related quality of life in patients with heart failure: a review of the literature. Eur J Cardiovasc Nurs 2006;5(1):5–15.

64. Moser DK, Heo S, Lee KS, et al. 'It could be worse... lot's worse!' Why health-related quality of life is better in older compared with younger individuals with heart failure. Age Ageing 2013; 42(5):626–32.

65. Hobbs FD, Kenkre JE, Roalfe AK, et al. Impact of heart failure and left ventricular systolic dysfunction on quality of life: a cross-sectional study comparing common chronic cardiac and medical disorders and a representative adult population. Eur Heart J 2002;23(23):1867–76.

66. Herr JK, Salyer J, Lyon DE, et al. Heart failure symptom relationships: a systematic review. J Cardiovasc Nurs 2013. [Epub ahead of print].

67. Moons P, Van Deyk K, De Geest S, et al. Is the severity of congenital heart disease associated with the quality of life and perceived health of adult patients? Heart 2005;91(9):1193–8.

68. Kovacs AH, Sears SF, Saidi AS. Biopsychosocial experiences of adults with congenital heart disease: review of the literature. Am Heart J 2005; 150(2):193–201.

69. Marino BS, Lipkin PH, Newburger JW, et al. Neurodevelopmental outcomes in children with congenital heart disease: evaluation and management: a scientific statement from the American Heart Association. Circulation 2012;126(9): 1143–72.

70. Bauer LC, Johnson JK, Pozehl BJ. Cognition in heart failure: an overview of the concepts and their measures. J Am Acad Nurse Pract 2011;23(11): 577–85.

71. Tobler D, Greutmann M, Colman JM, et al. End-of-life in adults with congenital heart disease: a call for early communication. Int J Cardiol 2012;155(3): 383–7.

72. Tobler D, Greutmann M, Colman JM, et al. Knowledge of and preference for advance care planning by adults with congenital heart disease. Am J Cardiol 2012;109(12):1797–800.

73. Tobler D, Greutmann M, Colman JM, et al. End-of-life care in hospitalized adults with complex congenital heart disease: care delayed, care denied. Palliat Med 2012;26(1):72–9.

74. Greutmann M, Tobler D, Colman JM, et al. Facilitators of and barriers to advance care planning in adult congenital heart disease. Congenit Heart Dis 2013;8(4):281–8.

75. Kovacs AH, Landzberg MJ, Goodlin SJ. Advance care planning and end-of-life management of adult patients with congenital heart disease. World J Pediatr Congenit Heart Surg 2013;4(1):62–9.

Biomarkers in Adult Congenital Heart Disease Heart Failure

Hideo Ohuchi, MD, PhD[a,b,*],
Gerhard-Paul Diller, MD, PhD, MSc[c]

KEYWORDS

- Adult congenital heart disease • Biomarker • Natriuretic peptide • Heart failure
- Ventricular dysfunction • Mortality

KEY POINTS

- Most adults with congenital heart disease (ACHD) show high levels of natriuretic peptides (NP) when compared with normal controls although the magnitude of elevation is less pronounced in patients with ACHD when compared with non-ACHD cardiac patients.
- Norepinephrine and NP levels were strongly related to outcome in studies that included many symptomatic patients, especially those with unrepaired ACHD, Eisenmenger syndrome, and pulmonary hypertension.
- Limited data are available regarding serial assessment of biomarkers, and such information could provide additional important information to help identify patients at risk, as demonstrated during patient follow-up and pregnancy. We provide an overview over the literature of biomarkers in ACHD, including possible associations with symptoms, ventricular function and outcome.

SPECIFIC PATHOPHYSIOLOGY IN ACHD

Major causes of heart failure (HF) in adults with acquired heart disease are myocardial ischemia, systemic hypertension, valvular disease and cardiomyopathies for left-sided HF, and idiopathic and thromboembolic pulmonary hypertension (PH) for right-sided HF. On the other hand, the cause of HF in adult congenital heart disease (ACHD) is different from that of non-ACHD, and the specific causes include single-ventricle physiology, such as Fontan circulation, non–left ventricular (LV) type morphology of the systemic ventricle, and various residual hemodynamic abnormalities, such as valve stenosis and/or regurgitation. In addition, cyanotic patients without definitive repair and those with Eisenmenger syndrome present with unique pathophysiology.

ASSESSMENT OF PATHOPHYSIOLOGY IN ACHD

The first step in managing ACHD HF patients is to understand their pathophysiology and to select the appropriate modalities for assessment. In addition to cardiac echocardiography, magnetic resonance imaging (MRI), and computed tomography (CT) for assessment of the cardiac structure and function, one should not forget that noncardiac global assessment of HF severity is also important for the prognosis and management strategy in both ACHD and non-ACHD HF patients. The major nonspecific assessment modalities include biomarkers and cardiopulmonary exercise testing, such information having become more relevant and established in daily practice in adult cardiac patients with non-ACHD. However,

[a] Department of Pediatric Cardiology, National Cerebral and Cardiovascular Center, 5-7-1 Fujishiro-dai, Suita, Osaka 565-8565, Japan; [b] Department of Adult Congenital Heart Disease, National Cerebral and Cardiovascular Center, 5-7-1 Fujishiro-dai, Suita, Osaka 565-8565, Japan; [c] Division of Adult Congenital and Valvular Heart Disease, Department of Cardiovascular Medicine, University Hospital Muenster, Albert-Schweitzer-Str. 33, Münster 48149, Germany
* Corresponding author. Department of Pediatric Cardiology, National Cerebral and Cardiovascular Center, 5-7-1 Fujishiro-dai, Suita, Osaka 565-8565, Japan.
E-mail address: hohuchi@hsp.ncvc.go.jp

Heart Failure Clin 10 (2014) 43–56
http://dx.doi.org/10.1016/j.hfc.2013.09.020
1551-7136/14/$ – see front matter © 2014 Elsevier Inc. All rights reserved.

there are limited data regarding these parameters, and the clinical significance of biomarkers remains largely unknown in ACHD.

CRITERIA FOR BIOMARKERS

Biomarkers of HF may be subdivided into 7 categories (**Box 1**),[1] and 3 criteria for biomarkers have been proposed. First, accurate, repeated measurements must be available to the clinician at a reasonable cost and with short turnaround times; second, the biomarker must provide information that is not already available from a careful clinical

---

> **Box 1**
> **Definitions and categorization of biomarkers in heart failure**
>
> *Definition*
> 1. Available to clinicians
> 2. The biomarker adds new information
> 3. The biomarker helps the clinician to manage patients
>
> *Category*
> 1. Inflammation
>
>   C-reactive protein, tumor necrosis factor-α, interleukin-6, etc
> 2. Oxidative stress
>
>   Oxidized low-density lipoproteins, myeloperoxidase, etc
> 3. Extracellular-matrix remodeling
>
>   Matrix metalloproteinases, plasma procollagen type III, etc
> 4. Neurohormones
>
>   Norepinephrine, renin, aldosterone, endothelin-1, etc
> 5. Myocyte injury
>
>   Troponins I and T, creatinine kinase MB fraction, etc
> 6. Myocyte stress
>
>   Atrial and brain natriuretic peptides, NT-proBNP, etc
> 7. New biomarkers
>
>   Adiponectin, asymmetric demethylarginine, etc
>
> *Data from* Braunwald E. Biomarkers in heart failure. N Engl J Med 2008;358:2149, with permission; and Morrow DA, de Lemos JA. Benchmarks for the assessment of novel cardiovascular biomarkers. Circulation 2007;115:950.

---

assessment; and third, knowledge of the measured level should aid in medical decision making.[2]

EVIDENCE OF BIOMARKERS IN ACHD

There has been large number of studies on circulating biomarkers in adult HF patients without ACHD. However, this evidence may not be always applicable to unique ACHD HF pathophysiology. This article subdivides documented studies into 6 categories, as follows: (1) studies of heterogeneous ACHD cohorts with various kinds of systemic ventricle (SV) (mixed group); (2) studies of ACHD patients with biventricular physiology with a morphologic right ventricle (RV) as a pulmonary ventricle (PV) (PRV group); (3) studies of ACHD with an RV as an SV (SRV group); (4) studies of adult patients with Fontan physiology (Fontan group); (5) studies of hypoxic ACHD without definitive repair, including Eisenmenger syndrome (Unrepaired group); and (6) studies of female ACHD patients during pregnancy and delivery (Pregnancy group) (**Table 1**).

Correlations between biomarkers and clinical variables and predictive and/or prognostic values of biomarkers in ACHD are summarized in **Tables 2** and **3**, respectively.

Mixed Group

Patients' characteristics
Heterogeneous ACHD patients with and without definitive repair were included in this category.[3–10] These studies consisted of 7 to 94 clinically stable patients with a mean age of 26.6 to 39.4 years, and a relatively large percentage of symptomatic ACHD patients, that is, New York Heart Association (NYHA) functional class II or higher (although those with NYHA class IV were rare). Ventricular function was assessed by echocardiography in all studies except 1,[3] and subjective visual assessment of SV function was used because of the difficulty in the measurement of SV volume. Several exclusion criteria were also applied variably, such as acute HF,[4,7] liver and/or renal dysfunction,[3,4,8] infection,[4] NYHA class IV,[10] and LV dysfunction.[3]

Biomarkers
All studies measured brain natriuretic peptide(s) (BNP), including one study of N-terminal pro-BNP (NT-proBNP),[10] and 3 studies measured atrial natriuretic peptide (ANP).[3,4,9] Catecholamines, hormones of the renin-angiotensin-aldosterone system (RAS) and asymmetric dimethylarginine were measured in 1 study each.[4,10] ACHD patients showed significantly higher levels of natriuretic peptides (NPs) compared with controls, and the

Table 1
Biomarkers in heart failure in adults with congenital heart disease

| | | | Biomarkers | | | | | | | | | | Patients | | | | | | Ventricular Function | | | |
| | | | Natriuretic Peptides | | | | Catecholamines | | RAS System | | ET-1 | Others | Cases | | | | | | | | | |
S.No	SV-Type Category	Authors,[Ref.]	ANP	NT-proANP	BNP	NT-proBNP	NE	E	PRA	PAC			Total	Female	Age (y)	NYHA I/II/III/IV	Pvo$_2$ (mL/kg/min)	Modality	SVEDVI (mL/m²)	SVEF/(Tei) [Visual EF]	PVEDVI (mL/m²)	PVEF/(Tei) (%)/—
1	Mixed	Tulevski et al,[3] 2001	○		○								21	9	26.6 ± 8.6	13/8/0/0		MRI/Echo		68.1 ± 11.0	65.3 ± 23.3	58.0 ± 12.0
		Bolger et al,[4] 2002	○		○		○	○	○	○	○		53	29	33.5 ± 1.5	11/31/10/1		Echo		[36/7/3]		
		Book et al,[5] 2005			○						○		8	3	27.3 ± 5.3	2.4 ± 0.9		Echo				
		Law et al,[6] 2005			○								7	—	—	—		—		[26.9 ± 14.8]		
		Perlowski et al,[7] 2007			○								54	31	39 ± 13	—		Echo				
		Trojnarska et al,[8] 2010			○								53	32	39.4 ± 14.3	4/36/13/0		Echo		[21/19/9]		
		Giannakoulas et al,[9] 2010	○		○								49	26	34 ± 11	11/28/10/0	15.5 ± 4.9	Echo				
		Tutarel et al,[10] 2012				○						○	94	39	30.2 ± 10.6	56/21/17/0		Echo		[52/33/7]		

(continued on next page)

Table 1
(continued)

S.No	SV-Type Category	Authors,Ref.	ANP	NT-proANP	BNP	NT-proBNP	NE	E	PRA	PAC	ET-1	Others	Total	Female	Age (y)	NYHA I/II/III/IV	Pvo₂ (mL/kg/min)	Modality	SVEDVI (mL/m²)	SVEF/(Tei) [Visual EF]	PVEDVI (mL/m²)	PVEF/(Tei) (%)/—
2	Pulmonary RV	Nagaya et al,[12] 1998	○		○								41	25	44 (20–68)			CT	56 ± 4 (ASD) 63 ± 4 (PH)	56 ± 3 (ASD) 57 ± 2 (PH)	165 ± 14 (ASD) 104 ± 6 (PH)	
		Nagaya et al,[13] 1998	○		○								31	19	46 (19–72)	10/20/1/0						
		Nagaya et al,[14] 2000	○		○		○	○					60	42	38 (15–69)	0/6/42/12		Echo				
		Brili et al,[15] 2005			○									25	—								
		Norozi et al,[16] 2005		○		○	○	○	○	○	○		50	26	27.8 ± 1.7	46/4/0/0		Echo		33 ± 1.4 (m)/34 ± 1 (f)		
		Norozi et al,[17] 2006				○							59	29	30 ± 8	32/25/2/0	25 ± 6	Echo		0.50 ± 0.09		(0.37 ± 0.1)
		Schoen et al,[18] 2007				○							20	12	43 ± 13	12/5/3/0		MRI/ Echo			127 ± 17	37 ± 9
		Festa et al,[19] 2007				○	○	○	○	○			70	26	21 ± 1	53/17/0/0	18.4 ± 1.6	MRI	76 ± 2	63 ± 1	140 ± 5	53 ± 1
		Koch et al,[20] 2010			○								130	53	16.1 ± 7.1	105/25/0/0		Echo				
		Oosterhof et al,[21] 2006			○								42	17	30 (17–57)	—		MRI				
		Westhoff-Bleck et al,[22] 2011				○							27	15	23.6 ± 2.9	1.9 ± 0.5 1.56 ± 0.5 (PVR)	26.6 ± 7.5	MRI	74.9 ± 15.8 83.1 ± 32.5 (PVR)	52.8 ± 8.2 59.2 ± 11.5 (PVR)	150.7 ± 27.7	47.6 ± 8.7

Biomarkers: Natriuretic Peptides (ANP, NT-proANP, BNP, NT-proBNP); Catecholamines (NE, E); RAS System (PRA, PAC); ET-1; Others. Patients: Cases (Total, Female). Ventricular Function.

No.	Group	Reference							n	n₂	Age	NYHA/sex		Modality			
3	Systemic RV (±Fontan)	Norozi et al,[23] 2005					○	○	33	5	23.4 ± 7.4			Echo			(0.63 ± 0.17)
		Dore et al,[24] 2005			○		○	○	29	8	30.3 ± 10.9			Echo			41.6 ± 9.3
		Chow et al,[25] 2008				○			44	—	19.7 ± 4.0	37/6/1/1		Echo			(0.48 ± 0.16)
		Vogt et al,[26] 2009				○			16	—	25.6 ± 3.7	7/4/5/0		Echo			
		Schaefer et al,[27] 2010					○		43	14	29 ± 4	—		MRI/Echo	77 ± 20		48 ± 8
		Plymen et al,[28] 2010					○		35	11	29 (18–40)	23/12/0/0		MRI	107 ± 27		51 ± 8
		Szymański et al,[29] 2011			○		○		42	11	20.8 ± 3.7	27/15 (II–IV)		Echo	20/42 (FAC ≤40%)		36.8 ± 7.8
		Winter et al,[30] 2008					○		47	17	35 (21–69)	—	(78.5% ± 23.9%)	MRI/CT/Echo			
		Koch et al,[31] 2008				○	○		48	14	19 ± 5 (9.6–37.7)	41/7/0/0		Echo			
		Garg et al,[32] 2008	○			○	○		24	8	24.6 (11.4–36.5)	14/6/4/0[a]	28.1 ± 7.5	MRI/RI	98.8 ± 27.8	49.1 ± 11.0	60.3 ± 8.4
		Larsson et al,[33] 2007				○	○		61	19	26 ± 8	36/26 (II–IV)		Echo			[23/12/26 (m-s)]
		Trojnarska et al,[34] 2010				○	○		40	24	28.8 ± 9.5	27/12/1/0	21.7 ± 5.9	—			
4	Fontan	Inai et al,[35] 2005	○		○	○	○		50	24	22.7 ± 7.0	41/9/0/0		Cath			56 ± 5
		Motoki et al,[36] 2009	○		○	○			68	28	25–53	1.7–2.6		Cath	80.6–170.6		57.1–63.3

(continued on next page)

Table 1
(continued)

S.No	SV-Type Category	Authors,Ref.	ANP	NT-proANP	BNP	NT-proBNP	NE	E	PRA	PAC	ET-1	Others	Total	Female	Age (y)	NYHA I/II/III/IV	Pvo₂ (mL/kg/min)	Modality	SVEDVI (mL/m²)	SVEF/(Tei) [Visual EF]	PVEDVI (mL/m²)	PVEF/(Tei) (%)/—
													Biomarkers → Natriuretic Peptides / Catecholamines / RAS System			**Patients** → Cases					**Ventricular Function**			
5	Unrepaired (± Eisenmenger)	Hopkins & Hall,[37] 1997		○									26	12	30 ± 8							
		Hopkins et al,[38] 2004		○		○							9	6	33 ± 12							
		Reardon et al,[39] 2012			○								53	23	44 ± 11.2			Cath/Echo		54 ± 9 (event−) 51 ± 10 (event+)		44 ± 9 (event−) 38 ± 13 (event+)
		Diller et al,[40] 2012			○								181	116	36.9 ± 12.1	19/48/111/3						
		Schuuring et al,[41] 2012				○						○	31	—	45 ± 12	I–II (9)/III–IV (22)		Echo				
		Saab & Aboulhosn,[42] 2013			○								13	8	38 ± 14	2.46		Cath/Echo		55		
6	Pregnancy	Tanous et al,[48] 2010		○									66	66	31 ± 5	54/10/2 ≥III		Echo				
		Kamiya et al,[49] 2012			○								25	25	31.3 ± 3.3 (event+) 30.0 ± 5.3 (event−)	23/1/1/0		Echo				

Visual EF consists of 3 categories (preserved/reduced/severely reduced). The symbol "○" indicates biomarkers that are assessed in the corresponding study.

Abbreviations: ANP, atrial natriuretic peptide; ASD, atrial septal defect; BNP, brain natriuretic peptide; Cath, cardiac catheterization; CT, computed tomography; E, epinephrine; Echo, echocardiogram; ET-1, endothelin-1; FAC, fractional area change; MRI, magnetic resonance imaging; NE, norepinephrine; NYHA, New York Heart Association functional class; PAC, plasma aldosterone; PRA, plasma renin activity; PVEDVI, pulmonary ventricular end-diastolic volume index; PVEF, pulmonary ventricular ejection fraction; Pvo₂, peak oxygen uptake; PVR, pulmonary valve replacement; RAS, renin-angiotensin-aldosterone; RI, radionuclide imaging; RV, morphologic right ventricle; SVEDVI, systemic ventricular end-diastolic volume index; SVEF, systemic ventricular ejection fraction.

NP levels were positively correlated with NYHA class[4,9,10] and inversely correlated with peak oxygen uptake (Pvo_2) in some studies.[4,8] Regarding the associations with ventricular function, NP levels were inversely correlated with the systolic function of the PV or SV.[3,4,9,10] Echocardiographic variables, such as Tei-index[7] and tissue Doppler findings,[6] were also associated with NP levels. In terms of the noncardiac variables, the NP level was correlated positively with age and inversely with arterial oxygen saturation (Spo_2).[8] Pulmonary function and Pvo_2 were also inversely correlated with the NP levels.[8] The norepinephrine level was higher in ACHD than in controls, and correlated with the NYHA classes and cardiothoracic ratio as well as the NP level.[4] The endothelin-1 level was also higher in the ACHD group and correlated with NYHA class, Pvo_2, cardiac size, and SV function, and these associations with clinical variables were the second strongest after the NP levels.[4] On the other hand, although the hormone levels of RAS were higher in the ACHD, there was a weak association with cardiopulmonary function.[4] Regarding the other biomarkers, one study demonstrated that asymmetric dimethylarginine level reflected the HF severity as did the NT-proBNP level, although it was not associated with ventricular function.[10] Regarding the diagnostic value, a BNP level of greater than 40 pg/mL predicted SV dysfunction,[6] and high levels of ANP and BNP predicted mortality in ACHD, with the statistically optimal cutoff values being 78 and 146 pg/mL, respectively.[9]

Note

Even if functional class was comparable, BNP level was lower in ACHD patients than in non-ACHD HF patients,[6] and similar findings were also demonstrated in pediatric and adolescent postoperative patients with CHD,[11] implying a unique HF pathophysiology in CHD patients regardless of age.

PRV Group

Patients' characteristics

This category includes patients with ventricular volume and/or pressure overload caused by atrial septal defect (ASD), those with idiopathic PH, and those with postoperative tetralogy of Fallot (TOF).[12–22] These studies consisted of 20 to 130 clinically stable patients. Ages at the time of study were lower in TOF patients, with a mean of 16 to 30 years, when compared with age in patients with an ASD and idiopathic PH, with a mean age of 38 to 46 years. Most patients with ASD[12,13,18] and TOF[15–17,20] were in NYHA class I or II, and NYHA class III or higher was rare. On the other hand, most patients were symptomatic in studies of idiopathic PH patients, including NYHA class IV patients.[12,14] In more than half of the studies, ventricular function was assessed by CT[12] or MRI[18,19,21,22] as well as echocardiography. Several exclusion criteria were also applied in some studies, such as acute HF, liver and/or renal dysfunction, arrhythmia, and LV dysfunction.[12–14,16–19]

Biomarkers

NP levels were measured in all studies, catecholamine levels in 3,[14,16,19] and RAS hormones in 2.[16,19] Higher levels of NP were found in the ACHD groups in general,[12,13,16,17,19] with even higher levels in those with PH,[13] whereas the catecholamine and RAS hormone levels did not differ from those in controls.[16,19] The NP and norepinephrine levels were correlated with NYHA class and Pvo_2[14,16,18–20] but the epinephrine and RAS hormone levels were not.[16] Regarding associations with ventricular function, despite a lack of association between LV function and biomarkers in all studies except 1,[21] a greater RV volume and a reduced RV systolic function were associated with higher levels of biomarkers.[12,15,16,18–21] As a result, the magnitude of pulmonary regurgitation was also positively correlated with NP levels.[16,20,21] NP levels were inversely correlated with the systolic function of the PV or SV.[3,4,9,10] Echocardiographic variables, such as the Tei-index[7] and tissue Doppler findings,[6] were also associated with NP levels. In particular, relatively strong correlations were observed between impaired hemodynamics and high levels of biomarkers in PH patients.[12–14,18] Regarding the diagnostic value, NP and norepinephrine levels were able to predict mortality in PH patients,[14] although there have been no studies as to whether biomarker(s) could predict the mortality of TOF patients. Apart from prognosis, a ratio of BNP to ANP of greater than 1.0,[13] NT-proBNP greater than 200 ng/L, and NT-proBNP greater than 105 to 148 ng/L was associated with the presence of PH, RV volume overload, and impaired exercise capacity, respectively.[17,19] Device ASD closure[18] and pulmonary valve replacement significantly decreased NP levels,[20,22] and the reduction in NP level was associated with the corresponding reduction in RV volume.[22] ANP level sensitively reflected an acute efficacy of PH treatment by nitric oxide, and long-term benefits resulted in decreases in both NP levels.[12] A cutoff BNP value of 150 pg/mL and the increase during follow-up predicted the mortality.[14]

Table 2

Correlations between biomarkers and clinical variables in heart failure in adults with congenital heart disease

S.No	SV-Type Category	Ref.	Biomarker	Unit	n	Value	Demographics		Functional Capacity		Systemic Ventricle			Pulmonary Ventricle		Hemodynamics						
							Age	Gender	NYHA	PvO2	EDV	EF/(Tei)	AVVR	EDV/Dd	EF/(Tei)	RAP	PVSP	PAP	CI	SpO2	PR	Qp/Qs
1	Mixed	3	ANP	pmol/L	21	7.3 ± 4.5						×		×	⊙		×					
			BNP	pmol/L		5.3 ± 3.5						×		×	⊙		×					
		4	ANP	pmol/L	53	56.6 ± 17.8			⊙	⊙		⊙										
			BNP	pmol/L		35.8 ± 7.7			⊙	○		○										
			NE	nmol/L		2.19 ± 0.09			⊙	×		○										
		7	BNP	pg/mL	54	—	⊙															
		8	BNP	pg/mL	53	122.4 ± 106.7			⊙	⊙		×/(○)			×/(⊙)					⊙		
		9	BNP	pg/mL	49	52.7 (39.1–115.4)						○										
		10	NT-proBNP	pg/mL	94	—			⊙			⊙										
2	Pulmonary RV	12	ANP	pg/mL	41	—					×	×		×	⊙	⊙		⊙	○			
			BNP	pg/mL		—					×	×		×	⊙	⊙		⊙	○			
		13	ANP	pg/mL	31	27 ± 4					×	×										○
			BNP	pg/mL		31 ± 5					×	×										
		14	ANP	pg/mL	60	—			○													
			BNP	pg/mL		—			○													
			NE	pg/mL		—			○													
		15	BNP	pg/mL	25	85.0 ± 87.0				×	×	×		⊙		⊙		⊙	⊙			
		16	NT-proANP	pg/mL	50	704 ± 62	×			⊙	×	×		×		⊙		⊙	⊙			
			NT-proBNP	pg/mL		147 ± 28 (m)/150 ± 23 (f)	×	×						○		×	×	×	○		⊙	
		17	NE	ng/L	59	452 ± 36	×				×	×										
			NT-proBNP	pg/mL		150 ± 141																
		18	NT-proBNP	ng/L	20	240 ± 93			○	○					×	○						○
		19	NT-proBNP	ng/L	70	218 ± 30				⊙	×	×		○	×		×				×	
		20	BNP	pg/mL	130	16 (11–30) (m)/37 (21–57) (f)		⊙	○	×				⊙							○	○
		21	BNP	pg/mL	42	—						⊙		⊙							⊙	

	Ref	Marker	Units	n	Value
3 Systemic RV (±Fontan)	23	NT-proBNP	pg/mL	33	240 ± 230
	24	NT-proBNP	pg/mL	29	257.7 ± 243.4
	25	BNP	pg/mL	44	19 (6–522)
	26	BNP	pg/mL	16	67 ± 12
	27	NT-proBNP	ng/L	43	200 ± 148
	28	NT-proBNP	pmol/L	35	25 (5–135, 38 ± 34)
	30	NT-proBNP	ng/L	47	269 (34–4476)
	31	BNP	pg/mL	48	—
	32	ANP	pg/mL	24	61.8 ± 43.3
	33	BNP	pg/mL	61	15.4 ± 18.2
		BNP	pmol/L		13 (1–52)
		NT-proBNP	ng/L		340 (49–1959)
	34	BNP	pg/mL	40	71.8 ± 74.4
4 Fontan	35	ANP	pg/mL	50	76 ± 10
		BNP	pg/mL		90.9 ± 14.3
		NE	pg/mL		380 ± 30
	36	BNP	pg/mL	68	32.9–227.2
5 Unrepaired (±Eisenmenger)	37	NT-proANP	pmol/L	26	1828 ± 1147
	38	NT-proANP	pmol/L	9	1817 ± 1553
		NT-proBNP	pmol/L		122 ± 140
	39	BNP	pg/mL	53	100 ± 157 (no-event)/ 322 ± 347 (event)[a]
	40	BNP	pg/mL	181	97.6 ± 150.3

Significance: ×, not significant; Δ, P<.1; ○, P<.05; ◉, P<.01.

Abbreviations: AVVR, atrioventricular valve regurgitation; CI, cardiac index; Dd, ventricular diastolic dimension; f, female; m, male; PAP, pulmonary artery pressure; PR, pulmonary regurgitation; PVSP, pulmonary ventricular systolic pressure; Qp/Qs, pulmonary to systemic flow ratio; Sp_{O_2}, arterial oxygen saturation. Other abbreviations are as in **Table 1**.

[a] Indicates P<.01 versus no-event group.

Table 3
Predictive and/or prognostic value of biomarkers in ACHD

S.No	SV-Type Category	Ref.	Biomarker	Unit	n	Power	Cutoff	Problems
1	Mixed	6	BNP	pg/mL	7	○	40	SV dysfunction
		8	BNP	pg/mL	53	×	—	PH(+)
		9	ANP	pg/mL	49	○	78	Mortality
			BNP	pg/mL		○	146	Mortality
2	Pulmonary RV	13	ANP	pg/mL	31	○	BNP/ANP >1.0	PH(+)
		14	ANP	pg/mL	60	○	—	Mortality
			BNP	pg/mL		○	150 (+FU increase)	Mortality
			NE	pg/mL		○	—	Mortality
		17	NT-proBNP	pg/mL	59	○	105	Pvo₂ <60%
		19	NT-proBNP	ng/L	70	○	148	Pvo₂ <20 (mL/kg/min)
		21	BNP	pg/mL	42	○	45	Corrected EF <30
3	Systemic RV (±Fontan)	25	BNP	pg/mL	44	○	36	SV Tei >0.45
		28	NT-proBNP	pmol/L	35	×	—	Renal dysfunction
		32	ANP	pg/mL	24	○	75	SVEF <40%
4	Fontan	35	ANP	pg/mL	50	×	—	Mortality
			BNP	pg/mL		×	—	Mortality
			NE	pg/mL		×	—	Mortality
5	Unrepaired (±Eisenmenger)	39	BNP	pg/mL	53	○	50	Morbidity (+mortality)
		40	BNP	pg/mL	181	○	100 (+FU increase)	Mortality
		41	NT-proBNP	ng/L	31	○	425	Mortality
			hsTnT	µg/L		○	0.014	Mortality
		42	BNP	pg/mL	13	Δ	200	SVEDP ≥12 (mm Hg)
6	Pregnancy	48	BNP	pg/mL	66	○	100	Cardiac event
		49	BNP	pg/mL	25	○	100	Cardiac event

Statistical significance: ×, not significant; Δ, maybe significant; ○, significant.
Abbreviations: FU, follow-up; PH, pulmonary hypertension; SVEDV, systemic ventricular end-diastolic pressure. Other abbreviations are as in **Tables 1** and **2**.

Note

Some adult TOF patients had impaired LV dysfunction as well as RV dysfunction. In addition, noncardiac complications, such as renal dysfunction, were not uncommon in these patients. Thus, evidence from studies with several exclusion criteria may not be applicable to real-world ACHD HF because these patients usually suffer from additional complications. As a consequence, future studies of HF in ACHD with a variety of complications may help to guide the management of these ACHD patients.

SRV Group

Patients' characteristics

Patients with transposition of the great arteries (TGA) after atrial switch operation and those with corrected TGA after functional repair were included in this category. Two studies included Fontan patients.[23–34] These studies consisted of 16 to 61 clinically stable patients with a mean age of 19 ± 5 to 30.3 ± 10.9 years, and most were in NYHA class II with few in NYHA class III or higher. Ventricular function was assessed by MRI[27,28,30,32] or CT[30] as well as echocardiography in most studies. Tei-index[23,25] and visual semi-quantitative assessment for SV function[33] were sometimes used. Several exclusion criteria were also applied in some studies, including acute HF, lung disease, and liver and/or renal dysfunction. Patients with PH and those of NYHA class III or higher were also excluded in some studies.[23,24,29,33,34]

Biomarkers

NP levels were measured in all studies except 1,[29] and catecholamines[24] and RAS hormones[24,29] were also assessed in a subset of studies. When compared with controls, ACHD showed high levels of BNP[25] and NT-proBNP,[23] and these levels were correlated with either NYHA class or Pv_{O_2} in most studies,[23,27,33,34] with the exception of 1 study in which BNP level was correlated with both NYHA class and Pv_{O_2}.[31] Therefore, associations of NP levels with NYHA class and Pv_{O_2} are inconsistent thus far. On the other hand, levels of BNP and NT-proBNP reflected impaired SV systolic function in most studies.[24,27,28] ANP level rather than BNP level reflected the SV function in one study.[32] Significant atrioventricular valve regurgitation was also associated with a high BNP level,[25,26,31] and angiotensin II level was correlated with SV systolic function only in female patients.[29] However, the association of catecholamine and RAS hormone levels with HF severity was only weak.[24,29] As for the noncardiac variables, age[31,33] and female gender[28,31] were related with a high level of BNP or NT-proBNP in some studies; however, these associations were not observed in the other studies.[28,33] In addition, a high level of aldosterone in female patients[29] was shown, and renal function[28] and body mass index[31] were not related with BNP or NT-proBNP level. One study demonstrated no association of BNP level with quality of life in these ACHD patients.[30] In terms of the diagnostic value, cutoff values of 36 pg/mL for BNP[25] and 75 pg/mL for ANP[32] predicted SV dysfunction, such as SV ejection fraction less than 40%. Impaired response of SV performance to dobutamine stress test was demonstrated in ACHD patients with a high BNP level.[26] On the other hand, there was little impact of PV (morphologic LV in this category of patients) function on the biomarkers,[28,29,32] except for one study in which greater RV dimension was related with a high BNP level.[25]

Note

Most studies did not include or specifically excluded severe HF ACHD patients in whom the benefits of biomarkers may be too small to stratify, as demonstrated in pediatric and adolescent patients with CHD.[11] Future studies with a relatively large number of symptomatic ACHD patients may clarify the clinical importance of biomarkers in practice.

Fontan Group

Patients' characteristics

Only 2 studies were included in this category, both of which consisted of 50 adult Fontan patients.[35,36] Their age ranged from 22.7 ± 7.0 to 53 years; the NYHA class was II or lower in most patients in their 20s whereas it was slightly

worse in patients presenting in their 30s, with a mean of 2.3.[36] SV function and hemodynamics were assessed by cardiac catheterization, and patients taking angiotensin-converting enzyme inhibitors and/or β-blockers were excluded from the study.[35]

Biomarkers

Various biomarkers were assessed in one study[35] and only BNP level was measured in the other study.[36] All of these biomarker levels were significantly higher in the ACHD patients.[35] No associations of biomarkers with NYHA class or Pv_{O_2} were shown.[35] BNP level was correlated with SV volume, end-diastolic pressure, cardiac index, and Sp_{O_2} in one study,[36] and levels of norepinephrine and angiotensin II were inversely correlated with SV systolic function, whereas ANP level inversely correlated with the cardiac index.[35] Regarding the prognostic value, no single biomarker was able to predict the mortality.[35] However, because the majority of Fontan patients were of the atriopulmonary connection type in one study,[35] the results may not be applicable to the modern cohort of adult Fontan patients.

Unrepaired Group

Patients' characteristics

Patients with Eisenmenger syndrome were included in all studies[37–41] except 1,[42] which consisted of heterogeneous SV morphologies. Of those, 2 studies concerned ACHD with Eisenmenger syndrome, including patients with Down syndrome.[39,40] The studies consisted of 9 to 181 clinically stable patients with a mean age of 30 ± 8 to 45 ± 12 years old. Their Sp_{O_2} ranged from 75% ± 7.9% to 86% ± 7%, and most patients were symptomatic. Cardiac catheterization and/ or echocardiography were used to assess the SV function, and patients with renal dysfunction were excluded in 2 studies.[38,41]

Biomarkers

All studies measured NP levels, NT-proANP in 2 studies,[37,38] NT-proBNP in 2,[38,41] and BNP in 3,[39,40,42] and the NP levels were significantly higher than normal values in ACHD patients.[37,38] High-sensitivity cardiac troponin T was measured in one study alongside NT-proBNP.[41] The BNP level did not correlate with NYHA class or 6-minute walk test distance, although older age was associated with a higher BNP level.[40] Hopkins and colleagues[38] demonstrated that hypoxia was an important determinant of high levels of NT-proANP and NT-proBNP, despite less volume loading to the atrial and/or ventricular wall. Regarding the diagnostic value, a BNP level higher than 200 pg/mL may identify patients with a high SV end-diastolic pressure of 12 mm Hg or higher.[42] For BNP, a value greater than the cutoff 50 pg/mL predicted the morbidity and mortality,[39] and values greater than 100 pg/mL or a significant increase during follow-up also predicted mortality.[40] High-sensitivity cardiac troponin T was also reported to be a predictor of mortality.[41]

Note

In normal people and non-ACHD patients, female gender,[43] renal dysfunction,[44] and anemia[45] are established determinants of a high BNP level, and obesity is associated with low BNP level.[46] In addition to these determinants, one should realize that hypoxia, which is a situation not uncommon in ACHD patients, is also responsible for high levels of NP.[37,38] Similar evidence was found in pediatric and adolescent total cavopulmonary connection–type Fontan patients.[47]

Pregnancy Group

Patients' characteristics

There have been 2 studies of biomarkers in pregnancy in which the most common underlying diagnosis was TOF.[48,49] Mean age was 30 years in both studies; most ACHD patients were in NYHA class I, followed by NYHA class II, with only 3 cases of NYHA class III. SV function during pregnancy and after delivery was assessed by echocardiography.

Biomarkers

In both studies, BNP levels during pregnancy were monitored, and the levels were significantly higher than those in normal controls.[48] Although associations between the BNP levels and NYHA class and Pvo$_2$ were not reported, SV function was preserved during pregnancy.[49] Regarding the diagnostic value, a peak BNP level of greater than 100 pg/mL was able to predict maternal cardiac events[48,49] and the negative predictive value was 100%,[48] although the baseline BNP levels were not associated with events.[49]

SUMMARY

Most individuals with ACHD, irrespective of symptoms and the role of the ventricles in supporting either the pulmonary or systemic circulation, show high levels of NP when compared with normal controls. The high NP levels largely reflect ventricular dysfunction caused by ventricular volume and/or pressure overload resulting from intracardiac shunting, pulmonary regurgitation, and atrioventricular valve regurgitation. In addition,

NP levels are related to patient age, gender, and hypoxia. The magnitude of NP-level elevation is less pronounced in patients with ACHD, although the exact mechanisms remain unknown. In terms of their prognostic value, norepinephrine and NP levels were relatively strongly related to outcome in studies that included many symptomatic patients, especially those with unrepaired ACHD, Eisenmenger syndrome, and PH. However, diagnostic and/or prognostic value of biomarkers is less consistent in other studies, probably because of the relatively small number of patients and small percentage of patients with severe HF included. In addition, such studies used many exclusion criteria and also obscured the role of biomarkers in the larger population; for example, although various biomarkers in adult Fontan patients may be elevated, their clinical significance remains unclear. Limited data are available regarding serial assessment of biomarkers, and such information could provide additional important information to help identify patients at risk, as demonstrated during patient follow-up and pregnancy.

REFERENCES

1. Braunwald E. Biomarkers in heart failure. N Engl J Med 2008;358:2148–59.
2. Morrow DA, de Lemos JA. Benchmarks for the assessment of novel cardiovascular biomarkers. Circulation 2007;115:949–52.
3. Tulevski II, Groenink M, van Der Wall EE, et al. Increased brain and atrial natriuretic peptides in patients with chronic right ventricular pressure overload: correlation between plasma neurohormones and right ventricular dysfunction. Heart 2001;86:27–30.
4. Bolger AP, Sharma R, Li W, et al. Neurohormonal activation and the chronic heart failure syndrome in adults with congenital heart disease. Circulation 2002;106:92–9.
5. Book WM, Hott BJ, McConnell M. B-type natriuretic peptide levels in adults with congenital heart disease and right ventricular failure. Am J Cardiol 2005;95:545–6.
6. Law YM, Keller BB, Feingold BM, et al. Usefulness of plasma B-type natriuretic peptide to identify ventricular dysfunction in pediatric and adult patients with congenital heart disease. Am J Cardiol 2005; 95:474–8.
7. Perlowski AA, Aboulhosn J, Castellon Y, et al. Relation of brain natriuretic peptide to myocardial performance index in adults with congenital heart disease. Am J Cardiol 2007;100:110–4.
8. Trojnarska O, Gwizdala A, Katarzynski S, et al. The BNP concentrations and exercise capacity

assessment with cardiopulmonary stress test in cyanotic adult patients with congenital heart diseases. Int J Cardiol 2010;139:241–7.

9. Giannakoulas G, Dimopoulos K, Bolger AP, et al. Usefulness of natriuretic peptide levels to predict mortality in adults with congenital heart disease. Am J Cardiol 2010;105:869–73.

10. Tutarel O, Denecke A, Bode-Böger SM, et al. Asymmetrical dimethylarginine—more sensitive than NT-proBNP to diagnose heart failure in adults with congenital heart disease. PLoS One 2012;7:e33795.

11. Ohuchi H, Takasugi H, Ohashi H, et al. Stratification of pediatric heart failure on the basis of neurohormonal and cardiac autonomic nervous activities in patients with congenital heart disease. Circulation 2003;108:2368–76.

12. Nagaya N, Nishikimi T, Okano Y, et al. Plasma brain natriuretic peptide levels increase in proportion to the extent of right ventricular dysfunction in pulmonary hypertension. J Am Coll Cardiol 1998;31:202–8.

13. Nagaya N, Nishikimi T, Uematsu M, et al. Secretion patterns of brain natriuretic peptide and atrial natriuretic peptide in patients with or without pulmonary hypertension complicating atrial septal defect. Am Heart J 1998;136:297–301.

14. Nagaya N, Nishikimi T, Uematsu M, et al. Plasma brain natriuretic peptide as a prognostic indicator in patients with primary pulmonary hypertension. Circulation 2000;102:865–70.

15. Brili S, Alexopoulos N, Latsios G, et al. Tissue Doppler imaging and brain natriuretic peptide levels in adults with repaired tetralogy of Fallot. J Am Soc Echocardiogr 2005;18:1149–54.

16. Norozi K, Buchhorn R, Kaiser C, et al. Plasma N-terminal pro-brain natriuretic peptide as a marker of right ventricular dysfunction in patients with tetralogy of Fallot after surgical repair. Chest 2005;128: 2563–70.

17. Norozi K, Buchhorn R, Bartmus D, et al. Elevated brain natriuretic peptide and reduced exercise capacity in adult patients operated on for tetralogy of Fallot is due to biventricular dysfunction as determined by the myocardial performance index. Am J Cardiol 2006;97:1377–82.

18. Schoen SP, Zimmermann T, Kittner T, et al. NT-proBNP correlates with right heart haemodynamic parameters and volumes in patients with atrial septal defects. Eur J Heart Fail 2007;9:660–6.

19. Festa P, Ait-Ali L, Prontera C, et al. Amino-terminal fragment of pro-brain natriuretic hormone identifies functional impairment and right ventricular overload in operated tetralogy of Fallot patients. Pediatr Cardiol 2007;28:339–45.

20. Koch AM, Zink S, Glöckler M, et al. Plasma levels of B-type natriuretic peptide in patients with tetralogy of Fallot after surgical repair. Int J Cardiol 2010; 143:130–4.

21. Oosterhof T, Tulevski II, Vliegen HW, et al. Effects of volume and/or pressure overload secondary to congenital heart disease (tetralogy of Fallot or pulmonary stenosis) on right ventricular function using cardiovascular magnetic resonance and B-type natriuretic peptide levels. Am J Cardiol 2006;97: 1051–5.

22. Westhoff-Bleck M, Girke S, Breymann T, et al. Pulmonary valve replacement in chronic pulmonary regurgitation in adults with congenital heart disease: impact of preoperative QRS-duration and NT-proBNP levels on postoperative right ventricular function. Int J Cardiol 2011;151:303–6.

23. Norozi K, Buchhorn R, Alpers V, et al. Relation of systemic ventricular function quantified by myocardial performance index (Tei) to cardiopulmonary exercise capacity in adults after Mustard procedure for transposition of the great arteries. Am J Cardiol 2005;96:1721–5.

24. Dore A, Houde C, Chan KL, et al. Angiotensin receptor blockade and exercise capacity in adults with systemic right ventricles: a multicenter, randomized, placebo-controlled clinical trial. Circulation 2005;112:2411–6.

25. Chow PC, Cheung EW, Chong CY, et al. Brain natriuretic peptide as a biomarker of systemic right ventricular function in patients with transposition of great arteries after atrial switch operation. Int J Cardiol 2008;127:192–7.

26. Vogt M, Kühn A, Wiese J, et al. Reduced contractile reserve of the systemic right ventricle under dobutamine stress is associated with increased brain natriuretic peptide levels in patients with complete transposition after atrial repair. Eur J Echocardiogr 2009;10:691–4.

27. Schaefer A, Tallone EM, Westhoff-Bleck M, et al. Relation of diastolic and systolic function, exercise capacity and brain natriuretic peptide in adults after Mustard procedure for transposition of the great arteries. Cardiology 2010;117:112–7.

28. Plymen CM, Hughes ML, Picaut N, et al. The relationship of systemic right ventricular function to ECG parameters and NT-proBNP levels in adults with transposition of the great arteries late after Senning or Mustard surgery. Heart 2010;96: 1569–73.

29. Szymański P, Klisiewicz A, Lubiszewska B, et al. Gender differences in angiotensin II and aldosterone secretion in patients with pressure overloaded systemic right ventricles are similar to those observed in systemic arterial hypertension. Int J Cardiol 2011;147:366–70.

30. Winter MM, Bouma BJ, van Dijk AP, et al. Relation of physical activity, cardiac function, exercise capacity, and quality of life in patients with a systemic right ventricle. Am J Cardiol 2008;102: 1258–62.

31. Koch AM, Zink S, Singer H. B-type natriuretic peptide in patients with systemic right ventricle. Cardiology 2008;110:1–7.

32. Garg R, Raman SV, Hoffman TM, et al. Serum markers of systemic right ventricular function and exercise performance. Pediatr Cardiol 2008;29:641–8.

33. Larsson DA, Meurling CJ, Holmqvist F, et al. The diagnostic and prognostic value of brain natriuretic peptides in adults with a systemic morphologically right ventricle or Fontan-type circulation. Int J Cardiol 2007;114:345–51.

34. Trojnarska O, Gwizdała A, Katarzyński S, et al. Evaluation of exercise capacity with cardiopulmonary exercise testing and BNP levels in adult patients with single or systemic right ventricles. Arch Med Sci 2010;6:192–7.

35. Inai K, Nakanishi T, Nakazawa M. Clinical correlation and prognostic predictive value of neurohumoral factors in patients late after the Fontan operation. Am Heart J 2005;150:588–94.

36. Motoki N, Ohuchi H, Miyazaki A, et al. Clinical profiles of adult patients with single ventricular physiology. Circ J 2009;73:1711–6.

37. Hopkins WE, Hall C. Paradoxical relationship between N-terminal proatrial natriuretic peptide and filling pressure in adults with cyanotic congenital heart disease. Circulation 1997;96:2215–20.

38. Hopkins WE, Chen Z, Fukagawa NK, et al. Increased atrial and brain natriuretic peptides in adults with cyanotic congenital heart disease: enhanced understanding of the relationship between hypoxia and natriuretic peptide secretion. Circulation 2004;109:2872–7.

39. Reardon LC, Williams RJ, Houser LS, et al. Usefulness of serum brain natriuretic peptide to predict adverse events in patients with the Eisenmenger syndrome. Am J Cardiol 2012;110:1523–6.

40. Diller GP, Alonso-Gonzalez R, Kempny A, et al. B-type natriuretic peptide concentrations in contemporary Eisenmenger syndrome patients: predictive value and response to disease targeting therapy. Heart 2012;98:736–42.

41. Schuuring MJ, van Riel AC, Vis JC, et al. High-sensitivity troponin T is associated with poor outcome in adults with pulmonary arterial hypertension due to congenital heart disease. Congenit Heart Dis, in press.

42. Saab FG, Aboulhosn JA. Hemodynamic characteristics of cyanotic adults with single-ventricle physiology without Fontan completion. Congenit Heart Dis 2013;8:124–30.

43. Redfield MM, Rodeheffer RJ, Jacobsen SJ, et al. Plasma brain natriuretic peptide concentration: impact of age and gender. J Am Coll Cardiol 2002;40:976–82.

44. Tsutamoto T, Wada A, Sakai H, et al. Relationship between renal function and plasma brain natriuretic peptide in patients with heart failure. J Am Coll Cardiol 2006;47:582–6.

45. Wold Knudsen C, Vik-Mo H, Omland T. Blood haemoglobin is an independent predictor of B-type natriuretic peptide (BNP). Clin Sci (Lond) 2005;109:69–74.

46. Wang TJ, Larson MG, Levy D, et al. Impact of obesity on plasma natriuretic peptide levels. Circulation 2004;109:594–600.

47. Ohuchi H, Takasugi H, Ohashi H, et al. Abnormalities of neurohormonal and cardiac autonomic nervous activities relate poorly to functional status in Fontan patients. Circulation 2004;110:2601–8.

48. Tanous D, Siu SC, Mason J, et al. B-type natriuretic peptide in pregnant women with heart disease. J Am Coll Cardiol 2010;56:1247–53.

49. Kamiya T, Iwamiya T, Neki R, et al. Outcome of pregnancy and effects on the right heart in women with repaired tetralogy of Fallot. Circ J 2012;76:957–63.

Diagnostic Tools for Arrhythmia Detection in Adults with Congenital Heart Disease and Heart Failure

Blandine Mondésert, MD[a], Anne M. Dubin, MD[b],
Paul Khairy, MD, PhD[a],*

KEYWORDS

- Arrhythmias • Electrophysiology • Heart failure • Adult congenital heart disease • Diagnostic testing

KEY POINTS

- Heart failure and arrhythmias are among the leading causes of morbidity and mortality in adults with congenital heart disease (CHD).
- The standard 12-lead electrocardiogram (ECG) remains the cornerstone for arrhythmia diagnosis and provides valuable information with regard to associated hemodynamic lesions and prognostic markers for sudden cardiac death.
- External loop recorders are helpful in diagnosing patients with suspected arrhythmias and monitoring those with known arrhythmias, and may be of value in routinely screening certain subpopulations, such as adults with tetralogy of Fallot.
- The prognostic value of signal-averaged ECG, heart rate variability, and microvolt T-wave alternans remain to be defined in adults with CHD and heart failure.
- Pacemakers and implantable cardioverter-defibrillators are equipped with a variety of features that may be helpful in diagnosing and quantifying arrhythmias, including data trends, stored intracardiac electrograms, and responses to antitachycardia pacing therapy.

INTRODUCTION

Progressively declining mortalities across the spectrum of cardiac birth defects are resulting in a growing and aging population of adults with congenital heart disease (CHD) of increasing complexity.[1] Heart failure and arrhythmias are among the leading causes of morbidity and mortality in this patient population, with a relationship that is bidirectional.[2–4] Heart failure can result in structural and electrophysiologic changes that alter the expression and function of a variety of membrane transport processes, thereby favoring arrhythmias.[5] In contrast, factors that predispose adults with CHD to arrhythmias, such as pressure or volume overload, hypoxemia, fibrosis, and surgical scars, may likewise be implicated in the pathophysiology of heart failure. Moreover, the well-recognized phenomenon of tachyarrhythmia-induced cardiomyopathy may be accentuated in patients with CHD and fragile physiologies, such as those with cyanosis, systemic right ventricles, or univentricular hearts.[6,7]

Financial Support: Dr P. Khairy is supported by a Canada Research Chair in Electrophysiology and Adult Congenital Heart Disease.

Conflict of Interest: Dr P. Khairy has received research funding for investigator-initiated grants from St. Jude Medical, Medtronic, and Boehringer-Ingelheim.

[a] Adult Congenital Center, Montreal Heart Institute, Université de Montréal, 5000 Bélanger Street East, Montreal, Québec H1T 1C8, Canada; [b] Department of Pediatric Cardiology, Lucile Packard Children's Hospital, Stanford University, 725 Welch Road, Suite 120, Palo Alto, CA 94304, USA

* Corresponding author.

E-mail address: paul.khairy@umontreal.ca

Heart Failure Clin 10 (2014) 57–67

http://dx.doi.org/10.1016/j.hfc.2013.09.009

1551-7136/14/$ – see front matter © 2014 Elsevier Inc. All rights reserved.

Given the high prevalence and potentially distressing consequences of arrhythmias in adults with CHD and heart failure, promptly recognizing rhythm disorders is an essential component of surveillance and follow-up.[8,9] This article discusses and appraises the electrophysiologic tools, both invasive and noninvasive, that are of potential diagnostic or prognostic value in adults with CHD and heart failure.

NONINVASIVE ELECTROPHYSIOLOGIC TOOLS
The 12-lead Electrocardiogram

The standard 12-lead electrocardiogram (ECG) is an indispensable tool for assessing adults with CHD and heart failure. It is critical in characterizing a broad spectrum of bradyarrhythmias and tachyarrhythmias, providing diagnostic clues in patients with previously undetected CHD (**Fig. 1**), and screening for associated hemodynamic complications, such as obstructive lesions. Typical ECG features in adults with common forms of CHD are summarized in **Table 1**.[10]

Moreover, the ECG can provide important prognostic information.[11–13] A wider QRS complex has been associated with increased risk of heart failure and sudden death in various congenital and noncongenital forms of heart disease. A QRS duration greater than 180 milliseconds is often retained in proposed risk stratification schemes for sudden death in patients with tetralogy of Fallot.[11,12,14,15] Correlations have also been described, albeit less consistently, between QRS duration and ventricular arrhythmias/sudden death in patients with complete transposition of the great arteries and

intra-atrial baffles.[13] In this patient population, associations have been reported between diastolic and systolic right ventricular volumes, N-terminal pro brain natriuretic peptide levels, and QRS duration.[16] In patients with Fontan surgery, QRS duration has been independently associated with peak oxygen capacity in multivariate analyses.[17] Associations between QT interval prolongation and increased mortality have also been described in diverse populations.[18,19] However, QRS duration and QT intervals are highly correlated, with the QRS complex constituting a sizable segment of the QT interval. As such, QT and JT dispersion, which quantify the difference between the longest and shortest respective intervals on a 12-lead ECG, are considered by some to more accurately reflect dispersion of repolarization. In patients with tetralogy of Fallot, the combination of prolonged QRS duration and increased QT[20] or JT dispersion[21] seems to more accurately predict ventricular arrhythmias than QRS duration alone.

External Loop Recorders

The value of routine serial ambulatory ECG monitoring (eg, 24-hour Holter recordings) remains debated in patients with CHD at large. Nevertheless, external loop recorders are generally considered helpful in evaluating patients with symptoms suggestive of arrhythmia (eg, palpitations, syncope), monitoring those with known arrhythmias (eg, sick sinus syndrome, paroxysmal atrial tachyarrhythmia), and assessing responses to therapy (eg, rate control in patients with permanent atrial tachyarrhythmias). Considering the high

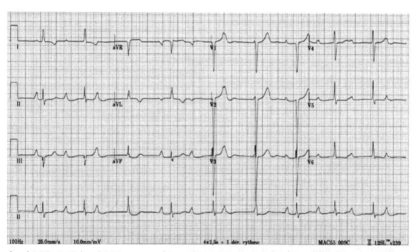

Fig. 1. Twelve-lead ECG. A 12-lead ECG was performed in a 38-year-old man with no known CHD who complained of dyspnea on exertion. Q waves over the right precordial lead (V1), absent septal q waves in V5 and V6, and abnormal Q waves in lead III suggest a diagnosis of congenitally corrected transposition of the great arteries with right-to-left septal depolarization. Complete atrioventricular block is noted.

prevalence of supraventricular and ventricular arrhythmias in adults with CHD and heart failure, external loop recorders are among the commonly prescribed diagnostic tools for arrhythmia detection.

In a recent retrospective study of adults with CHD, the prevalence of detected arrhythmias was 2-fold higher by Holter monitors than standard ECGs (31% vs 15%).[22] Arrhythmias consisted of isolated ectopy in 17%, supraventricular tachycardia in 12%, ventricular tachycardia in 7%, high-grade atrioventricular block in 5%, and pacemaker issues in 3%. A quarter of the patients with arrhythmias detected by Holter had no arrhythmias on ECG and 80% of patients with detected arrhythmias were asymptomatic. In symptomatic patients, 37% experienced similar symptoms during Holter monitoring, allowing a diagnosis to be established. A second series assessed Holter monitor results in 189 patients with tetralogy of Fallot (N = 100), Fontan surgery (N = 51), or transposition of the great arteries with atrial baffles (N = 38).[23] The test was considered clinically significant if it prompted a change in therapy. Using this definition, the investigators reported a modest (40%) sensitivity for routine monitoring and a high (96%) negative predictive value for future clinically significant arrhythmias. Relevant to adults with CHD, the diagnostic yield improved with older age.

Signal-averaged ECG

A signal-averaged ECG (SAECG) uses computer-based processing techniques to produce a high-resolution ECG capable of recording microvolt signals noninvasively from surface leads. Random noise that is not synchronized to the QRS complex is canceled out and smaller signals, such as ventricular late potentials, are retained. Such late potentials are thought to arise from areas of slow conduction around scar and are, therefore, considered to indicate an electrophysiologic substrate capable of sustaining potentially malignant reentrant ventricular tachyarrhythmias. Common parameters studied include the duration of the filtered QRS complex, duration of the terminal QRS complex less than 40 μV, and the root-mean-square amplitude of the terminal 40 milliseconds of the QRS complex (**Fig. 2**).

Late potentials were identified in 62% of 242 patients with CHD and ventriculotomy incisions.[24] Except for a scalar QRS duration greater than 180 milliseconds, no correlation was found between positive SAECG findings and risk factors for ventricular tachycardia. A series of 66 patients with tetralogy of Fallot consistently reported that a filtered QRS duration greater than 170 milliseconds

was associated with sustained ventricular tachycardia.[25] In contrast, a study of 31 patients with right ventriculotomy incisions or postrepair right bundle branch block found that a low-amplitude terminal root-mean-square voltage of 100 μV or less had 91% sensitivity and 70% specificity in predicting inducible sustained or nonsustained ventricular tachycardia.[26] Similar sensitivity but lower specificity was seen with QRS duration. The predictive value of a terminal low-amplitude QRS signal duration was weaker still. Moreover, the SAECG could not distinguish between sustained and nonsustained forms of inducible ventricular tachycardia. Given the lingering uncertainties regarding potential indications and their independent prognostic value, the SAECG is not yet considered a mainstream prognostic tool for adults with CHD.

Heart Rate Variability

The autonomic nervous system plays an important role in the pathophysiology of heart failure. Several markers of sympathovagal imbalances, as assessed by such tests as heart rate turbulence, baroreflex sensitivity, and heart rate variability (HRV), have been associated with adverse outcomes in patients with heart failure. Heart rate variability refers to beat-to-beat variations in heart rate, or the R-R interval.[27] In healthy individuals, R-R intervals vary with the respiratory cycle by shortening during inspiration and prolonging on expiration. Because these fluctuations are predominantly mediated by parasympathetic efferent activity, reduced HRV has primarily been attributed to a reduction in vagal tone.

In a series of 258 children with CHD, HRV was reduced in those with New York Heart Association (NYHA) functional class II to IV symptoms but was not associated with hemodynamic parameters.[28] Reductions in HRV span the spectrum of cyanotic and acyanotic forms of CHD.[29] One study found that HRV was reduced in children with CHD before surgery and declined after surgery, with marked impairment in patients with prolonged postoperative hospitalizations.[30] In the largest series to date of 383 postoperative patients with CHD, including 91 with Fontan surgery, impaired HRV predicted a combined end point consisting of hospitalizations and mortality in those with biventricular but not univentricular physiology.[31] Given the limited data, the role of HRV in risk stratifying adults with CHD and heart failure remains to be defined. Simpler methods that rely on 3 consecutive 12-lead 10-second ECGs have been proposed,[32] which may facilitate more widespread adoption if such information proves valuable in risk stratifying this patient population.

Table 1
Typical ECG features in common forms of adult CHD

Congenital Diagnosis	Rhythm	PR Interval	QRS Axis	QRS Configuration	Atrial Enlargement	Ventricular Hypertrophy	Particularities
Secundum atrial septal defect	NSR; ↑IART/AF with age	1° AVB 6%–19%	0°–180°; RAD; LAD in Holt-Oran or LAHB	rSr' or rsR' with RBBBi>RBBBc	RAE 35%	Uncommon	Crochetage pattern
Ventricular septal defect	NSR; PVCs	Normal or mild ↑; 1° AVB 10%	RAD with BVH; LAD 3%–15%	Normal or rsr'; possible RBBB	Possible RAE ± LAE	BVH 23%–61%; RVH with Eisenmenger	Katz-Wachtel phenomenon
AV canal defect	NSR; PVCs 30%	1° AVB >50%	Mod to extreme LAD; Normal with atypical	rSr' or rsR'	Possible LAE	Uncommon in partial; BVH in complete; RVH with Eisenmenger	Infero-posteriorly displaced AVN
Patent ductus arteriosus	NSR; ↑IART/AF with age	↑PR 10%–20%	Normal	Deep S V1, tall R V5 and V6	LAE with moderate PDA	Uncommon	Often either clinically silent or Eisenmenger
Pulmonary stenosis	NSR	Normal	Normal if mild; RAD with moderate/severe	Normal; severity	Possible RAE	RVH; Severity correlates with R:S in V1 and V6	Axis deviation correlates with RVP
Aortic coarctation	NSR	Normal	Normal or LAD	Normal	Possible LAE	LVH, especially by voltage criteria	Persistent RVH rare beyond infancy
Ebstein anomaly	NSR; possible EAR, SVT; AF/IART 40%	1° AVB common; short if WPW	Normal or LAD	Low-amplitude multiphasic atypical RBBB	RAE with Himalayan P waves	Diminutive RV	Accessory pathway common; Q II, III, aVF and V1–V4
Surgically repaired TOF	NSR; PVCs 10%; VT 12%	Normal or mild ↑	Normal or RAD; LAD 5%–10%	RBBB 90%	Peaked P waves; RAE possible	RVH possible if RVOT obstruction or PHT	QRS duration ± QTd predicts VT/SCD

L-TGA	NSR	1° AVB >50%; AVB 2%/y	LAD	Absence septal q; Q in III, aVF and right precordium	Not if no associated defects	Not if no associated defects	Anterior AVN; positive T precordial; WPW with Ebstein
D-TGA/intra-atrial baffle	Sinus bradycardia 60%; EAR; junctional; IART 25%	Normal	RAD	Absence of q, small r, deep S in left precordium	Possible RAE	RVH; diminutive LV	Possible AVB if VSD or TV surgery
UVH with Fontan	Sinus bradycardia 15%; EAR; junctional; IART >50%	Normal in TA; 1° AVB in DILV	LAD in single RV, TA, single LV with noninverted outlet	Variable; ↑↑ R and S amplitudes in limb and precordial leads	RAE in TA	RVH with single RV; possible LVH with single LV	Absent sinus node in LAI; AV block with L-loop or AVCD
Dextrocardia	NSR; P-wave axis 105°–165° with situs inversus	Normal	RAD	Inverse depolarization and repolarization	Not with situs inversus	LVH: tall R V1-V2; RVH: deep Q, small R V1 and tall R lateral	Situs solitus: normal P-wave axis and severe CHD
ALCAPA	NSR	Normal	Possible LAD	Pathologic ant-lat Q waves; possible ant-sept Q waves	Possible LAE	Selective hypertrophy of posterobasal LV	Possible ischemia

Abbreviations: AF, atrial fibrillation; ALCAPA, anomalous left coronary artery from the pulmonary artery; ant-lat, anterolateral; AV, atrioventricular; AVB, atrioventricular block; AVCD, atrioventricular canal defect; AVN, AV node; BVH, biventricular hypertrophy; CHD, congenital heart disease; DILV, double inlet left ventricle; D-TGA, complete transposition of the great arteries; EAR, ectopic atrial rhythm; IART, intra-atrial reentrant tachycardia; LAD, left axis deviation; LAE, left atrial enlargement; LAHB, left anterior hemiblock; LAI, left atrial isomerism; L-TGA, congenitally corrected transposition of the great arteries; LV, left ventricle; LVH, left ventricular hypertrophy; NSR, normal sinus rhythm; PDA, patent ductus arteriosus; PHT, pulmonary hypertension; PVC, premature ventricular contraction; QTd, QT dispersion; RAD, right axis deviation; RAE, right atrial enlargement; RBBB, right bundle branch block (i, incomplete; c, complete); RV, right ventricle; RVH, right ventricular hypertrophy; RVOT, right ventricular outflow tract; RVP, right ventricular pressure; SCD, sudden cardiac death; SVT, supraventricular tachycardia; TA, tricuspid atresia; TOF, tetralogy of Fallot; TV, tricuspid valve; UVH, univentricular heart; VSD, ventricular septal defect; VT, ventricular tachycardia; WPW, Wolff-Parkinson-White syndrome.

From Khairy P, Marelli AJ. Clinical use of electrocardiography in adults with congenital heart disease. Circulation 2007;116(23):2735; with permission.

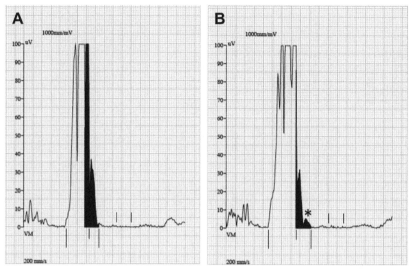

Fig. 2. (A) Normal SAECG tracing with a filtered QRS duration of 93 milliseconds (normal <114 milliseconds), a root-mean-square voltage in the last 40 milliseconds of 114 μV (normal >20 μV), and a filtered QRS duration less than 40 μV of 28 milliseconds (normal <38 milliseconds). (B) Abnormal SAECG consistent with late potentials (*asterisk*) characterized by a root-mean-square voltage in the last 40 milliseconds of 17 μV and a filtered QRS duration less than 40 μV of 39 milliseconds.

Microvolt T-wave Alternans

Microvolt T-wave alternans (TWA), an electrocardiographic phenomenon that indicates inhomogeneity of myocardial repolarization, is among the most promising up-and-coming noninvasive electrophysiologic prognostic tools. Studies have supported its value in risk stratifying patients with ischemic and nonischemic cardiomyopathy.[33,34] Guidelines from 2006 on the management of patients with ventricular arrhythmias and the prevention of sudden cardiac death include, as a class I indication, the possibility of requesting an ambulatory ECG to assess TWA.[35] Moreover, as a class IIA indication, it is deemed, "reasonable to use TWA to improve the diagnosis and risk stratification of patients with ventricular arrhythmias or who are at risk for developing life-threatening ventricular arrhythmias (level of evidence: A)."[35]

In a primarily pediatric population of 318 patients, 16% of whom had CHD, abnormal TWA was noted in 7% and was associated with ventricular arrhythmias and cardiac arrest.[36] In a recent cross-sectional study, microvolt TWA was more prevalent in the 102 patients with CHD and single-ventricle physiology or right ventricular disorders, including complete and congenitally corrected transposition of the great arteries, tetralogy of Fallot, and Ebstein anomaly, than in 52 controls of similar age (39% vs 2%).[37] Sustained ventricular tachyarrhythmias were more prevalent in those with abnormal microvolt TWA (19% vs 4%). Factors associated with abnormal microvolt TWA included lower oxygen saturation, higher NYHA functional class, and lower cardiopulmonary functional capacity.

Although the potential role of microvolt TWA remains unclear in adults with CHD and heart failure, the literature suggests that its strength lies in its high specificity and negative predictive value, whereas its sensitivity seems modest.

INVASIVE ELECTROPHYSIOLOGIC TOOLS
Implantable Loop Recorders

An implantable loop recorder (ILR; Reveal, Medtronic Inc, Minneapolis, MN; Confirm, St Jude Medical, Sylmar, CA; BioMonitor, Biotronik SE. Co. KG) is a single-lead ECG monitoring device that is placed subcutaneously. It offers longer term monitoring (from 3 to 6.4 years) than standard external loop recorders. Data are stored automatically according to programmed parameters for bradyarrhythmias and tachyarrhythmias and on patient activation. In general, ILRs are most commonly implanted in patients with syncope of unclear origin or with recurrent unexplained palpitations. ILRs have also been used in clinical trials to monitor response to therapy, such as following catheter ablation for atrial fibrillation.

In an early case-series of 4 patients with CHD and ILRs, a likely cause for symptoms was identified in 2 cases.[38] In a later retrospective cohort of 22 patients with CHD, the most frequent indication for an ILR was syncope followed by palpitations.[39] The ILR led to a diagnosis (either confirming or excluding arrhythmia) in 71%. From the ILR findings, 1 patient subsequently received a dual-chamber pacemaker and 2 had implantable cardioverter-defibrillators. ILRs were thought to be particularly helpful in patients with neurodevelopmental delay in whom accurate history was limited. ILRs have yet to be assessed in a population of adults with CHD and heart failure.

Electrophysiologic Testing

Electrophysiologic testing can measure properties of the conduction system and is considered the gold standard for diagnosing bradyarrhythmias and a variety of focal and reentrant tachyarrhythmias. As such, it is highly valued as a diagnostic tool for arrhythmias in selected adults with CHD and heart failure.[40] The prognostic value of programmed ventricular stimulation in this patient population remains a topic of active investigation. In a heterogeneous but selected series of 130

patients with CHD, sustained ventricular tachycardia was inducible in 25%.[41] In multivariate analyses, inducible ventricular tachycardia was associated with a 6-fold increased risk of mortality and a 3-fold higher risk of serious arrhythmic events. Nevertheless, one-third of patients with documented clinical ventricular tachycardia had negative studies, raising the possibility that prognostic value may vary according to the type of CHD.

In a multicenter, more homogenous cohort of 252 patients exclusively with surgically repaired tetralogy of Fallot, 35% had inducible sustained ventricular tachycardia,[42] a rate similar to patients after myocardial infarction with ejection fractions less than or equal to 40% and nonsustained ventricular tachycardia.[43] In multivariate analyses that adjusted for clinical, electrocardiographic, echocardiographic, and hemodynamic parameters, a positive test was associated with a 5-fold

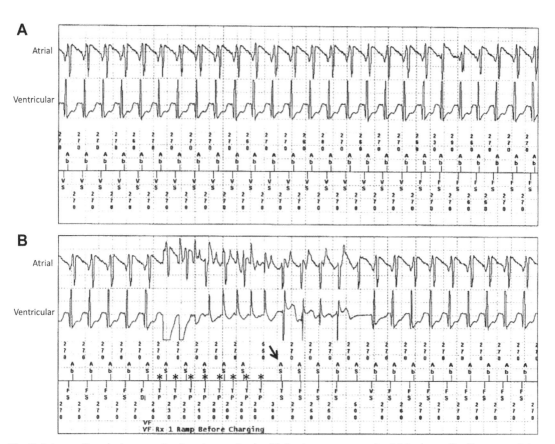

Fig. 3. Intracardiac electrogram tracings in a patient with Fontan surgery and a 1:1 tachycardia. Shown are intracardiac atrial and ventricular electrograms and marker channels in an adult with a univentricular heart and extracardiac Fontan. (*A*) Tachycardia with a 1:1 atrioventricular relationship (cycle length 270 milliseconds; ie, 222 beats/min). (*B*) The asterisks mark 8 beats of antitachycardia pacing (ATP) at decremental coupling intervals from 240 to 200 milliseconds. The ventricle is accelerated during ATP with the atrial rate remaining unchanged. On termination of ATP, an atrial beat (*arrow*) precedes the first ventricular beat. Dissociation of the ventricular rhythm from an unaltered rapid atrial rhythm is consistent with the diagnosis of an atrial tachyarrhythmia.

increased risk of subsequent clinical sustained ventricular tachyarrhythmia or sudden cardiac death.[42] Bayesian analyses suggest that programmed ventricular stimulation is most helpful in risk stratifying patients deemed at moderate risk of sudden death, and that its diagnostic yield is insufficient to justify routine screening in patients with tetralogy of Fallot at large.[44] It seems to be of value when used in conjunction with other markers in risk stratification schemes.[12,15,45] In contrast, limited data suggest that programmed ventricular stimulation is a poor predictor of clinical events in other patient populations, such as those with transposition of the great arteries and Mustard or Senning baffles.[46] Programmed ventricular stimulation may be of greatest interest in patients with CHD with potential scar-based reentrant ventricular tachycardia circuits (eg, ventriculotomy incisions, patches, or sutures).

Pacemakers and ICDs

In addition to providing the deliberate therapies to manage bradyarrhythmias and tachyarrhythmias, pacemakers and ICDs are equipped with a variety of arrhythmia detection algorithms and tools of potential interest for adults with CHD and heart failure.[47] For example, trended data, histograms, and detailed intracardiac electrogram recordings can identify asymptomatic arrhythmias, provide correlations between symptoms and underlying rhythms, quantify arrhythmia burden, assist in determining the need for therapy such as anticoagulants, monitor disease progression, and evaluate treatment efficacy.

Electrograms stored in ICDs may be particularly helpful in distinguishing atrial from ventricular tachyarrhythmias with a 1:1 atrioventricular relationship (eg, ventricular tachycardia with retrograde conduction vs sinus, atrial, or supraventricular reentrant tachycardia), a common scenario in young adults with CHD.[48,49] Discrimination algorithms are particularly useful in patients with CHD with ICDs placed for secondary prevention or on antiarrhythmic drug therapy in whom lower programmed cutoff rates expose them to a higher risk of inappropriate therapy for supraventricular tachycardia.[50] Although no study specific to CHD has addressed this issue, in a randomized trial of secondary-prevention dual-chamber ICDs, active discriminators were associated with a reduction of inappropriate shocks from 46% to 24% at 1 year, with no loss of sensitivity for detecting ventricular tachycardia.[51] With single-chamber discriminators, underdetection occurs in 0% to 0.4% of ventricular tachycardia episodes with stability, 0% to 2% with morphology, and 0.5% to 5% with onset criteria.[52] In addition, ventricular antitachycardia pacing (ATP) can provide valuable diagnostic clues in patients with 1:1 tachycardias by analyzing the atrial response[47,53]:

1. Dissociating the ventricular rhythm from a stable rapid atrial rhythm is consistent with a diagnosis of atrial tachycardia (**Fig. 3**).
2. An atrial cycle length that varies during ATP (ie, retrograde Wenckebach or block) indicates ventricular tachycardia or atrioventricular nodal reentrant tachycardia.

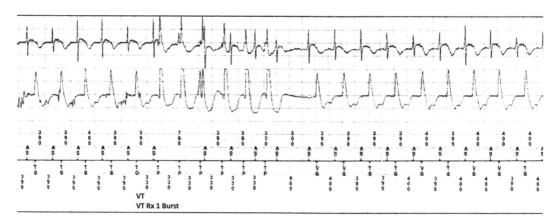

Fig. 4. A VAAV response during ATP in a 1:1 tachycardia. Shown from top to bottom are intracardiac atrial electrograms, ventricular electrograms, and telemetered marker channels. A 1:1 tachycardia is detected in the ventricular tachycardia (VT) zone, with a cycle length of 390 to 400 milliseconds. Antitachycardia ventricular pacing is delivered with a 6-beat drive train at 330 milliseconds. The last 3 beats result in ventricular capture, with the final 2 beats accelerating the atrial rhythm to the paced cycle length. The last paced beat (V) is followed by an AAV response, consistent with an atrial tachyarrhythmia. (*From* Mansour F, Khairy P. Programming ICDs in the modern era beyond out-of-the box settings. Pacing Clinic Electrophysiol 2011;34(4):517; with permission.)

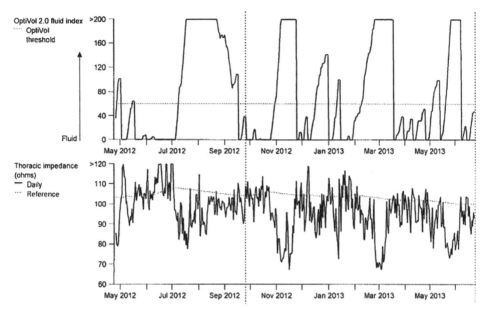

Fig. 5. OptiVol fluid index and thoracic impedance. The upper panel displays the OptiVol fluid index over time, which represents the accumulation of consecutive differences between daily measurements and the reference impedance. When the OptiVol level crosses the programmable threshold, indicated by the dotted line, it is considered a clinical event. The severity of the event is better assessed by reviewing the thoracic raw impedance graph in the lower panel. Decompensated heart failure is ostensibly indicated by an increase in the OptiVol fluid index to more than the programmed threshold along with a reduction in thoracic impedance that tracks below the dotted impedance reference line.

3. If the atrial cycle length accelerates to the ATP cycle length and arrhythmia is not interrupted on termination of ATP (so-called entrainment), the intervals following ATP should be analyzed
   a. VAAV: 2 consecutive atrial events following the last paced ventricular beat suggests atrial tachycardia (**Fig. 4**).[54]
   b. VVA: a ventricular event following the last paced ventricular beat suggests ventricular tachycardia.
   c. VAV: a VAV response is less helpful in distinguishing ventricular from supraventricular tachycardia.

   More specific to patients with heart failure, intrathoracic impedance monitoring (OptiVol, Medtronic Inc, Minneapolis, MN) was developed as a means of detecting transpulmonary fluid accumulation, which indicates pulmonary edema.[55] The objective is to identify subclinical physiologic changes and avert decompensated heart failure by prompting directed therapies. The OptiVol algorithm has been incorporated in Medtronic ICDs since 2007. Daily measurements are compared with the individual's baseline impedance and a continuous dynamic OptiVol fluid index value is computed (**Fig. 5**).[56] The usefulness of this algorithm remains questionable. Although early

studies suggested that such monitoring was associated with a reduction in heart failure–related hospitalizations, sensitivity and positive predictive values seem modest at best.[57,58] In a series of 47 children and patients with CHD, only 3 experienced exacerbations of heart failure.[59] A sensitivity of 33% was reported along with a low positive predictive value (≤4.4%) for heart failure exacerbations and arrhythmias.

REFERENCES

1. Khairy P, Ionescu-Ittu R, Mackie AS, et al. Changing mortality in congenital heart disease. J Am Coll Cardiol 2010;56:1149–57.
2. Escudero C, Khairy P, Sanatani S. Electrophysiologic considerations in congenital heart disease and their relationship to heart failure. Can J Cardiol 2013;29:821–9.
3. Oechslin EN, Harrison DA, Connelly MS, et al. Mode of death in adults with congenital heart disease. Am J Cardiol 2000;86:1111–6.
4. Zomer AC, Vaartjes I, van der Velde ET, et al. Heart failure admissions in adults with congenital heart disease; risk factors and prognosis. Int J Cardiol 2013;168:2487–93.
5. Nattel S, Khairy P, Schram G. Arrhythmogenic ionic remodeling: adaptive responses with maladaptive

consequences. Trends Cardiovasc Med 2001;11: 295–301.

6. Walsh EP, Cecchin F. Arrhythmias in adult patients with congenital heart disease. Circulation 2007; 115:534–45.

7. Abadir S, Khairy P. Electrophysiology and adult congenital heart disease: advances and options. Prog Cardiovasc Dis 2011;53:281–92.

8. Warnes CA, Williams RG, Bashore TM, et al. ACC/ AHA 2008 guidelines for the management of adults with congenital heart disease: executive summary. J Am Coll Cardiol 2008;52:1890–947.

9. Silversides CK, Marelli A, Beauchesne L, et al. Canadian Cardiovascular Society 2009 Consensus Conference on the management of adults with congenital heart disease: executive summary. Can J Cardiol 2010;26:143–50.

10. Khairy P, Marelli AJ. Clinical use of electrocardiography in adults with congenital heart disease. Circulation 2007;116:2734–46.

11. Gatzoulis MA, Balaji S, Webber SA, et al. Risk factors for arrhythmia and sudden cardiac death late after repair of tetralogy of Fallot: a multicentre study. Lancet 2000;356:975–81.

12. Khairy P, Harris L, Landzberg MJ, et al. Implantable cardioverter-defibrillators in tetralogy of Fallot. Circulation 2008;117:363–70.

13. Schwerzmann M, Salehian O, Harris L, et al. Ventricular arrhythmias and sudden death in adults after a Mustard operation for transposition of the great arteries. Eur Heart J 2009;30:1873–9.

14. Khairy P, Aboulhosn J, Gurvitz MZ, et al. Arrhythmia burden in adults with surgically repaired tetralogy of Fallot: a multi-institutional study. Circulation 2010;122:868–75.

15. Khairy P, Dore A, Poirier N, et al. Risk stratification in surgically repaired tetralogy of Fallot. Expert Rev Cardiovasc Ther 2009;7:755–62.

16. Plymen CM, Hughes ML, Picaut N, et al. The relationship of systemic right ventricular function to ECG parameters and NT-proBNP levels in adults with transposition of the great arteries late after Senning or Mustard surgery. Heart 2010;96:1569–73.

17. Westhoff-Bleck M, Norozi K, Schoof S, et al. QRS duration in Fontan circulation in adults: a predictor of aerobic capacity. Int J Cardiol 2009;132:375–81.

18. Robbins J, Nelson JC, Rautaharju PM, et al. The association between the length of the QT interval and mortality in the Cardiovascular Health Study. Am J Med 2003;115:689–94.

19. Vrtovec B, Delgado R, Zewail A, et al. Prolonged QTc interval and high B-type natriuretic peptide levels together predict mortality in patients with advanced heart failure. Circulation 2003;107: 1764–9.

20. Gatzoulis MA, Till JA, Redington AN. Depolarization-repolarization inhomogeneity after repair of tetralogy of Fallot. The substrate for malignant ventricular tachycardia? Circulation 1997;95:401.

21. Berul CI, Hill SL, Geggel RL, et al. Electrocardiographic markers of late sudden death risk in postoperative tetralogy of Fallot children. J Cardiovasc Electrophysiol 1997;8:1349–56.

22. Rodriguez FH, Moodie DS, Neeland M, et al. Identifying arrhythmias in adults with congenital heart disease by 24-h ambulatory electrocardiography. Pediatr Cardiol 2012;33:591–5.

23. Czosek RJ, Anderson J, Khoury PR, et al. Utility of ambulatory monitoring in patients with congenital heart disease. Am J Cardiol 2013;111:723–30.

24. Perloff JK, Middlekauf HR, Child JS, et al. Usefulness of post-ventriculotomy signal averaged electrocardiograms in congenital heart disease. Am J Cardiol 2006;98:1646–51.

25. Russo G, Folino AF, Mazzotti E, et al. Comparison between QRS duration at standard ECG and signal-averaging ECG for arrhythmic risk stratification after surgical repair of tetralogy of Fallot. J Cardiovasc Electrophysiol 2005;16:288–92.

26. Stelling JA, Danford DA, Kugler JD, et al. Late potentials and inducible ventricular tachycardia in surgically repaired congenital heart disease. Circulation 1990;82:1690.

27. Heart rate variability: standards of measurement, physiological interpretation and clinical use. Task Force of the European Society of Cardiology and the North American Society of Pacing and Electrophysiology. Circulation 1996;93:1043–65.

28. Massin M, von Bernuth G. Clinical and haemodynamic correlates of heart rate variability in children with congenital heart disease. Eur J Pediatr 1998; 157:967–71.

29. Aletti F, Ferrario M, de Jesus TB, et al. Heart rate variability in children with cyanotic and acyanotic congenital heart disease: analysis by spectral and non linear indices. Conf Proc IEEE Eng Med Biol Soc 2012;2012:4189–92.

30. Heragu NP, Scott WA. Heart rate variability in healthy children and in those with congenital heart disease both before and after operation. Am J Cardiol 1999;83:1654–7.

31. Ohuchi H, Negishi J, Miyake A, et al. Long-term prognostic value of cardiac autonomic nervous activity in postoperative patients with congenital heart disease. Int J Cardiol 2011;151:296–302.

32. Shah SA, Kambur T, Chan C, et al. Relation of short-term heart rate variability to incident heart failure (from the Multi-Ethnic Study of Atherosclerosis). Am J Cardiol 2013;112(4):533–40 PMID: 23683953.

33. Cutler MJ, Rosenbaum DS. Risk stratification for sudden cardiac death: is there a clinical role for T wave alternans? Heart Rhythm 2009;6: S56–61.

34. Cutler MJ, Rosenbaum DS. Explaining the clinical manifestations of T wave alternans in patients at risk for sudden cardiac death. Heart Rhythm 2009;6:S22–8.

35. Zipes DP, Camm AJ, Borggrefe M, et al. ACC/AHA/ESC 2006 guidelines for management of patients with ventricular arrhythmias and the prevention of sudden cardiac death. Circulation 2006;114: e385–484.

36. Alexander ME, Cecchin F, Huang KP, et al. Microvolt T-wave alternans with exercise in pediatrics and congenital heart disease: limitations and predictive value. Pacing Clin Electrophysiol 2006;29: 733–41.

37. Cieplucha A, Trojnarska O, Bartczak A, et al. Microvolt T wave alternans in adults with congenital heart diseases characterized by right ventricle pathology or single ventricle physiology: a case control study. BMC Cardiovasc Disord 2013;13:26.

38. Sanatani S, Peirone A, Chiu C, et al. Use of an implantable loop recorder in the evaluation of children with congenital heart disease. Am Heart J 2002;143:366–72.

39. Kenny D, Chakrabarti S, Ranasinghe A, et al. Single-centre use of implantable loop recorders in patients with congenital heart disease. Europace 2009;11:303–7.

40. Ermis P, Franklin W, Kim J, et al. Electrophysiology procedures in adults with congenital heart disease. Congenit Heart Dis 2012;7:344–8.

41. Alexander ME, Walsh EP, Saul JP, et al. Value of programmed ventricular stimulation in patients with congenital heart disease. J Cardiovasc Electrophysiol 1999;10:1033–44.

42. Khairy P, Landzberg MJ, Gatzoulis MA, et al. Value of programmed ventricular stimulation after tetralogy of Fallot repair: a multicenter study. Circulation 2004;109:1994–2000.

43. Buxton AE, Hafley GE, Lehmann MH, et al. Prediction of sustained ventricular tachycardia inducible by programmed stimulation in patients with coronary artery disease. Utility of clinical variables. Circulation 1999;99:1843–50.

44. Khairy P. Programmed ventricular stimulation for risk stratification in patients with tetralogy of Fallot: a Bayesian perspective. Nat Clin Pract Cardiovasc Med 2007;4:292–3.

45. Le Gloan L, Guerin P, Mercier LA, et al. Clinical assessment of arrhythmias in tetralogy of Fallot. Expert Rev Cardiovasc Ther 2010;8:189–97.

46. Khairy P, Harris L, Landzberg MJ, et al. Sudden death and defibrillators in transposition of the great arteries with intra-atrial baffles: a multicenter study. Circ Arrhythm Electrophysiol 2008;1:250–7.

47. Mansour F, Khairy P. Programming ICDs in the modern era beyond out-of-the box settings. Pacing Clin Electrophysiol 2011;34:506–20.

48. Wilkoff BL, Ousdigian KT, Sterns LD, et al. A comparison of empiric to physician-tailored programming of implantable cardioverter-defibrillators: results from the prospective randomized multicenter EMPIRIC trial. J Am Coll Cardiol 2006;48:330–9.

49. Arenal A, Ortiz M, Peinado R, et al. Differentiation of ventricular and supraventricular tachycardias based on the analysis of the first postpacing interval after sequential anti-tachycardia pacing in implantable cardioverter-defibrillator patients. Heart Rhythm 2007;4:316–22.

50. Khairy P, Mansour F. Implantable cardioverter-defibrillators in congenital heart disease: 10 programming tips. Heart Rhythm 2011;8:480–3.

51. Dorian P, Philippon F, Thibault B, et al. Randomized controlled study of detection enhancements versus rate-only detection to prevent inappropriate therapy in a dual-chamber implantable cardioverter-defibrillator. Heart Rhythm 2004;1:540–7.

52. Brugada J, Mont L, Figueiredo M, et al. Enhanced detection criteria in implantable defibrillators. J Cardiovasc Electrophysiol 1998;9:261–8.

53. Ridley DP, Gula LJ, Krahn AD, et al. Atrial response to ventricular antitachycardia pacing discriminates mechanism of 1:1 atrioventricular tachycardia. J Cardiovasc Electrophysiol 2005;16:601–5.

54. Issa ZF, Mansour IN. Diagnostic value of ICD anti-tachycardia pacing therapy. J Cardiovasc Electrophysiol 2007;18:548–9.

55. Yu CM, Wang L, Chau E, et al. Intrathoracic impedance monitoring in patients with heart failure: correlation with fluid status and feasibility of early warning preceding hospitalization. Circulation 2005;112:841–8.

56. Wang L. Fundamentals of intrathoracic impedance monitoring in heart failure. Am J Cardiol 2007;99: 3G–10G.

57. van Veldhuisen DJ, Braunschweig F, Conraads V, et al. Intrathoracic impedance monitoring, audible patient alerts, and outcome in patients with heart failure. Circulation 2011;124:1719–26.

58. Conraads VM, Tavazzi L, Santini M, et al. Sensitivity and positive predictive value of implantable intrathoracic impedance monitoring as a predictor of heart failure hospitalizations: the SENSE-HF trial. Eur Heart J 2011;32:2266–73.

59. Lapage MJ, von Alvensleben J, Dick M, et al. Utility of intrathoracic impedance monitoring in pediatric and congenital heart disease. Pacing Clin Electrophysiol 2013;36(8):994–9 PMID: 23594286.

Electrophysiologic Therapeutics in Heart Failure in Adult Congenital Heart Disease

Kara S. Motonaga, MD[a],*, Paul Khairy, MD, PhD[b],
Anne M. Dubin, MD[a]

KEYWORDS

- Arrhythmias • Electrophysiology • Heart failure • Adult congenital heart disease • Therapeutics
- Antiarrhythmics • Device therapy • Resynchronization

KEY POINTS

- Antiarrhythmic therapy is an important component of atrial arrhythmia management in the adult with congenital heart disease.
- Device therapy including conventional pacing, antitachycardia pacing, cardioversion, and defibrillation can be useful for atrial and ventricular arrhythmias in patients with congenital heart disease.
- Ablation of atrial and ventricular arrhythmias can decrease morbidity and mortality in this patient population. Advanced technologies including three-dimensional navigation systems and new energy sources can aid in successful ablation.
- Surgical interventions to improve hemodynamics or to interrupt arrhythmia circuits can be a useful therapeutic option in selected adults with congenital heart disease.

HEART FAILURE AND ARRHYTHMIAS IN ADULT CONGENITAL HEART DISEASE: SCOPE OF THE PROBLEM

With improvement in medical, interventional, and surgical therapies for congenital heart disease (CHD), most patients with CHD are surviving into adulthood such that there are now more adults living with CHD in the United States and Canada than there are patients with CHD younger than 18 years old.[1] Survival of the patient with adult CHD (ACHD) continues to improve with decreasing mortality rates that parallel those of the general population.[2]

Despite these successes, heart failure remains one of the most common causes of morbidity and mortality in ACHD.[3–6] In 2007, heart failure accounted for 20% of all ACHD hospital admissions in the United States.[7] Patients with ACHD with heart failure had a threefold increase in hospital mortality compared to those without heart failure.

Not surprisingly, most patients with ACHD with heart failure die from cardiovascular causes, especially pump failure and arrhythmias.[8] Fifty-two percent of patients with ACHD admitted with heart failure in the United States in 2007 also had arrhythmias.[8] Management of arrhythmias, therefore, is a critical component of caring for the patient with ACHD with heart failure.

These arrhythmias often result from surgical scars, as well as chronic volume and pressure

Financial Support: Dr P. Khairy is supported by a Canada Research Chair in Electrophysiology and Adult Congenital Heart Disease.
Conflict of Interest: Dr P. Khairy has received research funding for investigator-initiated grants from St. Jude Medical, Medtronic, and Boehringer-Ingelheim. Drs A.M. Dubin and K.S. Motonaga have received educational support from Medtronic Inc.
[a] Pediatric Cardiology, Stanford University, 750 Welch Road, Suite 325, Palo Alto, CA 94304, USA; [b] Adult Congenital Heart Center and Electrophysiology Service, Montreal Heart Institute, Université de Montréal, 5000 Belanger St E, Montreal, Quebec H1T 1C8, Canada
* Corresponding author. Stanford University, 750 Welch Road, Suite 325, Palo Alto, CA 94304.
E-mail address: sachie@stanford.edu

heartfailure.theclinics.com

loads, cyanosis, and chamber enlargement. Electrophysiologic therapeutic strategies in this population can include control of arrhythmias and prevention of sudden cardiac death (SCD) as well as preservation of cardiac function.

BRADYARRHYTHMIAS
Sinus Node Dysfunction

Congenital sinus node dysfunction may be seen in patients with CHD, such as those with heterotaxy with left atrial isomerism. These patients may lack a true sinus node altogether, which makes their heart rate dependent on slower atrial or junctional escape rhythms. More commonly, however, sinus node dysfunction is a result of surgical trauma to the sinoatrial node or its artery, which may occur during the atrial switch procedure (Mustard or Senning procedures) for d-transposition of the great arteries (d-TGA) or single-ventricle palliation with a Glenn or Fontan procedure.[9–12] In patients with Mustard procedures for d-TGA, symptomatic sinus node dysfunction is observed in 64% and 82% at 5 and 16 years of follow-up, respectively.[13]

Chronotropic incompetence may be poorly tolerated in patients with ACHD with compromised hemodynamics, especially those with a single ventricle or significant atrioventricular (AV) valve regurgitation. The likelihood of a patient developing intra-atrial reentrant tachycardia (IART) or atrial fibrillation is also increased significantly in this setting, which can result in the induction of secondary ventricular tachycardia and SCD.[9,14]

American College of Cardiology (ACC)/American Heart Association (AHA)/Heart Rhythm Society (HRS) 2012 guidelines recommend permanent pacing for symptomatic age-inappropriate bradycardia (class I, level of evidence B), tachy-brady syndrome with recurrent IART (class IIa, level of evidence C), sinus bradycardia in the setting of complex CHD with resting heart rate less than 40 bpm or pauses in ventricular rate longer than 3 seconds (class IIa, level of evidence C), or CHD and impaired hemodynamics caused by sinus bradycardia or loss of AV synchrony (class IIa, level of evidence C).[15]

AV Node Dysfunction

Patients with AV discordance have a 2% incidence of developing spontaneous AV block on an annual basis.[16] AV nodal conduction defects, however, are more commonly the sequelae of intracardiac repair (1%–3% of congenital heart surgeries), typically involving the ventricular septum.[17–20] In a study of adult patients with heart failure with a single or systemic right ventricle, 72% of symptomatic patients had a history of heart block. Of those who died with heart failure, 76% had second-degree AV block or higher and 62% required a pacemaker.

ACC/AHA/HRS 2012 guidelines recommend permanent pacing for advanced second-degree or third-degree AV block associated with symptomatic bradycardia, ventricular dysfunction, or low cardiac output (class I, level of evidence C), postoperative advanced second-degree or third-degree AV block that is not expected to resolve or that persists at least 7 days after cardiac surgery (class I, level of evidence B), or congenital third-degree AV block with a ventricular rate less than 70 bpm in the setting of CHD (class I, level of evidence C).

When permanent pacing is indicated, challenges include lack of or obstructed venous access, obstructed baffles or conduits, baffle leaks, difficulties in lead positioning, high rates of lead complications, and coexisting intracardiac shunts.[21–23] Single-site ventricular pacing, even from the subpulmonary left ventricle (LV) in this setting, results in an obligatory dyssynchronous ventricular contraction that may be associated with a reduction in ventricular performance over time. Pacemaker implantation has been proposed as a risk factor for mortality after the first heart failure admission in adults with CHD.[8,24]

Patients with CHD and devices face a lifelong prospect of potential device and lead-related complications, often requiring multiple reinterventions.[22] Given the high incidence of lead failure in an aging patient population, lead extraction procedures are increasingly required in adults with CHD.[25] Particular challenges are encountered in this population. In a cohort of 175 adults with attempted laser extraction of 270 leads, those with CHD were younger at implantation, had older leads at extraction, more right-sided implants, a higher proportion of active fixation leads, and had particular anatomic features including intracardiac shunting, leads in subpulmonary LVs, left atrial (LA) appendages, severely dilated and/or dysfunctional subpulmonary right ventricles (RVs), and partially obstructed baffles.[26] Despite these complexities, success rates (91%) and complication rates (6%) were similar to those in patients without CHD, although a longer procedural time was required.[26]

ATRIAL TACHYARRHYTHMIAS
Intra-atrial Reentrant Tachycardia

IART is the most common symptomatic sustained tachyarrhythmia in the ACHD population.[11,27] The terms intra-atrial reentrant tachycardia and incisional tachycardia have become customary labels for this arrhythmia to distinguish it from the typical variety of cavotricuspid isthmus (CTI) atrial flutter that occurs in structurally normal hearts.[28–30] Regions of fibrosis from suture lines or patches function in combination with natural conduction barriers (crista terminalis, valve orifices, and the superior and inferior caval orifices) to channel the wavefront of propagation along a macroreentrant loop.[31–33] Multiple coexisting IART pathways are possible, with varying circuits that are dependent, in part, on the anatomic defect and type of surgical repair.[34–36]

IART typically has a slower atrial rate (150–250 bpm) than typical CTI flutter, which may favor 1:1 conduction that can lead to hemodynamic instability and cardiac arrest in patients with ACHD with heart failure.[37] It is most often seen in older Fontan patients with atriopulmonary connections (up to 50%–60%) or lateral tunnels (20%–30%),[9,38–42] patients with Mustard or Senning atrial baffles for d-TGA (~30%),[10] or patients with tetralogy of Fallot (TOF; up to one-third),[43] but can also occur with repair of simple cardiac defects such as an atrial septal defect.[44,45] Other risk factors for IART include concomitant sinus node dysfunction (tachy-brady syndrome) and older age at time of heart surgery.[9]

Atrial Fibrillation

The prevalence of atrial fibrillation (AF) is increasing in the aging population with CHD and is significantly higher than in the general adult population with an earlier age of onset.[46] In patients with TOF, AF surpasses IART as the most common atrial tachyarrhythmia in patients older than 55 years of age.[47] AF is associated predominantly with markers of left-sided heart disease, lower LV ejection fraction, and LA dilation.[47,48] In addition, patients with ACHD with AF frequently have a previous history of IART.[46]

The specific cause and mechanism of AF in ACHD remain to be elucidated. Extrapolating from literature on AF in adults with structurally normal hearts, AF may be the result of random atrial microreentry.[49] It is likely related to atrial size, atrial myocardial fibrosis from pressure/volume loading or scarring related to surgery, and alterations in tissue refractoriness and/or automaticity.[49]

Hemodynamic instability can occur in the setting of a rapid ventricular response, particularly in patients with heart failure. Management principles are similar to AF encountered in other forms of adult heart disease, beginning with anticoagulation and ventricular rate control, and typically followed by electrical or medical cardioversion.

Acute treatment of IART and AF by electrical means (direct current cardioversion or overdrive pacing) or chemical means (class I or III antiarrhythmics) is effective, but maintenance of sinus rhythm in the long-term is challenging. Therapeutic options for recurrent atrial arrhythmias include (1) antiarrhythmic drugs, (2) catheter ablation, (3) pacemaker implantation for tachy-brady syndrome or to provide automatic atrial antitachycardia pacing (ATP), and (4) surgical intervention with a modified atrial maze or Cox-Maze operation. The choice must be tailored to the hemodynamic and electrophysiologic status of the individual patient.[27,50]

Pharmacologic Therapy for Atrial Arrhythmias

There is only minimal data on the efficacy and safety of antiarrhythmic drugs in the ACHD population, however, experience and extrapolation from adult series adds to information from smaller pediatric CHD series on antiarrhythmic therapy. Medications can be categorized into those that suppress arrhythmia versus those that are given for ventricular rate control. Selecting an appropriate antiarrhythmic therapy is a unique challenge and requires careful consideration of several factors in the ACHD heart failure population because of undesirable side effects (such as concomitant bradyarrhythmia, negative inotropic effects, and proarrhythmia effects that may be enhanced in the setting of heart failure).

Class II and class IV antiarrhythmic agents (AV nodal blocking agents)

β-Blockers and calcium channel blockers are primarily used for rate control as well as suppression of atrial ectopic beats that may act as triggers for atrial tachycardias. Calcium-channel blockers should be used with caution in patients with ACHD with heart failure because of negative inotropic effects. β-Blockers are the drug of choice for rate control in the setting of heart failure.[51] Both β-blockers and calcium channel blockers should be used cautiously in patients with the potential for sinus bradycardia or heart block.

Class I antiarrhythmic agents

Sodium channel blockers, which are often used to suppress atrial tachyarrhythmias, should be considered contraindicated in the patient with ACHD with heart failure because of their proarrhythmic potential and negative inotropic effects.[52] Proarrhythmia effects of flecainide and propafenone were significantly increased in pediatric patients with CHD as well as adult patients with heart failure, resulting in increased mortality.[53–55]

Class III antiarrhythmic agents

In contrast, class III antiarrhythmic agents may be considered in patients with CHD and heart failure.[56–58] Sotalol has been widely used in the management of atrial arrhythmias for several decades, including in patients with CHD.[56–60] The incidence of proarrhythmia side effects, however, has been as high as 10% in one pediatric cohort, including sinus bradycardia, heart block, torsades de pointes, and increased ventricular ectopy.[61] Sotalol should, therefore, be used with caution in the patient with ACHD with heart failure.

Another class III antiarrhythmic agent commonly used for chronic suppression of atrial tachyarrhythmias is amiodarone. Amiodarone is predominantly a potassium channel blocker but also exhibits α-receptor and β-receptor antagonism and results in prolongation of the QT interval. However, torsades de pointes is uncommon.[62] Amiodarone is typically well tolerated in patients with CHD and ventricular dysfunction with little or no negative inotropic effects.[63–65] Nevertheless, its use may be limited by the potential for noncardiac toxicity, which to some extent is dose and duration dependent. Abnormalities in thyroid function may be seen in up to one-third of patients with ACHD.[64] Risk factors for thyroid dysfunction in the patient with CHD include female gender, cyanotic CHD, previous Fontan repair, and an amiodarone dose greater than 200 mg/day.[66] Other adverse effects of amiodarone include hepatic dysfunction, pulmonary toxicity, photosensitivity, optic neuropathy, and neurologic changes.[62]

In general, maintenance of sinus rhythm with pharmacologic management of atrial flutter and AF alone is often problematic.[67–71] Amiodarone has consistently been shown to be more efficacious than other antiarrhythmic drugs with up to 75% to 85% suppression of AF and atrial flutter at 1 year,[67,68,71–74] but there remains a 50% recurrence rate by 3 to 5 years.[73,74]

Catheter Ablation for Atrial Arrhythmias

Catheter ablation is commonly used at many centers for intervention and treatment of atrial flutter and AF, particularly when antiarrhythmic drugs fail or are poorly tolerated. Advances in three-dimensional (3D) mapping techniques and catheter technologies have provided new optimism for arrhythmia management in adults with CHD. With a thorough understanding and appreciation for underlying structural disease, surgical barriers, tenuous physiology, and variations in conduction system anatomy, most arrhythmias can be safely and successfully ablated.[75,76] Particular challenges may be numerous including compromised vascular access because of previous venous cutdowns and/or multiple interventions during childhood. The chamber of interest may be formidably large, as in the atriopulmonary Fontan connections, with difficulties in ensuring optimal catheter contact and transmural lesions. Baffle or conduit obstructions and acute angles may impede access to areas of interest. Punctures across conduits or surgical patches may be required in TGA with intra-atrial baffles, univentricular hearts with total cavopulmonary connections, and surgically repaired atrial septal defects.

Many centers are now using catheter ablation as an early intervention for IART in preference to long-term drug therapy in patients with CHD.[34,77,78] Combining 3D electroanatomic mapping with good anatomic definition and traditional electrophysiologic maneuvers, acute success rates for IART ablation in CHD may exceed 80%.[34,77,78] Onset of new tachyarrhythmias and recurrences remain problematic, particularly among Fontan patients (nearly 40% at 2 years), who tend to have multiple IART circuits and thick and large atria.[77] Although far from perfect, ablation outcomes for IART are likely to improve with continued experience and seem superior to the degree of control obtained with medications alone. Even if IART episodes are not eliminated entirely by ablation, the procedure can reduce symptoms, improve quality of life, and eliminate the need for ongoing drug therapy.[77]

More recently, robotic systems for catheter ablation have been introduced into clinical practice.[79] With magnetic-guided systems, very soft and flexible ablation catheters can be navigated toward otherwise unattainable areas.[79–81] Initial series in patients with CHD have demonstrated the feasibility of ablating complex circuits across baffles and conduits with high (>85%) acute success rates with this technology.[82,83]

Catheter ablation for AF involves electrical isolation of the pulmonary veins from the left atrium. Risks include pulmonary vein stenosis, pericardial tamponade, stroke, and atrial-esophageal fistula formation.[84] Outcomes in ACHD remain to be defined. In a series of 36 patients with primarily simple CHD lesions compared with 355 controls without CHD, single procedural success at 300 days was achieved in 42% of patients with CHD compared with 53% of controls.[85] By 4 years of follow-up, the corresponding success rates were 27% and 36%, respectively. Adverse events were similar (15% vs 11%) except for more frequent vascular complications in patients with CHD (8% vs 1%, $P<.05$). The value of repeat interventions and the role of pulmonary vein isolation in patients with more complex forms of CHD remain to be studied.

Device Therapy for Atrial Arrhythmias

Pacemakers with advanced programming features that incorporate atrial tachycardia detection and automatic burst pacing to interrupt reentry may be beneficial for terminating atrial arrhythmias in select cases, with success rates in the order of 50%.[86–88] Multiple incisions, patches, or conduits reduce the efficacy by limiting entry into the culprit circuit, and finding the ideal pacing site can be technically challenging. A combined approach using radiofrequency ablation and mapping-guided lead implantation may be necessary.[89] Caution must be taken when using this therapy as ATP may also shift the cycle length to faster IART circuits or degenerate into AF.

Surgical Therapy for Atrial Arrhythmias

If the measures already discussed fail, or if the patient requires surgery for hemodynamic reasons, consideration should be given to concomitant surgical interventions for atrial arrhythmias. Techniques include epicardial and endocardial resection and atrial reduction, intraoperative radiofrequency or cryothermal ablation, and/or atrial incisions designed to cause conduction block between 2 anatomic barriers. Arrhythmia surgery has most often been used in patients with failing older-style atriopulmonary Fontan circulations undergoing conversion to the more contemporary extracardiac conduit or lateral tunnel Fontan. In conjunction with the anatomic conversion, a right-sided and/or left-sided maze procedure can be performed with relatively low rates of IART recurrence.[90–99] Although some CHD series have described prophylactic atrial incisions and cryoablation with a goal of prevention of atrial tachycardia,[100–102] the risk-benefit ratio may not always be favorable.[97]

There is considerable debate about whether surgery should be considered as primary therapy for atrial arrhythmias in the absence of underlying hemodynamic lesions such as Fontan obstruction.[22,103] Proponents of a primary surgical approach call attention to the markedly dilated and hypertrophied right atrium with reservations about the transmurality and contiguity of linear catheter ablation lesions, high recurrence rates after ablation, low perioperative mortality (1%), low late mortality (5%) and an 86% freedom from atrial reentrant tachyarrhythmias at 5 years.[91] In patients without other indications for Fontan conversion, supporters of transcatheter ablation for atrial arrhythmias emphasize its less invasive nature, very low associated morbidity and mortality, potential for longer-term arrhythmia-free survival in some, reduction of arrhythmia burden with improved quality of life in most, ease of repeat intervention if required, and the fact that catheter ablation does not preclude later surgical intervention for refractory arrhythmias.[76,77,104]

VENTRICULAR TACHYARRHYTHMIAS

SCD is among the leading causes of death (15%–26%) in patients with ACHD.[6,105,106] Patients with heart failure have the substrate and exposure to triggers for ventricular arrhythmias, such as myocardial scarring and stretching secondary to chronic volume and pressure loads, previous cardiac surgery, and intrinsic myocardial disease.[27,107,108] The progression of heart failure leads to structural and functional remodeling and results in heterogeneous fibrosis, hypertrophy, and ischemia. These cellular changes result in depolarization abnormalities and repolarization dispersion of cardiomyocytes that increase ventricular arrhythmia vulnerability.[109]

Ventricular tachycardia (VT) is well characterized in patients with repaired TOF, with a prevalence ranging from 3% to 14%[43,110–114] and an estimated annual incidence of SCD of 0.15%.[106,111] The mechanism for VT is typically macroreentry, involving narrow conduction corridors defined by regions of surgical scar in conjunction with natural conduction barriers such as the rim of a septal defect or the edge of a valve annulus.[115,116]

Pharmacologic Therapy for Ventricular Arrhythmias

Antiarrhythmic drugs are generally not considered first-line stand-alone therapy for ventricular arrhythmias in patients with CHD and heart failure. Nevertheless, they have an important role in decreasing the recurrence of ventricular arrhythmias and risk of shocks in implantable cardioverter defibrillator (ICD) recipients.

Class II antiarrhythmic agents

The benefits of β-blockers are well established in adults with heart failure in general and include improved functional capacity and overall survival.[117–120] Carvedilol is a nonselective α-adrenergic and β-adrenergic receptor blocker with additional afterload-reducing properties. Large-scale adult clinical studies as well as small retrospective pediatric studies have demonstrated reduction in mortality and hospitalizations with carvedilol in patients with heart failure.[118,121–125] There are no studies specifically evaluating the antiarrhythmic properties of carvedilol in patients with CHD and heart failure. However, in the Carvedilol Post-Infarct Survival Control in Left Ventricular Dysfunction (CAPRICORN) study, carvedilol reduced the incidence of malignant ventricular arrhythmias by 76% in adult patients after myocardial infarction with heart failure, demonstrating its potential antiarrhythmic effects.

Metoprolol is another commonly used β-blocker for heart failure with demonstrated efficacy,[117,126] including a 41% reduction in risk of sudden death.[126] However, the Carvedilol Or Metoprolol European Trial (COMET), in which carvedilol and metoprolol were randomly assigned to patients with heart failure, showed that carvedilol-treated patients experienced a 20% greater reduction in cardiovascular death and a 19% greater reduction in SCD than metoprolol-treated patients.[127,128] Different pharmacologic properties may account for the potential advantage of carvedilol over metoprolol in the treatment of patients with heart failure.

Class III antiarrhythmic agents

Amiodarone has been reported to suppress both PVCs and VT in patients with various forms of heart disease with an overall efficacy of 70%.[129] A meta-analysis of 13 randomized adult trials showed that amiodarone significantly reduced overall mortality by 13% and arrhythmic mortality and SCD by 29% after myocardial infarction or in patients with heart failure.[130]

Catheter Ablation for Ventricular Arrhythmias

Several recent case studies have addressed the role of catheter ablation in the treatment of VT in patients with CHD. These series have included a total of 74 patients with acute success rates ranging from 57% to 100% and recurrence rates as high as 40% (**Table 1**).[131–136] This is not surprising considering the difficulty of adequate lesion creation in a thick-walled chamber such as the RV in patients with TOF. Zeppenfeld and colleagues[135] performed 3D substrate mapping of the RV in patients with TOF and identified 4 anatomically defined isthmuses that were responsible for reentrant tachycardias. The most common isthmus (73%) was located between the superior aspect of the tricuspid valve annulus and scar/patch in the anterior RV outflow tract. Other isthmuses included the area between the pulmonary valve annulus and scar in the anterior RV outflow tract, the septal patch and the pulmonary valve annulus, and the septal patch and tricuspid valve annulus through the region of the ventriculo-infundibular fold.

The major challenges to VT ablation in CHD include difficulty inducing an electrically stable VT during ventricular stimulation, inducing nonclinical or hemodynamically unstable VT, higher-risk locations of substrates near the AV node or

coronary arteries, and anatomic obstacles such as venous obstruction or surgical patches that limit catheter access to the site of interest.[135,137] Given the high recurrence rate, catheter ablation of VT is predominantly used as a means to reduce the shock burden in patients with ICDs.

Cardiac Rhythm Management Device Therapy for Ventricular Arrhythmias

In the current era, the ICD is the mainstay therapy for primary and secondary prevention of SCD in adult patients with heart failure. ICDs are used with increasing frequency in the ACHD population even though most adults with CHD do not meet standard primary prevention indications, and there are no randomized controlled trials that demonstrate improved survival with ICDs in this population.

Even without the evidence of large randomized controlled trials, consensus guidelines (updated in 2012) outline reasonable courses of action.[15,138] Class I indications for ICD implantation in a patient with CHD includes aborted sudden cardiac arrest without a reversible cause (level of evidence B) and sustained VT after hemodynamic and electrophysiologic evaluation (level of evidence C). Class IIa indications include recurrent syncope of undetermined origin in the presence of either ventricular dysfunction or inducible ventricular arrhythmias at electrophysiologic study (level of evidence B).

Information on the outcomes of ICDs in adult patients with CHD is limited (**Table 2**).[37,139–146] In a multicenter study by Yap and colleagues[141] approximately 15 of 64 adult patients (23%) with CHD received a combined total of 46 appropriate shocks during a mean follow-up of 3.7 years. However, 26 of 64 adult patients (41%) with CHD received a combined total of 160 inappropriate shocks during the same period. All inappropriate shocks were caused by supraventricular tachycardia (including sinus tachycardia). There were 20 (31%) device-related reinterventions including 6 (9%) lead failures, which was the most common complication.

High rates of inappropriate shocks have consistently been reported as a result of coexisting supraventricular tachyarrhythmias and lead failures (see **Table 2**).[139,147,148] ICDs should be programmed carefully, bearing in mind the potential psychological burden of inappropriate discharges.[149] Strategies may include programming 2 VT detection zones with activation of ATP, programming higher defibrillation detection thresholds and/or prolonging time to detection, and the use of tailored supraventricular tachycardia discrimination algorithms to prevent unnecessary shocks.[141,149–154]

Table 1
Catheter ablation of ventricular tachycardia in adult patients with CHD

	Gonska et al,[131] 1996	Morwood et al,[132] 2004	Furushima et al,[133] 2006	Kriebel et al,[134] 2007	Zeppenfeld et al,[135] 2007	Tokuda et al,[136] 2012
Number of patients	16	14	7	10	11	16
Mean age (y)	34	21.6	25	29.1	43.7	52
Type of CHD	9 TOF 4 VSD 2 PS 1 d-TGA/ VSD	8 TOF 3 VSD 1 Ebstein anomaly 1 Single ventricle 1 Aortic stenosis	4 TOF 3 DORV	10 TOF	9 TOF 1 AVSD 1 d-TGA/VSD	8 TOF 3 VSD 1 d-TGA 1 DORV 1 PS 2 other
Used 3D mapping	No	Yes for some patients	No	Yes	Yes	Yes
Number of inducible VTs	16	20	14	13	15	—
No. of VTs Ablated per Patient						
1 VT	16 (100%)	9 (64%)	6 (86%)	8 (80%)	8 (73%)	—
2 VTs	—	4 (28%)	1 (14%)	2 (20%)	2 (18%)	—
≥3 VTs	—	1 (7%)	—	—	1 (9%)	—
Mean no. of VTs per patient	1	1.4	1.1	1.2	1.4	2.5
Acute Success per VT Induced						
Intention to treat	14/16 (88%)	10/20 (50%)	7/14 (50%)	11/13 (85%)	15/15 (100%)	—
When VT ablation attempted	14/16 (88%)	10/12 (83%)	4/8 (50%)	11/11 (100%)	15/15 (100%)	—
Acute success per patient when VT ablation attempted	14/16 (88%)	6/10 (60%)	4/7 (57%)	8/10 (80%)	11/11 (100%)	12/16 (75%)
Reason for Failure[a]						
Minimal/no ectopy	—	2 (20%)	—	—	—	—
High-risk location	—	1 (10%)	—	2 (15%)	—	—
Unstable	—	3 (30%)	—	—	—	—
Anatomic issues	—	2 (20%)	—	—	—	—
No reason identified	—	2 (20%)	—	—	—	—
Mean follow-up duration	16 mo	3.8 y	61 mo	35.4 mo	30.4 mo	4.4 y
Patients with recurrence of VT at follow-up[b]	1/14 (7%)	4/10 (40%)	0/4 (0%)	2/8 (25%)	1/11 (9%)	—

Abbreviations: 3D, three-dimensional; AVSD, atrioventricular septal defect; CHD, congenital heart disease; d-TGA, complete transposition of the great arteries; DORV, double outlet right ventricle; PS, pulmonary stenosis; TOF, tetralogy of Fallot; VSD, ventricular septal defect; VT, ventricular tachycardia.

[a] Percentage of failed ablations based on intention to treat.
[b] Recurrence rate in successfully ablated patients.
Data from Refs.[131–136]

Table 2
Outcomes of implantable cardioverter defibrillators in adult patients with CHD

	Alexander et al,[139] 2004	Dore et al,[140] 2004	Yap et al,[141] 2007	Khairy et al,[37] 2008	Khairy et al,[142] 2008	Witte et al,[143] 2008	Khanna et al,[144] 2011	Koyak et al,[145] 2012	Uyeda et al,[146] 2012
Number of patients	32	13	64	37	121	25	73	136	12
Age (y)	Mean 18	Mean 43	Mean 37	Mean 28	Median 33	Mean 24	Mean 41	Mean 41	Median 35
Follow-up duration	Median 1.4 y	Mean 29 mo	Median 3.7 y	Median 3.6 y	Median 3.7 y	Mean 695 d	Mean 2.2 y	Median 4.6 y	Median 2.9 y
Types of CHD	19 TOF 5 d-TGA 4 LVOTO 1 VSD 2 other	7 TOF 1 ccTGA 2 PS 1 VSD 1 other	40 TOF 7 d-TGA 5 DORV 3 VSD 6 other	37 d-TGA	121 TOF	25 TOF	32 TOF 12 ccTGA 7 d-TGA 5 PA/VSD 17 other	69 TOF 27 SD 18 ccTGA 22 other	5 TOF 2 ccTGA 1 d-TGA 4 other
Pre-ICD Events[a]									
Cardiac arrest, N (%)	10 (31)	4 (31)	13 (20)	10 (27)	16 (13)	—	4 (5)	31 (23)	5 (42)
Syncope/palpitations, N (%)	22 (69)	2 (15)	18 (28)	23 (62)	76 (63)	—	8 (11)	12 (9)	4 (33)
Sustained VT, N (%)	4 (13)	6 (46)	26 (41)	4 (11)	37 (31)	—	20 (27)	37 (27)	1 (8)
NSVT, N (%)	—	—	—	11 (30)	25 (21)	—	2 (3)	24 (18)	2 (17)
Indication for ICD									
Primary prevention, N (%)	18 (56)	3 (23)	25 (39)	23 (62)	68 (56)	7 (28)	47 (64)	68 (50)	2 (17)
Secondary prevention, N (%)	14 (44)	10 (77)	39 (61)	14 (38)	53 (44)	18 (72)	26 (36)	68 (50)	10 (83)
Programmed Stimulation Performed									
Number of patients, N (%)	30 (94)	11 (85)	44 (69)	17 (46)	86 (71)	17 (68)	—	85 (63)	11 (92)
Positive V-stimulation, N (%)[b]	23 (77)	8 (73)	38 (86)	9 (53)	62 (72)	—	—	63 (74)	11 (100)
Negative V-stimulation, N (%)[b]	6 (20)	3 (27)	6 (14)	8 (47)	24 (28)	—	—	18 (26)	—

Appropriate Shock									
Number of patients, N (%)	7 (22)	6 (46)	15 (23)	5 (14)	37 (31)	1 (4)	14 (19)	39 (29)	3 (25)
Time to first shock	Median 13 mo	Mean 13.8 mo	Median 2.3 y	—	—	—	Mean 1.9 y	—	Mean 9 mo
Number of shocks per patient	Mean 6	Mean 4	Median 1	Median 4	—	—	—	Mean 4	Median 2
Inappropriate Shock									
Number of patients, N (%)	8 (25)[c]	1 (8)	26 (41)	9 (24)	30 (25)	5 (20)	11 (15)	41 (30)	2 (17)
Time to first shock	Median 16 mo[c]	1 mo	Median 0.6 y	—	—	—	Mean 2.2 y	—	—
Number of shocks per patient	Mean 10[c]	—	Median 4	Mean 10	—	—	—	Mean 5	Mean 1
Cause of Inappropriate Shock[a]									
Lead issues/T-wave oversensing, N	9	1	—	48	6	10	—	38	—
Sinus tachycardia/SVT, N	12	—	26	30	24	—	11	3	2
Complications[d]									
Number of patients, N (%)	40 (53)[c]	—	19 (30)	14 (38)	36 (30)	2 (8)	10 (14)	40 (29)	—
Acute lead issues, N (%)	2 (3)[c]	—	2 (3)	5 (14)	4 (3)	1 (4)	1 (1)	2 (1)	—
Late lead issues, N (%)	16 (21)[c]	—	6 (9)	12 (32)	25 (21)	—	4 (5)	33 (24)	—

Abbreviations: ccTGA, congenitally corrected transposition of the great arteries; CHD, congenital heart disease; d-TGA, complete transposition of the great arteries; DORV, double outlet right ventricle; IART, INTRA-atrial reentrant tachycardia; ICD, implantable cardioverter defibrillator; LVOTO, left ventricular outflow tract obstruction; NSVT, nonsustained ventricular tachycardia; PA/VSD, pulmonary atresia, ventricular septal defect; PS, pulmonary stenosis; SD, septal defects; SVT, supraventricular tachycardia; TOF, tetralogy of Fallot; VSD, ventricular septal defect; VT, ventricular tachycardia.

[a] Nonexclusive events.
[b] Percentages of those who underwent programmed stimulation.
[c] Percentage of entire study population (N = 76), which included patients with CHD and primary electrical disease.
[d] Excluding inappropriate shocks.
Data from Refs.[37,139–146]

There are several technical challenges regarding the use of ICDs in patients with CHD that mandate careful planning before device implantation, including the complexity of the cardiac anatomy, associated extracardiac abnormalities, intracardiac shunting, and underdeveloped or obstructed venous access. Various transvenous, epicardial, intrathoracic, and subcutaneous lead implant techniques have been introduced to address these problems.[155–157] These approaches require some creativity and an understanding of anatomy and defibrillation vectors.[22]

An entirely subcutaneous ICD (S-ICD, Boston Scientific/Cameron Health) was recently approved for use in the United States in 2012 by the US Food and Drug Administration. This ICD system comprises a pulse generator placed in the midaxillary line and a subcutaneous electrode placed in the left parasternal position. This system has the advantage of avoiding transvenous access to the heart, which can be beneficial in patients with CHD with vascular access or intracardiac shunt issues.[79] Studies thus far have demonstrated that the S-ICD is able to reliably discriminate supraventricular tachycardia from VT and that its efficacy and safety seem comparable with standard transvenous ICD systems.[158–165] However, the inappropriate shock rate has been reported to be as high as 13% to 25%, mostly because of T-wave oversensing.[161–163,165] The major disadvantage of the S-ICD is that there is no integrated pacing capability. This would preclude any cardiac pacing for tachy-brady syndrome and ATP for atrial and/or ventricular arrhythmias, which are important therapeutic interventions in the ACHD population that have the potential to reduce shocks. In addition, the risk of erosion may be increased by the much larger pulse generator.[163] The configuration and placement of the shocking coil may also require particular attention in the setting of unusual cardiothoracic anatomies.[166] Long-term outcome data are currently unavailable for ACHD.[161,163,166,167] However, as this technology advances and experience grows, the S-ICD may become an important tool for appropriately selected patients with ACHD.

Surgical Therapy for Ventricular Arrhythmias

Surgical therapy for ventricular arrhythmias have primarily been reported in patients with TOF who require reoperations for pulmonary regurgitation and/or tricuspid regurgitation.[92,168] At the time of surgical pulmonary valve or RV-pulmonary artery conduit replacement, cryolesions can be laid down to create lines of conduction block across the isthmuses known to contribute to VT in this population.[135] Some centers perform preoperative electrophysiology studies in patients with TOF who will be undergoing surgical repair to assess their preoperative risk of ventricular arrhythmias or to map the ventricular arrhythmia for guidance of the surgical ablation; others perform intraoperative arrhythmia mapping.[92,110,168,169] Whether directed or empirical concomitant surgical ablation provides sufficient protection against sudden death remains uncertain. In one series of patients with TOF who underwent concomitant pulmonary valve replacement and cryolesions for ventricular arrhythmia, none of the 9 patients had recurrence of VT postoperatively.[168] However, in 2 other series, VT recurred in 10% to 20% despite surgical ablation.[110,169]

HEMODYNAMIC AUGMENTATION WITH CARDIAC RESYNCHRONIZATION

Cardiac resynchronization therapy (CRT) is an effective treatment for adult patients with LV failure and can result in improved cardiac function, LV reverse remodeling, decreased hospitalizations for heart failure, improved quality of life, and decreased overall mortality.[170–175]

In contrast to the adult CRT literature, there are currently no prospective randomized controlled trials evaluating CRT in patients with ACHD and there are no currently accepted guidelines for implementation of CRT in this population.[175,176] The typical scenario in adult heart failure of LV dysfunction with an LV ejection fraction (EF) of 35% or less and a QRS duration (QRSd) of 150 milliseconds or more with a left bundle branch block morphology is uncommon in patients with CHD. Therefore, the adult selection criteria for CRT cannot be easily translated to patients with ACHD.[177]

Information regarding outcomes of permanent CRT in patients with CHD is limited to case reports and several retrospective single and multicenter studies.[178–198] Dubin and colleagues[197] published the first multicenter retrospective survey in 2005, which included 103 patients (71% had CHD) from 22 international institutions who received CRT. After a median follow-up duration of 4 months, CRT resulted in a significant increase in EF by 13% and a decrease in QRSd by 40 milliseconds. Of the 18 patients listed for heart transplantation, 3 (17%) were removed from the list because of clinical improvement. There were 11 nonresponders (10.7%), defined as those who either had no change or a decrease in their EF. The overall mortality rate in this study was 5% (5 patients), including 3 caused by arrhythmic death.

Janousek and colleagues[198] published the second multicenter retrospective survey in 2009 and included 109 patients (80% had CHD) from 17 European centers who received CRT. This was the first study to identify predictors for responders versus nonresponders to CRT with multivariable analysis. Over a median follow-up duration of 7.5 months, CRT resulted in overall improvement in EF by 11.5%, decrease in QRSd by 30 milliseconds, decrease in the systemic ventricular end-diastolic dimension by a median of 1.1 z-scores, and improvement in New York Heart Association (NYHA) functional class. Four of the 10 patients (40%) originally listed for heart transplantation were removed from list after CRT. The presence of a systemic LV was the strongest multivariable predictor of improvement in cardiac function with CRT. Patients with a systemic LV and previous conventional pacing-induced dyssynchrony also showed major clinical improvement and reverse LV remodeling. There were 15 (18.5%) nonresponders (N = 81), defined as a lack of improvement in EF as well NYHA functional class. There were 7 deaths (6%), including 2 caused by ventricular arrhythmias, and CRT was discontinued in 7 patients for technical reasons or infection (6%).

The current CRT studies in patients with CHD demonstrate that CRT can benefit certain subsets of patients with CHD with a lower nonresponse rate (11%–23%) than the 30% nonresponse rate seen in the adult CRT literature.[170,171,195,197–200] CRT can also be safely used in patients with CHD, with similar complication rates as in the adult population (10%–29%).[195,197,198,201] The single most common major complication in the multicenter study by Dubin and colleagues[197] was coronary sinus lead issues, which were found in 5% to 18% of all transvenous pacemakers. This may be related to anatomic issues found in the CHD population. The overall mortality rate ranged from 5% to 8%, which is comparable with the 5% to 7% mortality rate reported in the adult trials.[170,195–198,200] Indications and outcomes should be carefully studied in a heterogeneous population with CHD, especially considering that recent trials have reported harmful effects of CRT in certain patient groups.[202]

CRT for the Failing LV

Between 45% and 78% of pediatric and patients with CHD in CRT studies have ventricular dyssynchrony and ventricular dysfunction related to conventional RV pacing.[195,197,198] The multicenter study by Janousek and colleagues[198] demonstrated the best response to CRT in patients with a systemic LV and pacing-related dyssynchrony who were upgraded to biventricular (BiV) pacing for CRT. CRT in this patient subgroup resulted in

major clinical improvement, LV reverse remodeling, and a significant decrease in QRSd representing successful correction of electrical dyssynchrony. Similar results were seen in adult patients with RV pacing-induced ventricular dysfunction after upgrading to a BiV CRT system.[203,204]

CRT for the Failing RV

Right ventricular heart failure is an important cause of late morbidity in CHD.[205] Thus, it is not surprising more than 70% of cases of CRT in the pediatric age group has been in the setting of CHD, with 30% to 40% involving the RV.[195,197,198] Several pacing strategies exist for CRT in patients with RV failure. Studies by Janousek and colleagues[206] and Dubin and colleagues[207,208] demonstrated that patients with 2-ventricle anatomy, right bundle branch block, and RV dysfunction (such as TOF) can be acutely, hemodynamically, and functionally improved with atrial synchronous single-site RV pacing for resynchronization. This strategy involves manipulation of the atrioventricular interval to apply the RV stimulus simultaneously with the native ventricular depolarization from the left bundle, thereby resulting in more synchronous electrical activation and maximum shortening of the QRS duration. Single-site RV pacing has the advantage of being technically straightforward for implantation, however, it may be difficult to maintain a stable degree of electrical fusion because of variations in intrinsic AV conduction over a wide range of activities and heart rates. In addition, a significantly prolonged baseline PR interval may prevent fusion between the paced and physiologic activation because of limitations in the maximum programmable AV interval on current pacemaker devices. In such cases, CRT with biventricular pacing may be necessary.

Thambo and colleagues[209,210] evaluated the effects of biventricular CRT in adults with TOF and RV dysfunction. Six months of chronic biventricular CRT demonstrated improvement in exercise tolerance, NYHA functional class, and LV EF as well as improvement in ventricular synchrony.[209] Therefore, although biventricular stimulation may involve a considerably more difficult implantation process, it allows for more consistently homogeneous ventricular activation when resynchronization of the failing RV with isolated RV pacing is not feasible or if concomitant LV dysfunction is present.

Patients with systemic RVs (such as ccTGA and d-TGA with intra-atrial baffles) represent another CHD population at risk for developing RV dysfunction.[211] Results of CRT in this patient population have been mixed. In a study by Janousek and colleagues in 2004,[190] 8 patients with systemic RVs underwent CRT with atrial synchronous simultaneous BiV pacing, which resulted in a decrease in QRSd and interventricular mechanical delay as well as improvement in RV function in all patients. The multicenter study by Dubin and colleagues in 2005[197] also demonstrated improvement in systemic RV EF with a decrease in QRSd and/or clinical improvement in 13 of 17 patients (77%) with systemic RVs. In contrast, Cecchin and colleagues[195] reported a poor response in the 9 patients with systemic RVs included in their 5-year single-center experience. Only 2 of these patients demonstrated a positive long-term response to CRT. The multicenter study by Janousek and colleagues in 2009[198] demonstrated a modest improvement in EF, QRSd, and NYHA classification and clinical improvement in 19 of 27 patients (70%) with systemic RVs. However, this response was significantly less pronounced than the positive response seen in the 62 patients with systemic LVs. The smaller benefit of CRT in the systemic RV population may be attributed to suboptimal myocardial fiber arrangement and abnormal ventricular contraction patterns when compared with both subpulmonary RVs and systemic LVs as well as decreased myocardial perfusion reserve, possibly resulting in chronic subendocardial ischemia.[212–217]

CRT for the Failing Single Ventricle

Because patients with single-ventricle physiology, by definition, do not have 2 separate ventricles, resynchronization must be achieved by multisite pacing of the functional single ventricle. This strategy of multisite pacing was first evaluated in the acute postoperative setting. Three unipolar temporary epicardial pacing leads were placed as far apart from each other on the ventricle as possible (right-sided free wall, left-sided free wall, and midline near the apex) to allow for simultaneous stimulation of both free walls. Zimmerman and colleagues[218] initially evaluated the acute effects of multisite pacing in 14 postoperative patients with single-ventricle physiology whereas Bacha and colleagues[219] later evaluated it in 26 postoperative patients. Both studies demonstrated that multisite ventricular pacing acutely resulted in improvement in systolic blood pressure, cardiac index, indices of dyssynchrony by echocardiography, and QRSd. Although the baseline QRSd was normal, multisite pacing further narrowed the QRSd in both studies.

Three studies of chronic CRT in patients with CHD have included a small number of patients with single-ventricle physiology demonstrating mixed results.[195,197,198] Cecchin and colleagues[195]

demonstrated improvement in NYHA classification by 2 to 3 points and/or increased EF by 10 units or more in 8 of 13 patients (62%) with single-ventricle physiology. The median baseline QRSd was prolonged at 129 milliseconds and decreased with multisite pacing to 116 milliseconds. The abnormal baseline QRSd may have been related to conventional pacing in 8 of 13 patients. The median baseline EF was 37%, which improved to 47% with multisite CRT. There was an overall positive response to CRT in 10 of the 11 patients with long-term follow-up. Two patients died; 1 as a result of progressive heart failure and 1 patient died suddenly and unexpectedly despite improvement both clinically and echocardiographically. Janousek and colleagues[198] also demonstrated improvement in NYHA functional class with multisite CRT in 3 of 4 patients (75%) with single-ventricle physiology included in their retrospective multicenter study. Dubin and colleagues,[197] however, did not find such promising results with clinical improvement in only 2 of 7 patients (29%) with single-ventricle physiology in their multicenter retrospective study, despite a significant decrease in mean QRSd by 45 milliseconds.

Although the small number of patients in these studies are insufficient to draw firm conclusions about the effect of CRT in patients with single-ventricle physiology, inconsistent responses may reflect the complex and heterogeneous structural abnormalities in this population and nonstandardized techniques. A better general understanding of electrical and mechanical interactions in patients with single-ventricle physiology is ultimately required for optimizing lead placement and CRT response depending on the anatomic substrate.

SUMMARY

Despite improvement in survival, heart failure and arrhythmias remain leading causes of morbidity and mortality in patients with ACHD. There are now several options available for the management of arrhythmias and ventricular dysfunction in patients with ACHD and heart failure. Ablation and device therapies continue to improve with advancing technologies. A combination of medical, surgical, and device therapies will likely be required and may be synergistic in decreasing the morbidity and mortality in the ACHD heart failure population.

REFERENCES

1. Marelli AJ, Mackie AS, Ionescu-Ittu R, et al. Congenital heart disease in the general population: changing prevalence and age distribution. Circulation 2007;115:163–72.

2. Khairy P, Ionescu-Ittu R, Mackie AS, et al. Changing mortality in congenital heart disease. J Am Coll Cardiol 2010;56:1149–57.

3. Zomer AC, Vaartjes I, Uiterwaal CS, et al. Circumstances of death in adult congenital heart disease. Int J Cardiol 2012;154:168–72.

4. Zomer AC, Uiterwaal CS, van der Velde ET, et al. Mortality in adult congenital heart disease: are national registries reliable for cause of death? Int J Cardiol 2011;152:212–7.

5. Verheugt CL, Uiterwaal CS, van der Velde ET, et al. Mortality in adult congenital heart disease. Eur Heart J 2010;31:1220–9.

6. Oechslin EN, Harrison DA, Connelly MS, et al. Mode of death in adults with congenital heart disease. Am J Cardiol 2000;86:1111–6.

7. Rodriguez FH 3rd, Moodie DS, Parekh DR, et al. Outcomes of heart failure-related hospitalization in adults with congenital heart disease in the united states. Congenit Heart Dis 2012. http://dx.doi.org/10.1111/chd.12019. [Epub ahead of print].

8. Zomer AC, Vaartjes I, van der Velde ET, et al. Heart failure admissions in adults with congenital heart disease; risk factors and prognosis. Int J Cardiol 2013. http://dx.doi.org/10.1016/j.ijcard.2013.03.003. [Epub ahead of print].

9. Fishberger SB, Wernovsky G, Gentles TL, et al. Factors that influence the development of atrial flutter after the Fontan operation. J Thorac Cardiovasc Surg 1997;113:80–6.

10. Flinn CJ, Wolff GS, Dick M 2nd, et al. Cardiac rhythm after the Mustard operation for complete transposition of the great arteries. N Engl J Med 1984;310:1635–8.

11. Ghai A, Harris L, Harrison DA, et al. Outcomes of late atrial tachyarrhythmias in adults after the Fontan operation. J Am Coll Cardiol 2001;37:585–92.

12. Manning PB, Mayer JE Jr, Wernovsky G, et al. Staged operation to Fontan increases the incidence of sinoatrial node dysfunction. J Thorac Cardiovasc Surg 1996;111:833–9 [discussion: 839–40].

13. Khairy P, Landzberg MJ, Lambert J, et al. Long-term outcomes after the atrial switch for surgical correction of transposition: a meta-analysis comparing the Mustard and Senning procedures. Cardiol Young 2004;14:284–92.

14. Kammeraad JA, van Deurzen CH, Sreeram N, et al. Predictors of sudden cardiac death after Mustard or Senning repair for transposition of the great arteries. J Am Coll Cardiol 2004;44:1095–102.

15. Epstein AE, DiMarco JP, Ellenbogen KA, et al. 2012 ACCF/AHA/HRS focused update incorporated into the ACCF/AHA/HRS 2008 guidelines for device-based therapy of cardiac rhythm abnormalities: a report of the American College of Cardiology Foundation/American Heart Association Task Force on Practice Guidelines and the Heart Rhythm Society. Circulation 2013;127:e283–352.

16. Huhta JC, Maloney JD, Ritter DG, et al. Complete atrioventricular block in patients with atrioventricular discordance. Circulation 1983;67:1374–7.

17. Anderson JB, Czosek RJ, Knilans TK, et al. Postoperative heart block in children with common forms of congenital heart disease: results from the KID database. J Cardiovasc Electrophysiol 2012;23:1349–54.

18. Gross GJ, Chiu CC, Hamilton RM, et al. Natural history of postoperative heart block in congenital heart disease: implications for pacing intervention. Heart Rhythm 2006;3:601–4.

19. Lillehei CW, Sellers RD, Bonnabeau RC, et al. Chronic postsurgical complete heart block. With particular reference to prognosis, management, and a new P-wave pacemaker. J Thorac Cardiovasc Surg 1963;46:436–56.

20. Weindling SN, Saul JP, Gamble WJ, et al. Duration of complete atrioventricular block after congenital heart disease surgery. Am J Cardiol 1998;82:525–7.

21. Bar-Cohen Y, Berul CI, Alexander ME, et al. Age, size, and lead factors alone do not predict venous obstruction in children and young adults with transvenous lead systems. J Cardiovasc Electrophysiol 2006;17:754–9.

22. Khairy P. EP challenges in adult congenital heart disease. Heart Rhythm 2008;5:1464–72.

23. Khairy P, Landzberg MJ, Gatzoulis MA, et al. Transvenous pacing leads and systemic thromboemboli in patients with intracardiac shunts: a multicenter study. Circulation 2006;113:2391–7.

24. Nothroff J, Norozi K, Alpers V, et al. Pacemaker implantation as a risk factor for heart failure in young adults with congenital heart disease. Pacing Clin Electrophysiol 2006;29:386–92.

25. Fortescue EB, Berul CI, Cecchin F, et al. Patient, procedural, and hardware factors associated with pacemaker lead failures in pediatrics and congenital heart disease. Heart Rhythm 2004;1:150–9.

26. Khairy P, Roux JF, Dubuc M, et al. Laser lead extraction in adult congenital heart disease. J Cardiovasc Electrophysiol 2007;18:507–11.

27. Walsh EP, Cecchin F. Arrhythmias in adult patients with congenital heart disease. Circulation 2007;115:534–45.

28. Nakagawa H, Shah N, Matsudaira K, et al. Characterization of reentrant circuit in macroreentrant right atrial tachycardia after surgical repair of congenital heart disease: isolated channels between scars allow "focal" ablation. Circulation 2001;103:699–709.

29. Kalman JM, VanHare GF, Olgin JE, et al. Ablation of 'incisional' reentrant atrial tachycardia complicating surgery for congenital heart disease. Use

of entrainment to define a critical isthmus of conduction. Circulation 1996;93:502–12.

30. Triedman JK, Jenkins KJ, Colan SD, et al. Intraatrial reentrant tachycardia after palliation of congenital heart disease: characterization of multiple macroreentrant circuits using fluoroscopically based three-dimensional endocardial mapping. J Cardiovasc Electrophysiol 1997;8:259–70.

31. Triedman JK, Alexander ME, Berul CI, et al. Electroanatomic mapping of entrained and exit zones in patients with repaired congenital heart disease and intra-atrial reentrant tachycardia. Circulation 2001;103:2060–5.

32. Love BA, Collins KK, Walsh EP, et al. Electroanatomic characterization of conduction barriers in sinus/atrially paced rhythm and association with intra-atrial reentrant tachycardia circuits following congenital heart disease surgery. J Cardiovasc Electrophysiol 2001;12:17–25.

33. Mandapati R, Walsh EP, Triedman JK. Pericaval and periannular intra-atrial reentrant tachycardias in patients with congenital heart disease. J Cardiovasc Electrophysiol 2003;14:119–25.

34. Collins KK, Love BA, Walsh EP, et al. Location of acutely successful radiofrequency catheter ablation of intraatrial reentrant tachycardia in patients with congenital heart disease. Am J Cardiol 2000; 86:969–74.

35. Delacretaz E, Ganz LI, Soejima K, et al. Multi atrial maco-re-entry circuits in adults with repaired congenital heart disease: entrainment mapping combined with three-dimensional electroanatomic mapping. J Am Coll Cardiol 2001;37:1665–76.

36. Akar JG, Kok LC, Haines DE, et al. Coexistence of type I atrial flutter and intra-atrial re-entrant tachycardia in patients with surgically corrected congenital heart disease. J Am Coll Cardiol 2001;38:377–84.

37. Khairy P, Harris L, Landzberg MJ, et al. Sudden death and defibrillators in transposition of the great arteries with intra-atrial baffles: a multicenter study. Circ Arrhythm Electrophysiol 2008;1:250–7.

38. Bartz PJ, Driscoll DJ, Dearani JA, et al. Early and late results of the modified Fontan operation for heterotaxy syndrome 30 years of experience in 142 patients. J Am Coll Cardiol 2006;48:2301–5.

39. Cecchin F, Johnsrude CL, Perry JC, et al. Effect of age and surgical technique on symptomatic arrhythmias after the Fontan procedure. Am J Cardiol 1995;76:386–91.

40. Gelatt M, Hamilton RM, McCrindle BW, et al. Risk factors for atrial tachyarrhythmias after the Fontan operation. J Am Coll Cardiol 1994;24:1735–41.

41. Nurnberg JH, Ovroutski S, Alexi-Meskishvili V, et al. New onset arrhythmias after the extracardiac conduit Fontan operation compared with the intraatrial lateral tunnel procedure: early and midterm

results. Ann Thorac Surg 2004;78:1979–88 [discussion: 1988].

42. Weber HS, Hellenbrand WE, Kleinman CS, et al. Predictors of rhythm disturbances and subsequent morbidity after the Fontan operation. Am J Cardiol 1989;64:762–7.

43. Roos-Hesselink J, Perlroth MG, McGhie J, et al. Atrial arrhythmias in adults after repair of tetralogy of Fallot. Correlations with clinical, exercise, and echocardiographic findings. Circulation 1995;91: 2214–9.

44. Li W, Somerville J. Atrial flutter in grown-up congenital heart (GUCH) patients. Clinical characteristics of affected population. Int J Cardiol 2000;75: 129–37 [discussion: 138–9].

45. Wong T, Davlouros PA, Li W, et al. Mechano-electrical interaction late after Fontan operation: relation between P-wave duration and dispersion, right atrial size, and atrial arrhythmias. Circulation 2004;109:2319–25.

46. Do D. Prevalence of atrial fibrillation in adult congenital heart disease [abstract]. Heart Rhythm 2013;10:S45.

47. Khairy P, Aboulhosn J, Gurvitz MZ, et al. Arrhythmia burden in adults with surgically repaired tetralogy of Fallot: a multi-institutional study. Circulation 2010;122:868–75.

48. Kirsh JA, Walsh EP, Triedman JK. Prevalence of and risk factors for atrial fibrillation and intra-atrial reentrant tachycardia among patients with congenital heart disease. Am J Cardiol 2002;90:338–40.

49. Fuster V, Ryden LE, Cannom DS, et al. 2011 ACCF/AHA/HRS focused updates incorporated into the ACC/AHA/ESC 2006 guidelines for the management of patients with atrial fibrillation: a report of the American College of Cardiology Foundation/American Heart Association Task Force on Practice Guidelines developed in partnership with the European Society of Cardiology and in collaboration with the European Heart Rhythm Association and the Heart Rhythm Society. J Am Coll Cardiol 2011;57:e101–98.

50. Walsh EP. Interventional electrophysiology in patients with congenital heart disease. Circulation 2007;115:3224–34.

51. Yancy CW, Jessup M, Bozkurt B, et al. 2013 ACCF/AHA guideline for the management of heart failure: a report of the American College of Cardiology Foundation/American Heart Association Task Force on Practice Guidelines. Circulation 2013. http://dx.doi.org/10.1161/CIR.0b013e31829e8776. [Epub ahead of print].

52. Pratt CM, Moye LA. The cardiac arrhythmia suppression trial: background, interim results and implications. Am J Cardiol 1990;65:20B–9B.

53. Echt DS, Liebson PR, Mitchell LB, et al. Mortality and morbidity in patients receiving encainide,

flecainide, or placebo. The Cardiac Arrhythmia Suppression Trial. N Engl J Med 1991;324:781–8.

54. Fish FA, Gillette PC, Benson DW Jr. Proarrhythmia, cardiac arrest and death in young patients receiving encainide and flecainide. The Pediatric Electrophysiology Group. J Am Coll Cardiol 1991; 18:356–65.

55. Janousek J, Paul T. Safety of oral propafenone in the treatment of arrhythmias in infants and children (European retrospective multicenter study). Working Group on Pediatric Arrhythmias and Electrophysiology of the Association of European Pediatric Cardiologists. Am J Cardiol 1998;81: 1121–4.

56. Tanel RE, Walsh EP, Lulu JA, et al. Sotalol for refractory arrhythmias in pediatric and young adult patients: initial efficacy and long-term outcome. Am Heart J 1995;130:791–7.

57. Beaufort-Krol GC, Bink-Boelkens MT. Sotalol for atrial tachycardias after surgery for congenital heart disease. Pacing Clin Electrophysiol 1997; 20:2125–9.

58. Beaufort-Krol GC, Bink-Boelkens MT. Effectiveness of sotalol for atrial flutter in children after surgery for congenital heart disease. Am J Cardiol 1997;79: 92–4.

59. Miyazaki A, Ohuchi H, Kurosaki K, et al. Efficacy and safety of sotalol for refractory tachyarrhythmias in congenital heart disease. Circ J 2008;72: 1998–2003.

60. Rao SO, Boramanand NK, Burton DA, et al. Atrial tachycardias in young adults and adolescents with congenital heart disease: conversion using single dose oral sotalol. Int J Cardiol 2009;136: 253–7.

61. Pfammatter JP, Paul T, Lehmann C, et al. Efficacy and proarrhythmia of oral sotalol in pediatric patients. J Am Coll Cardiol 1995;26:1002–7.

62. Zimetbaum P. Amiodarone for atrial fibrillation. N Engl J Med 2007;356:935–41.

63. Coumel P, Fidelle J. Amiodarone in the treatment of cardiac arrhythmias in children: one hundred thirty-five cases. Am Heart J 1980;100:1063–9.

64. Villain E. Amiodarone as treatment for atrial tachycardias after surgery. Pacing Clin Electrophysiol 1997;20:2130–2.

65. Singh SN, Fletcher RD, Fisher SG, et al. Amiodarone in patients with congestive heart failure and asymptomatic ventricular arrhythmia. Survival trial of antiarrhythmic therapy in congestive heart failure. N Engl J Med 1995;333:77–82.

66. Thorne SA, Barnes I, Cullinan P, et al. Amiodarone-associated thyroid dysfunction: risk factors in adults with congenital heart disease. Circulation 1999;100:149–54.

67. Roy D, Talajic M, Dorian P, et al. Amiodarone to prevent recurrence of atrial fibrillation. Canadian Trial

of Atrial Fibrillation Investigators. N Engl J Med 2000;342:913–20.

68. Singh BN, Singh SN, Reda DJ, et al. Amiodarone versus sotalol for atrial fibrillation. N Engl J Med 2005;352:1861–72.

69. Perry JC, Garson A Jr. Flecainide acetate for treatment of tachyarrhythmias in children: review of world literature on efficacy, safety, and dosing. Am Heart J 1992;124:1614–21.

70. Zarembski DG, Nolan PE Jr, Slack MK, et al. Treatment of resistant atrial fibrillation. A meta-analysis comparing amiodarone and flecainide. Arch Intern Med 1995;155:1885–91.

71. Naccarelli GV, Wolbrette DL, Khan M, et al. Old and new antiarrhythmic drugs for converting and maintaining sinus rhythm in atrial fibrillation: comparative efficacy and results of trials. Am J Cardiol 2003;91:15D–26D.

72. Kochiadakis GE, Marketou ME, Igoumenidis NE, et al. Amiodarone, sotalol, or propafenone in atrial fibrillation: which is preferred to maintain normal sinus rhythm? Pacing Clin Electrophysiol 2000;23: 1883–7.

73. Chun SH, Sager PT, Stevenson WG, et al. Long-term efficacy of amiodarone for the maintenance of normal sinus rhythm in patients with refractory atrial fibrillation or flutter. Am J Cardiol 1995;76:47–50.

74. Gosselink A, Crijns HM, Van Gelder IC, et al. Low-dose amiodarone for maintenance of sinus rhythm after cardioversion of atrial fibrillation or flutter. JAMA 1992;267:3289–93.

75. Khairy P, Balaji S. Cardiac arrhythmias in congenital heart diseases. Indian Pacing Electrophysiol J 2009;9:299–317.

76. Triedman JK, DeLucca JM, Alexander ME, et al. Prospective trial of electroanatomically guided, irrigated catheter ablation of atrial tachycardia in patients with congenital heart disease. Heart Rhythm 2005;2:700–5.

77. Triedman JK, Alexander ME, Love BA, et al. Influence of patient factors and ablative technologies on outcomes of radiofrequency ablation of intra-atrial re-entrant tachycardia in patients with congenital heart disease. J Am Coll Cardiol 2002; 39:1827–35.

78. Triedman JK, Bergau DM, Saul JP, et al. Efficacy of radiofrequency ablation for control of intra-atrial reentrant tachycardia in patients with congenital heart disease. J Am Coll Cardiol 1997;30:1032–8.

79. Mondesert B, Abadir S, Khairy P. Arrhythmias in adult congenital heart disease: the year in review. Curr Opin Cardiol 2013;28:354–9.

80. Ernst S. Robotic approach to catheter ablation. Curr Opin Cardiol 2008;23:28–31.

81. Wu J, Pflaumer A, Deisenhofer I, et al. Mapping of intraatrial reentrant tachycardias by remote

magnetic navigation in patients with d-transposition of the great arteries after Mustard or Senning procedure. J Cardiovasc Electrophysiol 2008;19: 1153–9.

82. Wu J, Pflaumer A, Deisenhofer I, et al. Mapping of atrial tachycardia by remote magnetic navigation in postoperative patients with congenital heart disease. J Cardiovasc Electrophysiol 2010;21:751–9.

83. Ernst S, Babu-Narayan SV, Keegan J, et al. Remote-controlled magnetic navigation and ablation with 3D image integration as an alternative approach in patients with intra-atrial baffle anatomy. Circ Arrhythm Electrophysiol 2012;5:131–9.

84. Calkins H, Kuck KH, Cappato R, et al. 2012 HRS/EHRA/ECAS expert consensus statement on catheter and surgical ablation of atrial fibrillation: recommendations for patient selection, procedural techniques, patient management and follow-up, definitions, endpoints, and research trial design. Europace 2012;14:528–606.

85. Philip F, Muhammad KI, Agarwal S, et al. Pulmonary vein isolation for the treatment of drug-refractory atrial fibrillation in adults with congenital heart disease. Congenit Heart Dis 2012;7:392–9.

86. Rhodes LA, Walsh EP, Gamble WJ, et al. Benefits and potential risks of atrial antitachycardia pacing after repair of congenital heart disease. Pacing Clin Electrophysiol 1995;18:1005–16.

87. Ragonese P, Drago F, Guccione P, et al. Permanent overdrive atrial pacing in the chronic management of recurrent postoperative atrial reentrant tachycardia in patients with complex congenital heart disease. Pacing Clin Electrophysiol 1997;20: 2917–23.

88. Stephenson EA, Casavant D, Tuzi J, et al. Efficacy of atrial antitachycardia pacing using the Medtronic AT500 pacemaker in patients with congenital heart disease. Am J Cardiol 2003;92:871–6.

89. El Yaman MM, Asirvatham SJ, Kapa S, et al. Methods to access the surgically excluded cavotricuspid isthmus for complete ablation of typical atrial flutter in patients with congenital heart defects. Heart Rhythm 2009;6:949–56.

90. Mavroudis C, Backer CL, Deal BJ, et al. Total cavopulmonary conversion and maze procedure for patients with failure of the Fontan operation. J Thorac Cardiovasc Surg 2001;122:863–71.

91. Backer CL, Tsao S, Deal BJ, et al. Maze procedure in single ventricle patients. Semin Thorac Cardiovasc Surg Pediatr Card Surg Annu 2008;11:44–8.

92. Deal BJ, Mavroudis C, Backer CL. Beyond Fontan conversion: surgical therapy of arrhythmias including patients with associated complex congenital heart disease. Ann Thorac Surg 2003; 76:542–53 [discussion: 553–4].

93. Deal BJ, Mavroudis C, Backer CL, et al. Impact of arrhythmia circuit cryoablation during Fontan conversion for refractory atrial tachycardia. Am J Cardiol 1999;83:563–8.

94. Mavroudis C, Backer CL, Deal BJ, et al. Fontan conversion to cavopulmonary connection and arrhythmia circuit cryoblation. J Thorac Cardiovasc Surg 1998;115:547–56.

95. Mavroudis C, Deal BJ, Backer CL. The beneficial effects of total cavopulmonary conversion and arrhythmia surgery for the failed Fontan. Semin Thorac Cardiovasc Surg Pediatr Card Surg Annu 2002;5:12–24.

96. Mavroudis C, Deal BJ, Backer CL. Arrhythmia surgery in association with complex congenital heart repairs excluding patients with Fontan conversion. Semin Thorac Cardiovasc Surg Pediatr Card Surg Annu 2003;6:33–50.

97. Mavroudis C, Deal BJ, Backer CL. Surgery for arrhythmias in children. Int J Cardiol 2004; 97(Suppl 1):39–51.

98. Mavroudis C, Deal BJ, Backer CL, et al. 111 Fontan conversions with arrhythmia surgery: surgical lessons and outcomes. Ann Thorac Surg 2007;84: 1457–66.

99. Mavroudis C, Deal BJ, Backer CL, et al. Arrhythmia surgery in patients with and without congenital heart disease. Ann Thorac Surg 2008;86:857–68.

100. Collins KK, Rhee EK, Delucca JM, et al. Modification to the Fontan procedure for the prophylaxis of intra-atrial reentrant tachycardia: short-term results of a prospective randomized blinded trial. J Thorac Cardiovasc Surg 2004;127:721–9.

101. Sheikh AM, Tang AT, Roman K, et al. The failing Fontan circulation: successful conversion of atriopulmonary connections. J Thorac Cardiovasc Surg 2004;128:60–6.

102. Weinstein S, Cua C, Chan D, et al. Outcome of symptomatic patients undergoing extracardiac Fontan conversion and cryoablation. J Thorac Cardiovasc Surg 2003;126:529–36.

103. Therrien J, Dore A, Gersony W, et al. CCS consensus conference 2001 update: recommendations for the management of adults with congenital heart disease. Part I. Can J Cardiol 2001;17: 940–59.

104. Khairy P, Poirier N, Mercier LA. Univentricular heart. Circulation 2007;115:800–12.

105. Nieminen HP, Jokinen EV, Sairanen HI. Causes of late deaths after pediatric cardiac surgery: a population-based study. J Am Coll Cardiol 2007; 50:1263–71.

106. Silka MJ, Hardy BG, Menashe VD, et al. A population-based prospective evaluation of risk of sudden cardiac death after operation for common congenital heart defects. J Am Coll Cardiol 1998;32:245–51.

107. Sullivan ID, Presbitero P, Gooch VM, et al. Is ventricular arrhythmia in repaired tetralogy of Fallot

an effect of operation or a consequence of the course of the disease? A prospective study. Br Heart J 1987;58:40–4.

108. Deanfield JE, Ho SY, Anderson RH, et al. Late sudden death after repair of tetralogy of Fallot: a clinicopathologic study. Circulation 1983;67:626–31.

109. Shiga T, Kasanuki H. Drug therapy for ventricular tachyarrhythmia in heart failure. Circ J 2007; 71(Suppl A):A90–6.

110. Harrison DA, Harris L, Siu SC, et al. Sustained ventricular tachycardia in adult patients late after repair of tetralogy of Fallot. J Am Coll Cardiol 1997;30:1368–73.

111. Murphy JG, Gersh BJ, Mair DD, et al. Long-term outcome in patients undergoing surgical repair of tetralogy of Fallot. N Engl J Med 1993;329:593–9.

112. Gatzoulis MA, Till JA, Somerville J, et al. Mechanoelectrical interaction in tetralogy of Fallot. QRS prolongation relates to right ventricular size and predicts malignant ventricular arrhythmias and sudden death. Circulation 1995;92:231–7.

113. Gatzoulis MA, Balaji S, Webber SA, et al. Risk factors for arrhythmia and sudden cardiac death late after repair of tetralogy of Fallot: a multicentre study. Lancet 2000;356:975–81.

114. Berul CI, Hill SL, Geggel RL, et al. Electrocardiographic markers of late sudden death risk in postoperative tetralogy of Fallot children. J Cardiovasc Electrophysiol 1997;8:1349–56.

115. Horowitz LN, Vetter VL, Harken AH, et al. Electrophysiologic characteristics of sustained ventricular tachycardia occurring after repair of tetralogy of Fallot. Am J Cardiol 1980;46:446–52.

116. Downar E, Harris L, Kimber S, et al. Ventricular tachycardia after surgical repair of tetralogy of Fallot: results of intraoperative mapping studies. J Am Coll Cardiol 1992;20:648–55.

117. Hjalmarson A, Goldstein S, Fagerberg B, et al. Effects of controlled-release metoprolol on total mortality, hospitalizations, and well-being in patients with heart failure: the Metoprolol CR/XL Randomized Intervention Trial in congestive heart failure (MERIT-HF). MERIT-HF Study Group. JAMA 2000; 283:1295–302.

118. Packer M, Coats AJ, Fowler MB, et al. Effect of carvedilol on survival in severe chronic heart failure. N Engl J Med 2001;344:1651–8.

119. Connolly SJ. Meta-analysis of antiarrhythmic drug trials. Am J Cardiol 1999;84:90R–3R.

120. Teo KK, Yusuf S, Furberg CD. Effects of prophylactic antiarrhythmic drug therapy in acute myocardial infarction. An overview of results from randomized controlled trials. JAMA 1993;270:1589–95.

121. Rusconi P, Gomez-Marin O, Rossique-Gonzalez M, et al. Carvedilol in children with cardiomyopathy: 3-year experience at a single institution. J Heart Lung Transplant 2004;23:832–8.

122. Azeka E, Franchini Ramires JA, Valler C, et al. Delisting of infants and children from the heart transplantation waiting list after carvedilol treatment. J Am Coll Cardiol 2002;40:2034–8.

123. Bruns LA, Chrisant MK, Lamour JM, et al. Carvedilol as therapy in pediatric heart failure: an initial multicenter experience. J Pediatr 2001; 138:505–11.

124. Packer M, Bristow MR, Cohn JN, et al. The effect of carvedilol on morbidity and mortality in patients with chronic heart failure. U.S. Carvedilol Heart Failure Study Group. N Engl J Med 1996;334: 1349–55.

125. Packer M, Fowler MB, Roecker EB, et al. Effect of carvedilol on the morbidity of patients with severe chronic heart failure: results of the Carvedilol Prospective Randomized Cumulative Survival (COPERNICUS) study. Circulation 2002;106: 2194–9.

126. Hjalmarson A, Fagerberg B. MERIT-HF mortality and morbidity data. Basic Res Cardiol 2000; 95(Suppl 1):I98–103.

127. Poole-Wilson PA, Swedberg K, Cleland JG, et al. Comparison of carvedilol and metoprolol on clinical outcomes in patients with chronic heart failure in the Carvedilol or Metoprolol European Trial (COMET): randomised controlled trial. Lancet 2003;362:7–13.

128. Torp-Pedersen C, Poole-Wilson PA, Swedberg K, et al. Effects of metoprolol and carvedilol on cause-specific mortality and morbidity in patients with chronic heart failure–COMET. Am Heart J 2005;149:370–6.

129. Connolly SJ. Evidence-based analysis of amiodarone efficacy and safety. Circulation 1999;100: 2025–34.

130. Effect of prophylactic amiodarone on mortality after acute myocardial infarction and in congestive heart failure: meta-analysis of individual data from 6500 patients in randomised trials. Amiodarone Trials Meta-Analysis Investigators. Lancet 1997;350: 1417–24.

131. Gonska BD, Cao K, Raab J, et al. Radiofrequency catheter ablation of right ventricular tachycardia late after repair of congenital heart defects. Circulation 1996;94:1902–8.

132. Morwood JG, Triedman JK, Berul CI, et al. Radiofrequency catheter ablation of ventricular tachycardia in children and young adults with congenital heart disease. Heart Rhythm 2004;1: 301–8.

133. Furushima H, Chinushi M, Sugiura H, et al. Ventricular tachycardia late after repair of congenital heart disease: efficacy of combination therapy with radiofrequency catheter ablation and class III antiarrhythmic agents and long-term outcome. J Electrocardiol 2006;39:219–24.

134. Kriebel T, Saul JP, Schneider H, et al. Noncontact mapping and radiofrequency catheter ablation of fast and hemodynamically unstable ventricular tachycardia after surgical repair of tetralogy of Fallot. J Am Coll Cardiol 2007;50:2162–8.

135. Zeppenfeld K, Schalij MJ, Bartelings MM, et al. Catheter ablation of ventricular tachycardia after repair of congenital heart disease: electroanatomic identification of the critical right ventricular isthmus. Circulation 2007;116:2241–52.

136. Tokuda M, Tedrow UB, Kojodjojo P, et al. Catheter ablation of ventricular tachycardia in nonischemic heart disease. Circ Arrhythm Electrophysiol 2012; 5:992–1000.

137. Khairy P, Stevenson WG. Catheter ablation in tetralogy of Fallot. Heart Rhythm 2009;6:1069–74.

138. Epstein AE, DiMarco JP, Ellenbogen KA, et al. ACC/AHA/HRS 2008 guidelines for device-based therapy of cardiac rhythm abnormalities: a report of the American College of Cardiology/American Heart Association Task Force on Practice Guidelines (writing committee to revise the ACC/AHA/NASPE 2002 guideline update for implantation of cardiac pacemakers and antiarrhythmia devices): developed in collaboration with the American Association for Thoracic Surgery and Society of Thoracic Surgeons. Circulation 2008; 117:e350–408.

139. Alexander ME, Cecchin F, Walsh EP, et al. Implications of implantable cardioverter defibrillator therapy in congenital heart disease and pediatrics. J Cardiovasc Electrophysiol 2004;15:72–6.

140. Dore A, Santagata P, Dubuc M, et al. Implantable cardioverter defibrillators in adults with congenital heart disease: a single center experience. Pacing Clin Electrophysiol 2004;27:47–51.

141. Yap SC, Roos-Hesselink JW, Hoendermis ES, et al. Outcome of implantable cardioverter defibrillators in adults with congenital heart disease: a multicentre study. Eur Heart J 2007;28:1854–61.

142. Khairy P, Harris L, Landzberg MJ, et al. Implantable cardioverter-defibrillators in tetralogy of Fallot. Circulation 2008;117:363–70.

143. Witte KK, Pepper CB, Cowan JC, et al. Implantable cardioverter-defibrillator therapy in adult patients with tetralogy of Fallot. Europace 2008;10:926–30.

144. Khanna AD, Warnes CA, Phillips SD, et al. Single-center experience with implantable cardioverter–defibrillators in adults with complex congenital heart disease. Am J Cardiol 2011;108:729–34.

145. Koyak Z, de Groot JR, Van Gelder IC, et al. Implantable cardioverter defibrillator therapy in adults with congenital heart disease: who is at risk of shocks? Circ Arrhythm Electrophysiol 2012;5:101–10.

146. Uyeda T, Inoue K, Sato J, et al. Outcome of implantable cardioverter defibrillator therapy for congenital heart disease. Pediatr Int 2012;54: 379–82.

147. Korte T, Koditz H, Niehaus M, et al. High incidence of appropriate and inappropriate ICD therapies in children and adolescents with implantable cardioverter defibrillator. Pacing Clin Electrophysiol 2004;27:924–32.

148. Berul CI, Van Hare GF, Kertesz NJ, et al. Results of a multicenter retrospective implantable cardioverter-defibrillator registry of pediatric and congenital heart disease patients. J Am Coll Cardiol 2008;51: 1685–91.

149. Khairy P, Mansour F. Implantable cardioverter-defibrillators in congenital heart disease: 10 programming tips. Heart Rhythm 2011;8:480–3.

150. Lee CH, Nam GB, Park HG, et al. Effects of antiarrhythmic drugs on inappropriate shocks in patients with implantable cardioverter defibrillators. Circ J 2008;72:102–5.

151. Connolly SJ, Dorian P, Roberts RS, et al. Comparison of beta-blockers, amiodarone plus beta-blockers, or sotalol for prevention of shocks from implantable cardioverter defibrillators: the OPTIC study: a randomized trial. JAMA 2006;295:165–71.

152. Ferreira-Gonzalez I, Dos-Subira L, Guyatt GH. Adjunctive antiarrhythmic drug therapy in patients with implantable cardioverter defibrillators: a systematic review. Eur Heart J 2007;28:469–77.

153. Wathen MS, DeGroot PJ, Sweeney MO, et al. Prospective randomized multicenter trial of empirical antitachycardia pacing versus shocks for spontaneous rapid ventricular tachycardia in patients with implantable cardioverter-defibrillators: pacing fast ventricular tachycardia reduces shock therapies (PainFREE Rx II) trial results. Circulation 2004;110:2591–6.

154. Wathen M. Implantable cardioverter defibrillator shock reduction using new antitachycardia pacing therapies. Am Heart J 2007;153:44–52.

155. Stephenson EA, Batra AS, Knilans TK, et al. A multicenter experience with novel implantable cardioverter defibrillator configurations in the pediatric and congenital heart disease population. J Cardiovasc Electrophysiol 2006;17:41–6.

156. Kaltman JR, Gaynor JW, Rhodes LA, et al. Subcutaneous array with active can implantable cardioverter defibrillator configuration: a follow-up study. Congenit Heart Dis 2007;2:125–9.

157. Tomaske M, Pretre R, Rahn M, et al. Epicardial and pleural lead ICD systems in children and adolescents maintain functionality over 5 years. Europace 2008;10:1152–6.

158. Bardy GH, Smith WM, Hood MA, et al. An entirely subcutaneous implantable cardioverter-defibrillator. N Engl J Med 2010;363:36–44.

159. Dabiri Abkenari L, Theuns DA, Valk SD, et al. Clinical experience with a novel subcutaneous

implantable defibrillator system in a single center. Clin Res Cardiol 2011;100:737–44.

160. Gold MR, Theuns DA, Knight BP, et al. Head-to-head comparison of arrhythmia discrimination performance of subcutaneous and transvenous ICD arrhythmia detection algorithms: the START study. J Cardiovasc Electrophysiol 2012;23:359–66.

161. Kobe J, Reinke F, Meyer C, et al. Implantation and follow-up of totally subcutaneous versus conventional implantable cardioverter-defibrillators: a multicenter case-control study. Heart Rhythm 2013;10:29–36.

162. Olde Nordkamp LR, Dabiri Abkenari L, Boersma LV, et al. The entirely subcutaneous implantable cardioverter-defibrillator: initial clinical experience in a large Dutch cohort. J Am Coll Cardiol 2012;60:1933–9.

163. Jarman JW, Lascelles K, Wong T, et al. Clinical experience of entirely subcutaneous implantable cardioverter-defibrillators in children and adults: cause for caution. Eur Heart J 2012;33:1351–9.

164. Aydin A, Hartel F, Schluter M, et al. Shock efficacy of subcutaneous implantable cardioverter-defibrillator for prevention of sudden cardiac death: initial multicenter experience. Circ Arrhythm Electrophysiol 2012;5:913–9.

165. Weiss R, Knight BP, Gold MR, et al. Safety and efficacy of a totally subcutaneous implantable-cardioverter defibrillator. Circulation 2013;128:944–53.

166. Peters B, Will A, Berger F, et al. Implantation of a fully subcutaneous ICD in a patient with single ventricle morphology and Eisenmenger physiology. Acta Cardiol 2012;67:473–5.

167. Calvo N, Arguedas H, Lopez G, et al. Totally subcutaneous ICD implantation as an alternative to the conventional ICD in a patient with a congenital cardiopathy. Rev Esp Cardiol 2013;66:827–9.

168. Therrien J, Siu SC, Harris L, et al. Impact of pulmonary valve replacement on arrhythmia propensity late after repair of tetralogy of Fallot. Circulation 2001;103:2489–94.

169. Karamlou T, Silber I, Lao R, et al. Outcomes after late reoperation in patients with repaired tetralogy of Fallot: the impact of arrhythmia and arrhythmia surgery. Ann Thorac Surg 2006;81:1786–93 [discussion: 1793].

170. Abraham WT, Fisher WG, Smith AL, et al, Miracle Study Group. Multicenter InSync Randomized Clinical Evaluation. Cardiac resynchronization in chronic heart failure. N Engl J Med 2002;346:1845–53.

171. Cazeau S, Leclercq C, Lavergne T, et al. Effects of multisite biventricular pacing in patients with heart failure and intraventricular conduction delay. N Engl J Med 2001;344:873–80.

172. Higgins SL, Hummel JD, Niazi IK, et al. Cardiac resynchronization therapy for the treatment of heart failure in patients with intraventricular conduction delay and malignant ventricular tachyarrhythmias. J Am Coll Cardiol 2003;42:1454–9.

173. Bristow MR, Saxon LA, Boehmer J, et al. Cardiac-resynchronization therapy with or without an implantable defibrillator in advanced chronic heart failure. N Engl J Med 2004;350:2140–50.

174. Cleland JG, Daubert JC, Erdmann E, et al. The effect of cardiac resynchronization on morbidity and mortality in heart failure. N Engl J Med 2005;352:1539–49.

175. Linde C, Ellenbogen K, McAlister FA. Cardiac resynchronization therapy (CRT): clinical trials, guidelines, and target populations. Heart Rhythm 2012;9:S3–13.

176. Stahlberg M, Lund LH, Zabarovskaja S, et al. Cardiac resynchronization therapy: a breakthrough in heart failure management. J Intern Med 2012;272:330–43.

177. Alexander ME, Berul CI, Fortescue EB, et al. Who is eligible for cardiac resynchronization therapy in pediatric cardiology? [abstract]. Heart Rhythm 2004;1:S122–3.

178. Rodriguez-Cruz E, Karpawich PP, Lieberman RA, et al. Biventricular pacing as alternative therapy for dilated cardiomyopathy associated with congenital heart disease. Pacing Clin Electrophysiol 2001;24:235–7.

179. Roofthooft MT, Blom NA, Rijlaarsdam ME, et al. Resynchronization therapy after congenital heart surgery to improve left ventricular function. Pacing Clin Electrophysiol 2003;26:2042–4.

180. Blom NA, Bax JJ, Ottenkamp J, et al. Transvenous biventricular pacing in a child after congenital heart surgery as an alternative therapy for congestive heart failure. J Cardiovasc Electrophysiol 2003;14:1110–2.

181. Senzaki H, Kyo S, Matsumoto K, et al. Cardiac resynchronization therapy in a patient with single ventricle and intracardiac conduction delay. J Thorac Cardiovasc Surg 2004;127:287–8.

182. Janousek J, Tomek V, Chaloupecky V, et al. Dilated cardiomyopathy associated with dual-chamber pacing in infants: improvement through either left ventricular cardiac resynchronization or programming the pacemaker off allowing intrinsic normal conduction. J Cardiovasc Electrophysiol 2004;15:470–4.

183. Cowburn PJ, Parker JD, Cameron DA, et al. Cardiac resynchronization therapy: retiming the failing right ventricle. J Cardiovasc Electrophysiol 2005;16:439–43.

184. Kakavand B, Douglas WI, Manfredi JA, et al. Successful management of acute failure of the

systemic right ventricle with cardiac resynchronization therapy. Pediatr Cardiol 2006;27:612–3.

185. van Beek E, Backx A, Singh S. Cardiac resynchronization as therapy for congestive cardiac failure in children dependent on chronic cardiac pacing. Cardiol Young 2006;16:187–9.

186. Chen CA, Wang SS, Chiu SN, et al. Left ventricular reverse remodeling after successful cardiac resynchronization therapy in a 3-year-old girl with idiopathic dilated cardiomyopathy. Int J Cardiol 2007;117:e7–9.

187. Gonzalez MB, Schweigel J, Kostelka M, et al. Cardiac resynchronization in a child with dilated cardiomyopathy and borderline QRS duration: speckle tracking guided lead placement. Pacing Clin Electrophysiol 2009;32:683–7.

188. Ortega M, Merino JL, Blanco FV, et al. Cardiac resynchronization therapy in an infant with double outlet right ventricle and mechanical dyssynchrony. J Cardiovasc Electrophysiol 2012;23:781–3.

189. Hauser J, Michel-Behnke I, Khazen C, et al. Successful cardiac resynchronization therapy in a 1.5-year-old girl with dilated cardiomyopathy and functional mitral regurgitation. Int J Cardiol 2013;167:e83–4.

190. Janousek J, Tomek V, Chaloupecky VA, et al. Cardiac resynchronization therapy: a novel adjunct to the treatment and prevention of systemic right ventricular failure. J Am Coll Cardiol 2004;44:1927–31.

191. Strieper M, Karpawich P, Frias P, et al. Initial experience with cardiac resynchronization therapy for ventricular dysfunction in young patients with surgically operated congenital heart disease. Am J Cardiol 2004;94:1352–4.

192. Moak JP, Hasbani K, Ramwell C, et al. Dilated cardiomyopathy following right ventricular pacing for AV block in young patients: resolution after upgrading to biventricular pacing systems. J Cardiovasc Electrophysiol 2006;17:1068–71.

193. Khairy P, Fournier A, Thibault B, et al. Cardiac resynchronization therapy in congenital heart disease. Int J Cardiol 2006;109:160–8.

194. Jauvert G, Rousseau-Paziaud J, Villain E, et al. Effects of cardiac resynchronization therapy on echocardiographic indices, functional capacity, and clinical outcomes of patients with a systemic right ventricle. Europace 2009;11:184–90.

195. Cecchin F, Frangini PA, Brown DW, et al. Cardiac resynchronization therapy (and multisite pacing) in pediatrics and congenital heart disease: five years experience in a single institution. J Cardiovasc Electrophysiol 2009;20:58–65.

196. Perera JL, Motonaga KS, Miyake CY, et al. Does pediatric CRT increase the risk of ventricular tachycardia? [abstract]. Heart Rhythm 2013;10:S210–1.

197. Dubin AM, Janousek J, Rhee E, et al. Resynchronization therapy in pediatric and congenital heart disease patients: an international multicenter study. J Am Coll Cardiol 2005;46:2277–83.

198. Janousek J, Gebauer RA, Abdul-Khaliq H, et al, Working Group for Cardiac Dysrhythmias and Electrophysiology of the Association for European Paediatric Cardiology. Cardiac resynchronisation therapy in paediatric and congenital heart disease: differential effects in various anatomical and functional substrates. Heart 2009;95:1165–71.

199. Moss AJ, Hall WJ, Cannom DS, et al. Cardiac-resynchronization therapy for the prevention of heart-failure events. N Engl J Med 2009;361:1329–38.

200. Young JB, Abraham WT, Smith AL, et al. Combined cardiac resynchronization and implantable cardioversion defibrillation in advanced chronic heart failure: the miracle ICD trial. JAMA 2003;289:2685–94.

201. Bhatta L, Luck JC, Wolbrette DL, et al. Complications of biventricular pacing. Curr Opin Cardiol 2004;19:31–5.

202. Thibault B, Harel F, Ducharme A, et al. Cardiac resynchronization therapy in patients with heart failure and a QRS complex <120 milliseconds: the evaluation of resynchronization therapy for heart failure (LESSER-EARTH) trial. Circulation 2013;127:873–81.

203. Valls-Bertault V, Fatemi M, Gilard M, et al. Assessment of upgrading to biventricular pacing in patients with right ventricular pacing and congestive heart failure after atrioventricular junctional ablation for chronic atrial fibrillation. Europace 2004;6:438–43.

204. Leon AR, Greenberg JM, Kanuru N, et al. Cardiac resynchronization in patients with congestive heart failure and chronic atrial fibrillation: effect of upgrading to biventricular pacing after chronic right ventricular pacing. J Am Coll Cardiol 2002;39:1258–63.

205. Helbing WA, Rebergen SA, Maliepaard C, et al. Quantification of right ventricular function with magnetic resonance imaging in children with normal hearts and with congenital heart disease. Am Heart J 1995;130:828–37.

206. Janousek J, Vojtovic P, Hucin B, et al. Resynchronization pacing is a useful adjunct to the management of acute heart failure after surgery for congenital heart defects. Am J Cardiol 2001;88:145–52.

207. Dubin AM, Feinstein JA, Reddy VM, et al. Electrical resynchronization: a novel therapy for the failing right ventricle. Circulation 2003;107:2287–9.

208. Dubin AM, Hanisch D, Chin C, et al. A prospective pilot study of right ventricular resynchronization [abstract]. Heart Rhythm 2008;5:S42.

209. Thambo JB, De Guillebon M, Xhaet O, et al. Biventricular pacing in patients with tetralogy of

Fallot: non-invasive epicardial mapping and clinical impact. Int J Cardiol 2011;30:30.

210. Thambo JB, Dos Santos P, De Guillebon M, et al. Biventricular stimulation improves right and left ventricular function after tetralogy of Fallot repair: acute animal and clinical studies. Heart Rhythm 2010;7:344–50.

211. Rosenthal D, Chrisant MR, Edens E, et al. International Society for Heart and Lung Transplantation: practice guidelines for management of heart failure in children. J Heart Lung Transplant 2004; 23:1313–33.

212. Lubiszewska B, Gosiewska E, Hoffman P, et al. Myocardial perfusion and function of the systemic right ventricle in patients after atrial switch procedure for complete transposition: long-term follow-up. J Am Coll Cardiol 2000;36:1365–70.

213. Millane T, Bernard EJ, Jaeggi E, et al. Role of ischemia and infarction in late right ventricular dysfunction after atrial repair of transposition of the great arteries. J Am Coll Cardiol 2000;35: 1661–8.

214. Pettersen E, Helle-Valle T, Edvardsen T, et al. Contraction pattern of the systemic right ventricle shift from longitudinal to circumferential shortening and absent global ventricular torsion. J Am Coll Cardiol 2007;49:2450–6.

215. Redington AN, Rigby ML, Oldershaw P, et al. Right ventricular function 10 years after the Mustard operation for transposition of the great arteries: analysis of size, shape, and wall motion. Br Heart J 1989;62:455–61.

216. Fogel MA, Weinberg PM, Fellows KE, et al. A study in ventricular-ventricular interaction. Single right ventricles compared with systemic right ventricles in a dual-chamber circulation. Circulation 1995; 92:219–30.

217. Singh TP, Humes RA, Muzik O, et al. Myocardial flow reserve in patients with a systemic right ventricle after atrial switch repair. J Am Coll Cardiol 2001;37:2120–5.

218. Zimmerman FJ, Starr JP, Koenig PR, et al. Acute hemodynamic benefit of multisite ventricular pacing after congenital heart surgery. Ann Thorac Surg 2003;75:1775–80.

219. Bacha EA, Zimmerman FJ, Mor-Avi V, et al. Ventricular resynchronization by multisite pacing improves myocardial performance in the postoperative single-ventricle patient. Ann Thorac Surg 2004;78: 1678–83.

The Exceptional and Far-Flung Manifestations of Heart Failure in Eisenmenger Syndrome

Alexander R. Opotowsky, MD, MPH[a],
Michael J. Landzberg, MD[a], Maurice Beghetti, MD[b],*

KEYWORDS

- Congenital heart disease • Pulmonary hypertension • Eisenmenger syndrome
- Systemic-to-pulmonary arterial shunts

KEY POINTS

- Eisenmenger syndrome is defined as pulmonary hypertension with high pulmonary vascular resistance and consequently reversed or bidirectional shunt through any large communication between the pulmonary and systemic circulations.
- Despite extensive multi-system dysfunction related primarily to hypoxemia and erythrocytosis, the prognosis for patients with ES is better than for those with pulmonary arterial hypertension who do not have a patent shunt.
- Clinical congestive heart failure due to primary cardiac dysfunction is relatively uncommon, though symptoms of dyspnea and fatigue are frequent.
- Recent studies have demonstrated the safety and modest efficacy of pulmonary vasodilators to improve exercise capacity and functional status in highly symptomatic patients with Eisenmenger syndrome. Their role in less symptomatic patients, as well as impact on specific clinical outcomes, remain unclear.
- While the potential to 'treat and repair' patients with Eisenmenger syndrome remains an exhilarating prospect, historical precedent argues for an extremely cautious approach, appreciating a clear distinction between acute success and clinical benefit.

INTRODUCTION

Congenital heart disease (CHD) is the most common inborn defect with an incidence of approximately 1% at birth. Dramatic advances in diagnosis and, in particular, treatment of CHD allow almost 95% of patients to reach adulthood,[1] resulting in a growing population of adults with repaired or palliated CHD. These patients have a high burden of heart failure, arrhythmia, and pulmonary vascular disease (PVD).[2–5]

CHD comprise a heterogeneous group of abnormal structures, communications, and connections between the cardiac chambers and vessels with different hemodynamic consequences, hence, varying need for follow-up and intervention. Systemic to pulmonary shunts (ie, ventricular septal defect [VSD], atrial septal defect [ASD], atrioventricular septal defect, and patent ductus arteriosus [PDA]) account for approximately 60% of CHD.

a Boston Adult Congenital Heart and Pulmonary Hypertension Service, Boston Children's Hospital and Brigham and Women's Hospital, Harvard Medical School, 300 Longwood Avenue, Boston, MA 02115, USA; b Pediatric Cardiology Unit, Department of the Child and Adolescent, Children's Hospital, University of Geneva, 6 rue Willy Donzé, Geneva 14 1211, Switzerland
* Corresponding author.
E-mail address: maurice.beghetti@hcuge.ch

Heart Failure Clin 10 (2014) 91–104
http://dx.doi.org/10.1016/j.hfc.2013.09.005
1551-7136/14/$ – see front matter © 2014 Elsevier Inc. All rights reserved.

Pulmonary hypertension (PH) is a major complicating factor of systemic to pulmonary shunt either by causing increased morbidity and mortality during or immediately after surgical repair or by preventing complete repair for those with increased pulmonary vascular resistance (PVR) and advanced PVD.[6]

In 1897, Victor Eisenmenger described a patient who suffered from cyanosis and dyspnea since infancy who died of massive hemoptysis at 32 years of age.[7] A postmortem examination revealed a large VSD and severe pulmonary vascular remodeling, although the underlying pathophysiology was not recognized in early reports, with a focus on the anatomic features of an Eisenmenger VSD with a dextroposed aorta overriding the right ventricle (RV) leading to right-to-left flow.[8] Almost 60 years later, Paul Wood coined the, term *Eisenmenger syndrome (ES)*, fundamentally defined as "pulmonary hypertension at systemic level, due to a high pulmonary vascular resistance (>800 dyn s/cm^5), with reversed or bidirectional shunt through...any large communication between the two circulations."[9,10]

ES represents the most advanced form of PH associated with CHD. The signs and symptoms of ES result from low blood oxygen saturation and include cyanosis, dyspnea, fatigue, dizziness, syncope, and arrhythmia. In general, patients with ES have reduced life expectancy, although many survive into their third or fourth decade, with some even surviving into their seventh decade. Of all patients with CHD, Diller and colleagues[11] reported that those with ES are the most severely compromised in terms of exercise intolerance. Exercise intolerance in these patients has been identified as a predictor of hospitalization or death, independent of age, gender, World Health Organization functional class, or underlying cardiac defect. Anecdotal evidence suggests that patients with ES adapt their lifestyle around their exercise capabilities and tend to underemphasize objective limitation. This review focuses on epidemiology and classification; pathophysiology, with an emphasis on the complex multisystem manifestation of heart failure in these patients; and treatment of ES.

EPIDEMIOLOGY AND CLASSIFICATION
Epidemiology

Advances in pediatric cardiology, especially surgery, have increased the numbers of CHD patients surviving into adulthood and have helped to prevent the onset of ES in the developed world, resulting in a greater than 50% reduction in the prevalence of ES over the past 50 years. The occurrence of ES has decreased from approximately 8% in the 1950s to approximately 1% to 2% in the current era.[12] The true prevalence of ES is unknown, however, because some patients are not followed in centers of expertise from which prevalence data derive. Historical data suggest that ES occurs in approximately 8% of patients with CHD in general but in approximately 10% to 12% in a presence of a left-to-right shunt.[13] Recent reports by CONgenital CORvitia (CONCOR), a Netherlands registry, suggest a prevalence of PH-CHD of 4.6%, among which 1% had ES.[12] In the Euro Heart Survey, 531 patients with PH were reported among the 1900 adults with CHD; of these 531, 231 had ES.[14] Another approach is to analyze how many patients are reported in the current PH registries. In the adult registries, the prevalence of PH-CHD varies from 11% in a French registry to 23% to 27% in a Scottish registry.[15,16] This difference may be attributed to study design, recruitment, and inclusion criteria. The percentage in pediatric registries is higher, with number approaching 45%.[17,18] These registries, however, include PH associated with CHD which does not fulfill the definition of ES (ie, reversed shunt and cyanosis) but some other forms of PH-CHD according to the classification (**Box 1**) and some also likely include patients with PH but normal PVR. A recent specific ES registry originating from Belgium has estimated the prevalence as 11 per million adults.[19] Patients with chromosomal abnormalities are less likely to undergo early repair and more likely to have cyanosis and PH in adulthood.[20]

Classification

Structural changes in the pulmonary vasculature in all forms of pulmonary arterial hypertension (PAH), group 1 of the current World Health Organization classification scheme, including ES, are qualitatively similar, although there is some variation in the distribution and prevalence of pathologic changes within different underlying causes. According to a classification scheme proposed at the Dana Point conference published in 2009, PAH resulting from CHD is grouped with idiopathic PAH, drug-related PAH, PAH associated with connective tissue diseases, and HIV-related PAH.[21] CHD, however, comprises, as discussed previously, a heterogeneous spectrum of pathology that may differ from other forms of PH with regards to cardiac anatomy, hemodynamics, and natural history. This group includes many defects that have different evolutions and this is of importance. One major difference is between pre-tricuspid and post-tricuspid shunts, with the latter developing PVD more rapidly. This is one reason why subclassifications have been developed to better define

Box 1
The European Society of Cardiology proposed clinical classification of congenital, systemic-to-pulmonary shunts associated with pulmonary arterial hypertension

A. Eisenmenger syndrome (ES)

> ES includes all systemic-to-pulmonary shunts due to large defects, leading to a severe increase in PVR and resulting in a reversed (pulmonary-to-systemic) or bidirectional shunt. Cyanosis, erythrocytosis, and multiple organ involvement are present.

B. PAH associated with systemic-to-pulmonary shunts

> In these patients with moderate to large defects, the increase in PVR is mild to moderate, systemic-to-pulmonary shunt is still largely present, and no cyanosis is present at rest.

C. PAH with small defects

> In cases of small defects (in adults, usually VSDs<1 cm and ASDs<2 cm of effective diameter assessed by echocardiography) the clinical picture is similar to idiopathic PAH.

D. PAH after corrective cardiac surgery

> In these cases, CHD has been corrected but PAH is either still present immediately after surgery or has recurred several months or years after surgery in the absence of significant postoperative residual congenital lesions or defects that originate as a sequela to previous surgery.

Adapted from Galie N, Hoeper MM, Humbert M, et al. Guidelines for the diagnosis and treatment of pulmonary hypertension: the Task Force for the Diagnosis and Treatment of Pulmonary Hypertension of the European Society of Cardiology (ESC) and the European Respiratory Society (ERS), endorsed by the International Society of Heart and Lung Transplantation (ISHLT). Eur Heart J 2009;30(20):2498; with permission.

PH-CHD patients. Subclassifications have been suggested by Galie,[22] Schulze Neick,[23] and van Albada and Berger,[24] taking into account several factors important to describe the lesions and factors important in the development of PVD, such as type and size of defects, hemodynamics, presence of extracardiac anomalies, and repair status (unrepaired, palliated, or repaired). Based on these suggestions and further understanding of the disease, specific classifications have been introduced in the clinical classification of PH.[25,26]

These modifications include a specific subclassifications for PH-CHD, allowing for a simple clinical classification of congenital systemic to pulmonary shunt, including ES, PAH-CHD with elevated PVR considered inoperable, PAH with small defects that are not considered the cause of PAH, and PAH after successful corrective surgery (see **Box 1**). A more extensive pathologic and pathophysiologic classification has also been published that should satisfy both CHD experts and nonexperts (**Box 2**), defining major characteristics of the systemic to pulmonary shunt.

Pathophysiology of the Eisenmenger Syndrome: Cardiac Breathlessness Without Congestive Heart Failure

In the presence of a normal pulmonary vascular bed, systemic vascular resistance is higher than PVR, systemic arterial pressure is higher than pulmonary arterial pressure, and subsystemic ventricular compliance is lower than subpulmonary ventricular compliance. As such, blood shunts from left to right across any permissive defect (ie, ASD, VSD, or PDA). In the setting of a large defect, a considerable volume of blood shunts in this manner. For reasons not entirely understood, this additional load variably results in pulmonary vascular remodeling. The timing and extent of remodeling is variable. Although there is enormous heterogeneity in presentation, extensive pulmonary vascular remodeling is more common and occurs earlier in patients with PDA or VSD than in those with atrial level (or other pre-tricuspid) shunts and is modestly correlated with lesion size. Early remodeling (eg, medial hypertrophy) may be reversible but a subset of patients develops marked and currently irreversible pulmonary vascular remodeling, including extensive intimal proliferation, fibrosis, plexiform lesions, and arteriolar occlusion indistinguishable from findings in idiopathic PAH. Patients usually undergo repair prior to development of such remodeling if identified, and there are no recent natural history studies of cellular changes preceding the final result of this level of extensive remodeling; as a result, the fundamental mechanisms are not well understood.

Although these are the hallmarks and defining features of ES, complications and long-term prognosis are often proximately more related to dysfunction in other organ systems as a consequence of chronic hypoxemia and erythrocytosis. Symptoms and signs of congestive heart failure, such as dependent edema, are common, but they are usually mild, relatively stable, and readily managed with diuretic therapy. Important systolic ventricular dysfunction is uncommon. Effort

---

Box 2
European Society of Cardiology proposed anatomic-pathophysiologic classification of congenital systemic-to-pulmonary shunts associated with pulmonary arterial hypertension

Type

  Simple pretricuspid shunts

    ASD

      Ostium secundum

      Sinus venosus

      Ostium primum

    Total or partial unobstructed anomalous pulmonary venous return

  Simple post-tricuspid shunts

    VSD

    PDA

  Combined shunts

    Describe combination and define predominant defect

  Complex congenital heart disease

    Complete atrioventricular septal defect

    Truncus arteriosus

    Single ventricle physiology with unobstructed pulmonary blood flow

    Transposition of the great arteries with VSD (without pulmonary stenosis) and/or PDA

    Other

Dimension (specify for each defect if more than one congenital heart defect exists)

  Hemodynamic (specify Qp:Qs)

    Restrictive (pressure gradient across the defect)

    Nonrestrictive

  Anatomic

    Small to moderate (ASD<2.0 cm and VSD<1.0 cm)

    Large (ASD≥2.0 cm and VSD≥1.0 cm)

Direction of shunt

  Predominantly systemic-to-pulmonary

  Predominantly pulmonary-to-systemic

  Bidirectional

Associated cardiac and extracardiac abnormalities

Repair status

  Unoperated

  Palliated (specify type of operation[s], age at surgery)

  Repaired (specify type of operation[s], age at surgery)

Adapted from Galie N, Hoeper MM, Humbert M, et al. Guidelines for the diagnosis and treatment of pulmonary hypertension: the Task Force for the Diagnosis and Treatment of Pulmonary Hypertension of the European Society of Cardiology (ESC) and the European Respiratory Society (ERS), endorsed by the International Society of Heart and Lung Transplantation (ISHLT). Eur Heart J 2009;30(20):2499; with permission.

intolerance and functional limitation, however, are essentially ubiquitous. As described by Wood, "Apart from breathlessness, the chief symptoms of the Eisenmenger syndrome are angina pectoris, hemoptysis, and congestive heart failure, in that order of onset." Only approximately 10% of patients in Wood's series of 127 patients were deemed to have congestive heart failure.[9] Though more recent reports suggest a higher incidence of symptomatic heart failure,[27,28] understanding the multisystem dysfunction and compensation in ES is integral to considering the distinct underpinnings of dyspnea and volume retention in this distinct syndrome.

Wood elegantly reasoned that oxygenation of blood flowing past the head and neck arterial oxygen sensors was a major contributor, based on the observation that patients with PDA, compared with those who have an ASD or VSD, had less severe effort intolerance (Fig. 1).[9,10] Although this is a major contributor to effort intolerance in patients with ES, there are other contributors, including limited systemic cardiac output reserve, increased red cell mass, and deconditioning.

Systemic arterial oxygen saturation ($Sao_2\%$) is a complex function of hemoglobin concentration, systemic cardiac output, pulmonary blood flow, effectiveness of oxygenation in the lungs (pulmonary venous oxygen saturation), distribution of systemic blood flow, and oxygen extraction in the periphery (Fig. 2).[29] Furthermore, $Sao_2\%$ is not the only important measure of systemic oxygen status, because both oxygen content (cO_2) and the partial pressure of oxygen (Po_2) have important specific significance. Oxygen content, a function of hemoglobin concentration, Po_2, and Sao_2, represents the absolute amount of oxygen carried per unit of blood and represents the most important variable when considering adequacy of tissue oxygen delivery. Some homeostatic mechanisms, however, respond primarily to Po_2.

Appreciation of the complexity of these interactions and the lack of an apparent single therapeutic goal (eg, higher $Sao_2\%$) leads logically to a conclusion that effectiveness of therapies cannot be intuited or theoretically derived by their impact on one variable. For example, although generally thought contraindicated because of a fear of systemic arterial desaturation, small cautious studies of primarily systemic vasodilators, such as nifedipine and enalapril, in select patients with ES and other cyanotic CHD suggest they may actually improve functional status without worsening hypoxemia.[30–32] More relevant to current clinical practice, the concern that pulmonary vasodilators are nonselective and also dilate the systemic circulation may be misplaced. If both systemic and

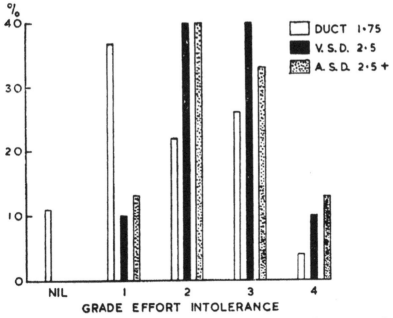

Degree of effort intolerance in the three main groups of Eisenmenger's syndrome.

Fig. 1. Paul Wood's observation that patients with PDA had less prominent effort intolerance than those with ASD or VSD. DUCT, patent ductus arteriosus. (*From* Wood P. The Eisenmenger syndrome or pulmonary hypertension with reversed central shunt. I. Br Med J 1958;2(5098):705; with permission.)

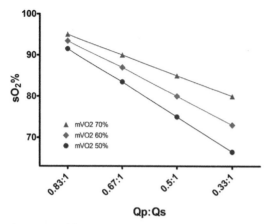

Fig. 2. Simplified diagram showing the dependence of Sao₂% on both Qp:Qs, and mixed systemic venous saturation, itself a function of systemic cardiac output, pulmonary venous saturation, systemic arterial oxygen saturation, and hemoglobin concentration. Pulmonary venous blood is assumed to be fully saturated. mVO2, mixed venous oxygen saturation.

pulmonary flows are increased, even with a lower ratio of pulmonary flow to systemic flow (Qp:Qs), the result may be higher systemic Sao₂% and less effort intolerance due to the effect on saturation and also to the higher systemic cardiac output itself (ie, increased tissue oxygen delivery). Conversely, lower hemoglobin concentrations seen with some medications (eg, endothelin receptor antagonists) may limit their effectiveness.

Perhaps the most insidious effect of the fear of systemic vasodilation is the pervasive recommendation that patients with ES avoid moderately intense or more strenuous physical activity.[33] With exertion, hypoxemia does worsen for patients with ES, as it does in general for people with some degree of resting hypoxemia. There are potential risks to physical activity, but documentation of harm is anecdotal or hypothetical. The adverse effects of aerobic deconditioning are real, however, and undoubtedly have a major impact on quality of life. The benefits of regular moderately strenuous aerobic activity have been demonstrated for a diverse array of diseases long thought to contraindicate physical activity, including PAH, acquired heart failure, and chronic lung disease. Therefore there does not seem to be any reason patients with ES should respond differently to chronic, frequent, moderately strenuous aerobic conditioning.

CONSEQUENCES OF CHRONIC HYPOXEMIA

This discussion of multisystem pathophysiology in ES includes data from both ES and, when the physiology is expected to be similar (mainly when primary mechanisms are likely hypoxemia and erythrocytosis), other forms of cyanotic congenital heart disease.

Secondary Erythrocytosis and Hematologic Abnormalities

Erythrocytosis, a direct response to chronic hypoxemia, is the hallmark hematologic abnormality of ES. Elevated red cell mass provides enhanced tissue oxygen delivery but also causes increased viscosity and endothelial shear stress. Historically, high hemoglobin concentration was viewed as the cause of many of the hyperviscosity symptoms experienced by ES patients as well as a major contributor to adverse outcomes. Phlebotomy was, within this framework, recommended to lower hemoglobin concentration in order to improve symptoms and perhaps outcomes. Studies have confirmed an improvement in symptoms and exercise capacity after phlebotomy over days to weeks.[34] Acute normalization of hematocrit has benefits in terms of coagulation and renal function (discussed later). Over the past 3 decades, however, clinical investigators have developed a deeper appreciation of the relationship between hemoglobin concentration, red cell morphology, viscosity, and symptoms. Repeated phlebotomy often results in iron deficiency and consequently less deformable microcytic red cells, paradoxically increasing viscosity.[35] Iron deficiency is independently associated with a higher incidence of cerebrovascular accidents and overall risk of adverse outcomes (discussed below).

Other components of blood are also affected. ES is associated with an increased propensity to both bleeding and thrombosis. An intuitive explanation is that whole blood is diluted because a greater proportion by volume is accounted for by red cells. Although dilution may apply to a subset of loosely regulated circulating markers, it is of limited explanatory value. Erythrocytosis itself, via its effects on viscosity, may predispose to microvascular obstruction but that does not readily explain macroscopic thromboembolism. One potential mechanism is that increased red cell concentration results in a high shear stress vascular environment, with consequent effects on the endothelium and platelets.[36] Platelet count is, on average, lower among cyanotic patients, inversely correlates with hematocrit, and increases after phlebotomy.[36,37] Platelet aggregation in response to adenosine diphosphate and other factors is decreased, a finding also inversely correlated with the severity of erythrocytosis.[38] Several hematological characteristics seem to favor increased bleeding as well, such as a paucity of large von Willebrand factor multimers,[39,40] although similar findings have also been reported for noncyanotic CHD and acquired valve disease.[41,42] Which of these abnormalities is most associated with clinical bleeding or thrombosis is unclear, making reliable extrapolation to therapeutic recommendations difficult.

Vascular Function

Endothelial function, in both the pulmonary and systemic circulation, is also abnormal in patients with ES. Several investigators have reported on endothelial function and circulating endothelial markers and cells,[43,44] and there is evidence of impaired endothelium-dependent relaxation.[45,46] This may be directly related to erythrocytosis or hypoxemia, but it is also in the context of increased inflammation in cyanotic congenital heart disease, as reflected by higher levels of serum C-reactive protein and interleukin 6.[43,47] Existing small studies, however, have not addressed whether these findings are associated with functional status or outcomes.

Pulmonary and Ventilatory Effects

Patients with cyanotic CHD, including those with ES, have reduced aerobic exercise capacity. Peak oxygen consumption ($\dot{V}O_2$) is reduced, and oxygen uptake kinetics are abnormal, with blunted phase I response to exercise. Phase I refers to the initial approximately 20 seconds of exercise, before venous blood from exercising muscle returns to the pulmonary circulation. The increase in $\dot{V}O_2$ seen during this period, therefore, is due to increased pulmonary blood flow and not to a decrease in venous PO_2. The blunted response in ES reflects impaired augmentation of pulmonary blood flow.[48] Even at low levels of steady work, patients with ES are more dependent on increased heart rate to maintain cardiac output, given limited augmentation of pulmonary blood flow. Minute ventilation ($\dot{V}e$):volume of expired CO_2 per minute ($\dot{V}CO_2$) is also elevated; consequently, both resting and exercise ventilatory demands are increased in order to maintain acid-base homeostasis.[49–51] This is in part related to underlying PVD but mainly due directly to right-to-left shunting, permitting venous blood high in CO_2 with lower pH to bypass the lungs. Despite elevated $\dot{V}e$ and $\dot{V}e$:$\dot{V}CO_2$ and low end-tidal CO_2 ($PETCO_2$), arterial pH and CO_2 remain normal. Thus, ventilation is appropriate as a response to shunting, presumably controlled by arterial chemoreceptors. Treatment with an endothelin receptor antagonist in adults with ES improves ventilatory efficiency, whereas peak $\dot{V}O_2$ is not affected, likely reflective of decreased right-to-left shunting.[52]

As discussed previously, exercise-related decreases in peripheral arterial $Sao_2\%$ are a function of increased oxygen extraction, more right-to-left shunting, and, potentially, decreased pulmonary venous oxygen saturation. Investigators have demonstrated a decrease in PO_2 and $Sao_2\%$ in the supine relative to sitting position, which is prevented by supplemental oxygen.[50] This argues against intracardiac shunting as the sole cause of hypoxemia in these patients. There is a high burden of nocturnal hypoxemia episodes mainly during rapid eye movement sleep in the absence of obstructive or central apnea. The frequency of nocturnal hypoxemia correlates with hematocrit, although iron status was unknown for the population studied.[53] Despite these findings, a small 2-year trial failed to demonstrate benefit of nocturnal oxygen supplementation.[54]

Renal Function and Uric Acid Metabolism

Renal dysfunction is common in ES. Glomerular filtration rate is variably impaired, clinically apparent as elevated serum creatinine concentration.[55] Glomerular filtration rate, however, is usually only mildly reduced.[19] While renal plasma flow is low there is a high filtration fraction,[56] presumably reflecting efferent arteriolar constriction or as a consequence of the direct effect of glomerular filtration to increase blood viscosity in the efferent arterioles.[57–59]

Most relevant, perhaps, to the understanding of heart failure in patients with ES is the presence of abnormal renal fluid handling. Isovolumic phlebotomy, with a decrease in hematocrit to normal, does not affect glomerular filtration rate but filtration fraction declines. The latter is associated with spontaneous diuresis, although this finding is not universal in all patients.[60] Additionally, a subset of patients demonstrates an inability to excrete a water load or appropriately concentrate urine.[61]

Serum uric acid concentration is elevated in ES, related to reduced renal excretion with a small contribution of increased production in the setting of tissue hypoxia and cell turnover.[61–63] Oya and colleagues[62] reported that elevated serum uric acid concentration was associated with increased mortality (hazard ratio [HR] 1.6; 95% CI, 1.3–2.7) independently of clinical factors and other serum markers. Renal dysfunction itself is also independently associated with increased mortality in ES.[55,64]

Other Selected Miscellaneous Findings

In addition to the findings discussed previously, there is a range of findings and events, both incidental and potentially medically important, for which ES patients are at increased risk. A subset is discussed, but there are many others not discussed, including a propensity to calcium bilirubinate gallstones,[65] particular ophthalmologic findings[66,67] and pheochromocytoma.[68]

Immune and Infectious Issues

The most notable consistently reported infectious complication in patients with ES and other cyanotic heart disease patients is cerebral abscess.[69] Logically, this could be explained by the presence of right-to-left shunt flow bypassing pulmonary circulation filtration. If this were the only mechanism, a similar relative increase in the incidence of other systemic infections might be expected, but this does not seem to be the case with exceptions (eg, endocarditis and sinusitis).[70] Mechanisms may include the effect of cyanosis on the immune system and on normal barriers to central nervous system infection. For example, acute and sub-acute hypoxia causes greater permeability of the blood-brain barrier, although the applicability to chronic cyanosis due to heart disease is not defined.[71]

Coronary Circulation

ES is associated with impressive remodeling of the large extramural coronary vessels and coronary microcirculation, and evidence suggests these patients are resistant to developing atherosclerotic disease.[72–75] This is especially remarkable in that other characteristics (ie, endothelial dysfunction, elevated serum glucose, renal dysfunction, elevated uric acid, and systemic inflammation) are usually associated with an increased risk for atherosclerosis. Intermittent hypoxemia may have possible proatherogenic effects in other diseases and local hypoxia plays a role in the development of atherosclerotic plaques.[76,77] Blood lipid profiles seem slightly more favorable in ES patients, but, given the modest difference and the specific findings on the circulation, it seems unlikely to account for the apparent absence of coronary atherosclerosis.[78]

THE RIGHT VENTRICLE IN EISENMENGER SYNDROME

The RV in patients with ES is notable for several reasons, although interest derives mainly from its apparent resilience in the face of markedly elevated afterload. Most of the characteristics of patients with ES listed thus far seem likely to predispose to worse outcomes than observed among patients with PAH without a right-to-left shunt. It is not entirely clear why the opposite is

true, but favorable differences in RV remodeling and ventricular interaction seem to play a role. First, the RV is universally hypertrophied, with wall thickness generally equal to left ventricular wall thickness.[79] Some investigators have suggested this may be because of a lack of RV regression after birth (preservation of a fetal pattern), but patients with atrial level shunts who develop elevated PVR much later in life have generally similar findings and prognosis. A second characteristic is that the ventricular septum is generally neutral throughout the cardiac cycle, whereas in PAH without a shunt there is mid- to end-systolic bowing of the septum toward the left side, impeding diastolic filling and limiting cardiac output. Echocardiography has been helpful in better understanding RV adaptation in ES. Although longitudinal function seems impaired in ES, similarly to PAH without shunt, both RV and LV wall thicknesses are greater, the RV is modestly smaller whereas the LV is conversely larger, and short-axis function is better preserved resulting in an improved myocardial performance index.[80] Finally, shunting at any level provides a relief valve for the right heart; although not intuitive, right-to-left shunting at any level serves to decrease both RV preload and afterload (eg, the pulmonary circulation is more compliant at lower filling volume). As a result of these factors and other yet-to-be-defined factors, right heart failure per se is an uncommon finding, and right atrial pressure is usually normal or close to it.

Treatment

Treatment options for ES remain limited by the recognition that multiple contributors exist to PAH and multisystem organ dysfunction in ES and by the few data specific to the varied and particular physiologies involved in producing limited capacitance and compliance as well as elevated PVR coupled with failure of the subpulmonary cardiovascular chambers.

Benefits of a formal program of exercise training initiated by experienced clinicians have been suggested in a small nonrandomized cohort study of a mixed population of PAH-CHD, half of whom had ES[81]; extension of these findings falls largely to first principles until more robust study is accomplished.

Use of nocturnal supplemental oxygen in patients with ES (who on average had a >10% increase in Sao$_2$% with nasal cannulae oxygen administration) did not improve functional capacity, quality of life, or survival in a small prospective study by experienced investigators of 10 ES patients living at altitude.[54] Nocturnal oxygen did not improve secondary erythrocytosis, underscoring multiple potential confounders and calling into question the ability to extend these findings without further detailed investigation.

The nonspecific symptoms of fatigue, muscle weakness, and headache seen in adults with ES are similar to symptoms of iron deficiency. Past practice of venesection to reduce secondary erythrocytosis served to worsen already existing low iron stores and further compromised oxygen tissue delivery, reduced functional capacity, and increased rather than decreased the risk of stroke.[82,83] Demonstration phase study of 3 months of iron supplementation in adults with ES with measured iron deficiency (generally determined by transferrin saturation of <10%–20% rather than by depending solely on low serum ferritin which may vary in relationship to fluctuation in inflammatory state) correlated use of iron with improved quality of life and increase of 6-minute walk distance with rise in hemoglobin concentration.[84] Although iron repletion in the setting of iron deficiency seems justified in ES, further study of the adaptive and pathologic interactions between chronic cyanosis, secondary erythrocytosis, iron metabolism and utilization, and organ and tissue perfusion seems warranted prior to determining optimal hemoglobin for such patients.[85]

Results of observational cohort studies of targeted therapies for PAH in patients with ES (nifedipine,[30,31,86] intravenous prostaglandin and similar molecules,[87] bosentan,[88–97] ambrisentan,[98] sildenafil,[99–102] and tadalafil[103]) have demonstrated mixed results, although largely suggesting some degree of short- and intermediate-term clinical benefit (walk distance and quality of life) or improved hemodynamics; other studies have challenged these benefits or have suggested limitation in the sustaining of such effects. Findings have been equivalent for ES associated with Down syndrome. Overall, such investigation largely has served as exploratory analyses, underscoring the need to understand and control for the multiple features contributing to phenotypic expression of subpulmonary cardiovascular chamber failure as well as lack of knowledge regarding disease formation and progression; registry trials assessing risks for progression of ES are ongoing.

Randomized trials of medical PAH therapy for ES have focused on those with simple anatomic defects. Initial trials involving sildenafil[104] and tadalafil[103] demonstrated promise. Bosentan[105–107] has been most widely studied in randomized trials, with current guidelines of care for ES reflecting the positive short- and intermediate-term safety and benefit (improved hemodynamics and 6-minute walk distance) of bosentan in the Eisenmenger population. Translation of these results into practice is reflected in the retrospective, single-center, propensity-score adjusted analysis of a large cohort of adults with ES, demonstrating targeted PAH therapy for ES as the first medical intervention to significantly reduce mortality in this population.[108,109] More contemporary studies, however, including a larger proportion of treated patients with longer follow-up time, have found that although advanced PAH therapy seems to deliver a sustained improvement in functional status as measured by functional class, Sao_2%, and 6 minute walk test distance,[108,110] there is no clear mortality benefit (univariate HR 0.9; 95% CI, 0.43–1.88; $P = .8$).[110]

Information on combination targeted PAH therapy for adults with ES has largely been anecdotal and experiential, with a single randomized controlled crossover trial suggesting limited benefit of mild increase in systemic arterial Sao_2% with bosentan and sildenafil.[111,112]

There are anecdotal reports of mechanical catheter-based and surgical therapies potentially appropriate for adults with ES, including limitation of pulmonary blood flow by placement of a pulmonary artery band in the setting of persistent intracardiac shunting,[113,114] redirecting ventricular inflow via baffle creation to allow differential streaming of oxygenated blood (palliative Mustard baffle),[115] lowering subpulmonary ventricular afterload by creation of descending aorta to left pulmonary artery (Potts) shunt in the absence of other intravascular shunting,[116–118] and aggressive targeted medical PAH therapy in the presence of intracardiac shunting and severely elevated PVR followed by subsequent shunt closure (treat and repair).[119,120] These treatments remain in the realm of innovative therapy and should be considered only on protocol and when alternative therapies are failing. Transplantation, either lung or heart-lung, is an option for a subset of patients,[121,122] although the relatively good intermediate-term prognosis makes it a challenge to identify ES patients who do not have extensive multiorgan dysfunction whose outlook would improve with transplant and its associated risks.[123]

Future Aspects

There is still significant progress to make in understanding the pathophysiology of ES and the best approach to therapy. For this small population, this can be accomplished only through development of multicenter and multinational registries and trials. It must be understood why some patients develop ES early in life whereas others develop lesions slowly, if ever, in the presence of the same anatomy. Even though progress has been achieved in the treatment of ES, including the first positive randomized controlled trial performed using a specific therapy for PAH, much remains to be done. Anticoagulation remains controversial for ES, given the combined prothrombotic and bleeding propensity (described previously). Likewise, no consensus has been reached on the utility of standard oxygen supplementation. The role of advanced therapies must also be better studied, in particular, combination therapy.

SUMMARY

Significant advances have been achieved during the past decade, and the approach to ES has transitioned from a do-not-harm clinical philosophy and a scientifically largely neglected entity to a multiorgan disease that requires dedicated diagnostic procedures and specific and expert therapeutic approaches. The desire to actively improve the quality and longevity of life for these patients, however, must be balanced against the known high risk of many previously heralded interventions and the real potential that today's silver bullets may as problematic as those of yesteryear when submitted to extensive scrutiny. That said, development of targeted pulmonary vascular therapies has not only changed therapy but also renewed interest in ES. This will hopefully translate into innovations to improve the functional status and longevity of patients with ES. The seductive dream of treat and repair is in the mind of all physicians caring for these patients but the way remains long and fraught. Progress has been made and undoubtedly will continue, but lack of proper caution risks reliving the experiences that led Paul Wood to note that, "surgical repair of the defect has been responsible in recent years for more deaths in the ES than any other agent except haemoptysis."[10]

REFERENCES

1. Warnes CA, Liberthson R, Danielson GK, et al. Task force 1: the changing profile of congenital heart disease in adult life. J Am Coll Cardiol 2001; 37(5):1170–5.
2. Marelli AJ, Mackie AS, Ionescu-Ittu R, et al. Congenital heart disease in the general population: changing prevalence and age distribution. Circulation 2007;115(2):163–72.
3. Opotowsky AR, Siddiqi OK, Webb GD. Trends in hospitalizations for adults with congenital heart disease in the U.S. J Am Coll Cardiol 2009;54(5): 460–7.
4. Rodriguez FH 3rd, Moodie DS, Parekh DR, et al. Outcomes of Heart Failure-Related Hospitalization in Adults with Congenital Heart Disease in the United States. Congenit Heart Dis 2012. [Epub ahead of print].
5. O'Leary JM, Siddiqi OK, de Ferranti S, et al. The Changing Demographics of Congenital Heart Disease Hospitalizations in the United States, 1998 Through 2010. JAMA 2013;309(10):984–6.
6. Beghetti M. Congenital heart disease and pulmonary hypertension. Rev Port Cardiol 2004;23(2): 273–81.
7. Eisenmenger V. Die angeborenen defekte der kammerscheidwand des herzens. Z Klin Med 1897; 32(Suppl 11):1–28.
8. Taussig HB. Congenital Malformations of the Heart: The Commonwealth Fund; 1947.
9. Wood P. The Eisenmenger syndrome or pulmonary hypertension with reversed central shunt. I. Br Med J 1958;2(5098):701–9.
10. Wood P. The Eisenmenger syndrome or pulmonary hypertension with reversed central shunt. Br Med J 1958;2(5099):755–62.
11. Diller GP, Dimopoulos K, Okonko D, et al. Exercise intolerance in adult congenital heart disease: comparative severity, correlates, and prognostic implication. Circulation 2005;112(6):828–35.
12. Duffels MG, Engelfriet PM, Berger RM, et al. Pulmonary arterial hypertension in congenital heart disease: an epidemiologic perspective from a Dutch registry. Int J Cardiol 2007;120(2):198–204.
13. Duffels M, van Loon L, Berger R, et al. Pulmonary arterial hypertension associated with a congenital heart defect: advanced medium-term medical treatment stabilizes clinical condition. Congenit Heart Dis 2007;2(4):242–9.
14. Engelfriet PM, Duffels MG, Moller T, et al. Pulmonary arterial hypertension in adults born with a heart septal defect: the Euro Heart Survey on adult congenital heart disease. Heart 2007;93(6):682–7.
15. Peacock AJ, Murphy NF, McMurray JJ, et al. An epidemiological study of pulmonary arterial hypertension. Eur Respir J 2007;30(1):104–9.
16. Humbert M, Sitbon O, Chaouat A, et al. Pulmonary arterial hypertension in France: results from a national registry. Am J Respir Crit Care Med 2006; 173(9):1023–30.
17. Berger RM, Beghetti M, Humpl T, et al. Clinical features of paediatric pulmonary hypertension: a registry study. Lancet 2012;379(9815):537–46.
18. Barst RJ, McGoon MD, Elliott CG, et al. Survival in childhood pulmonary arterial hypertension: insights from the registry to evaluate early and long-term pulmonary arterial hypertension disease management. Circulation 2012;125(1):113–22.
19. Van de Bruaene A, Delcroix M, Pasquet A, et al. The Belgian Eisenmenger syndrome registry:

implications for treatment strategies? Acta Cardiol 2009;64(4):447–53.

20. Baraona F, Gurvitz M, Landzberg MJ, et al. Hospitalizations and mortality in the United States for adults with Down syndrome and congenital heart disease. Am J Cardiol 2013;111(7):1046–51.

21. Simonneau G, Robbins IM, Beghetti M, et al. Updated clinical classification of pulmonary hypertension. J Am Coll Cardiol 2009;54(Suppl 1): S43–54.

22. Galie N, Manes A, Palazzini M, et al. Management of pulmonary arterial hypertension associated with congenital systemic-to-pulmonary shunts and Eisenmenger's syndrome. Drugs 2008;68(8): 1049–66.

23. Schulze-Neick I, Beghetti M. Classifying pulmonary hypertension in the setting of the congenitally malformed heart–cleaning up a dog's dinner. Cardiol Young 2008;18(1):22–5.

24. van Albada ME, Berger RM. Pulmonary arterial hypertension in congenital cardiac disease–the need for refinement of the Evian-Venice classification. Cardiol Young 2008;18(1):10–7.

25. McLaughlin VV, Archer SL, Badesch DB, et al. ACCF/AHA 2009 expert consensus document on pulmonary hypertension: a report of the American College of Cardiology Foundation Task Force on Expert Consensus Documents and the American Heart Association: developed in collaboration with the American College of Chest Physicians, American Thoracic Society, Inc., and the Pulmonary Hypertension Association. Circulation 2009;119(16): 2250–94.

26. Galie N, Hoeper MM, Humbert M, et al. Guidelines for the diagnosis and treatment of pulmonary hypertension: the Task Force for the Diagnosis and Treatment of Pulmonary Hypertension of the European Society of Cardiology (ESC) and the European Respiratory Society (ERS), endorsed by the International Society of Heart and Lung Transplantation (ISHLT). Eur Heart J 2009;30(20):2493–537.

27. Oya H, Nagaya N, Uematsu M, et al. Poor prognosis and related factors in adults with Eisenmenger syndrome. Am Heart J 2002;143(4):739–44.

28. Diller GP, Dimopoulos K, Broberg CS, et al. Presentation, survival prospects, and predictors of death in Eisenmenger syndrome: a combined retrospective and case-control study. Eur Heart J 2006; 27(14):1737–42.

29. Barnea O, Austin EH, Richman B, et al. Balancing the circulation: theoretic optimization of pulmonary/systemic flow ratio in hypoplastic left heart syndrome. J Am Coll Cardiol 1994;24(5):1376–81.

30. Wong CK, Lau CP, Leung WH, et al. The use of nifedipine in patients with Eisenmenger's syndrome complicating patency of the arterial duct. Int J Cardiol 1989;25(2):173–8.

31. Wong CK, Yeung DW, Lau CP, et al. Improvement of exercise capacity after nifedipine in patients with Eisenmenger syndrome complicating ventricular septal defect. Clin Cardiol 1991;14(12):957–61.

32. Hopkins WE, Kelly DP. Angiotensin-converting enzyme inhibitors in adults with cyanotic congenital heart disease. Am J Cardiol 1996;77(5):439–40.

33. Warnes CA, Williams RG, Bashore TM, et al. ACC/ AHA 2008 guidelines for the management of adults with congenital heart disease: a report of the American College of Cardiology/American Heart Association Task Force on Practice Guidelines (Writing Committee to Develop Guidelines on the Management of Adults With Congenital Heart Disease). Developed in Collaboration With the American Society of Echocardiography, Heart Rhythm Society, International Society for Adult Congenital Heart Disease, Society for Cardiovascular Angiography and Interventions, and Society of Thoracic Surgeons. J Am Coll Cardiol 2008; 52(23):e1–121.

34. Oldershaw PJ, Sutton MG. Haemodynamic effects of haematocrit reduction in patients with polycythaemia secondary to cyanotic congenital heart disease. Br Heart J 1980;44(5):584–8.

35. Van de Pette JE, Guthrie DL, Pearson TC. Whole blood viscosity in polycythaemia: the effect of iron deficiency at a range of haemoglobin and packed cell volumes. Br J Haematol 1986;63(2):369–75.

36. Horigome H, Hiramatsu Y, Shigeta O, et al. Overproduction of platelet microparticles in cyanotic congenital heart disease with polycythemia. J Am Coll Cardiol 2002;39(6):1072–7.

37. Maurer HM, McCue CM, Robertson LW, et al. Correction of platelet dysfunction and bleeding in cyanotic congenital heart disease by simple red cell volume reduction. Am J Cardiol 1975;35(6): 831–5.

38. Mauer HM, McCue CM, Caul J, et al. Impairment in platelet aggregation in congenital heart disease. Blood 1972;40(2):207–16.

39. Territo MC, Perloff JK, Rosove MH, et al. Acquired Von Willebrand Factor Abnormalities in Adults with Congenital Heart Disease: Dependence Upon Cardiopulmonary Pathophysiological Subtype. Clin Appl Thromb Hemost 1998;4(4):257–61.

40. Rabinovitch M, Andrew M, Thom H, et al. Abnormal endothelial factor VIII associated with pulmonary hypertension and congenital heart defects. Circulation 1987;76(5):1043–52.

41. Gill JC, Wilson AD, Endres-Brooks J, et al. Loss of the largest von Willebrand factor multimers from the plasma of patients with congenital cardiac defects. Blood 1986;67(3):758–61.

42. Vincentelli A, Susen S, Le Tourneau T, et al. Acquired von Willebrand syndrome in aortic stenosis. N Engl J Med 2003;349(4):343–9.

43. Diller GP, van Eijl S, Okonko DO, et al. Circulating endothelial progenitor cells in patients with Eisenmenger syndrome and idiopathic pulmonary arterial hypertension. Circulation 2008; 117(23):3020–30.

44. Smadja DM, Gaussem P, Mauge L, et al. Circulating endothelial cells: a new candidate biomarker of irreversible pulmonary hypertension secondary to congenital heart disease. Circulation 2009; 119(3):374–81.

45. Dinh Xuan AT, Higenbottam TW, Clelland C, et al. Impairment of pulmonary endothelium-dependent relaxation in patients with Eisenmenger's syndrome. Br J Pharmacol 1990;99(1):9–10.

46. Oechslin E, Kiowski W, Schindler R, et al. Systemic endothelial dysfunction in adults with cyanotic congenital heart disease. Circulation 2005;112(8): 1106–12.

47. Martinez-Quintana E, Rodriguez-Gonzalez F, Fabregas-Brouard M, et al. Serum and 24-hour urine analysis in adult cyanotic and noncyanotic congenital heart disease patients. Congenit Heart Dis 2009;4(3):147–52.

48. Sietsema KE, Cooper DM, Perloff JK, et al. Dynamics of oxygen uptake during exercise in adults with cyanotic congenital heart disease. Circulation 1986;73(6):1137–44.

49. Dimopoulos K, Okonko DO, Diller GP, et al. Abnormal ventilatory response to exercise in adults with congenital heart disease relates to cyanosis and predicts survival. Circulation 2006;113(24): 2796–802.

50. Sandoval J, Alvarado P, Martinez-Guerra ML, et al. Effect of body position changes on pulmonary gas exchange in Eisenmenger's syndrome. Am J Respir Crit Care Med 1999;159(4 Pt 1):1070–3.

51. Sietsema KE, Cooper DM, Perloff JK, et al. Control of ventilation during exercise in patients with central venous-to-systemic arterial shunts. J Appl Physiol 1988;64(1):234–42.

52. Yang-Ting S, Aboulhosn J, Sun XG, et al. Effects of pulmonary vasodilator therapy on ventilatory efficiency during exercise in adults with Eisenmenger syndrome. Congenit Heart Dis 2011;6(2): 139–46.

53. Ramakrishnan S, Juneja R, Bardolei N, et al. Nocturnal hypoxaemia in patients with Eisenmenger syndrome: a cohort study. BMJ Open 2013;3(3). Available at: http://www.biomedsearch.com/attachments/00/23/48/29/23482988/bmjopen-2012-002039.pdf.

54. Sandoval J, Aguirre JS, Pulido T, et al. Nocturnal oxygen therapy in patients with the Eisenmenger syndrome. Am J Respir Crit Care Med 2001; 164(9):1682–7.

55. Dimopoulos K, Diller GP, Koltsida E, et al. Prevalence, predictors, and prognostic value of renal dysfunction in adults with congenital heart disease. Circulation 2008;117(18):2320–8.

56. Scott HW Jr, Elliott SR 2nd. Renal hemodynamics in congenital cyanotic heart disease. Bull Johns Hopkins Hosp 1950;86(1):58–71.

57. Malizia E. Renal function and hemodynamics in primary and secondary polycythemia. Acta Med Scand 1956;154(5):399–406.

58. Thron CD, Chen J, Leiter JC, et al. Renovascular adaptive changes in chronic hypoxic polycythemia. Kidney Int 1998;54(6):2014–20.

59. Dittrich S, Kurschat K, Lange PE. Abnormal rheology in cyanotic congenital heart disease–a factor in non-immune nephropathy. Scand J Urol Nephrol 2001;35(5):411–5.

60. Wilcox CS, Payne J, Harrison BD. Renal function in patients with chronic hypoxaemia and cor pulmonale following reversal of polycythaemia. Nephron 1982;30(2):173–7.

61. Ross EA, Perloff JK, Danovitch GM, et al. Renal function and urate metabolism in late survivors with cyanotic congenital heart disease. Circulation 1986;73(3):396–400.

62. Oya H, Nagaya N, Satoh T, et al. Haemodynamic correlates and prognostic significance of serum uric acid in adult patients with Eisenmenger syndrome. Heart 2000;84(1):53–8.

63. Hayabuchi Y, Matsuoka S, Akita H, et al. Hyperuricaemia in cyanotic congenital heart disease. Eur J Pediatr 1993;152(11):873–6.

64. Daliento L, Somerville J, Presbitero P, et al. Eisenmenger syndrome. Factors relating to deterioration and death. Eur Heart J 1998;19(12):1845–55.

65. Niwa K, Perloff JK, Kaplan S, et al. Eisenmenger syndrome in adults: ventricular septal defect, truncus arteriosus, univentricular heart. J Am Coll Cardiol 1999;34(1):223–32.

66. Traustason S, Jensen AS, Arvidsson HS, et al. Retinal oxygen saturation in patients with systemic hypoxemia. Invest Ophthalmol Vis Sci 2011;52(8): 5064–7.

67. Petersen RA, Rosenthal A. Retinopathy and papilledema in cyanotic congenital heart disease. Pediatrics 1972;49(2):243–9.

68. Rutter TW, Mullin V. Pheochromocytoma in a patient with Eisenmenger's complex. Anesth Analg 1991; 73(4):496–8.

69. Lumbiganon P, Chaikitpinyo A. Antibiotics for brain abscesses in people with cyanotic congenital heart disease. Cochrane Database Syst Rev 2013;(3):CD004469.

70. Rosenthal A, Fellows KE. Acute infectious sinusitis in cyanotic congenital heart disease. Pediatrics 1973;52(5):692–6.

71. Kaur C, Ling EA. Blood brain barrier in hypoxic-ischemic conditions. Curr Neurovasc Res 2008; 5(1):71–81.

72. Dedkov EI, Perloff JK, Tomanek RJ, et al. The coronary microcirculation in cyanotic congenital heart disease. Circulation 2006;114(3):196–200.

73. Perloff JK. The coronary circulation in cyanotic congenital heart disease. Int J Cardiol 2004; 97(Suppl 1):79–86.

74. Chugh R, Perloff JK, Fishbein M, et al. Extramural coronary arteries in adults with cyanotic congenital heart disease. Am J Cardiol 2004;94(10): 1355–7.

75. Fyfe A, Perloff JK, Niwa K, et al. Cyanotic congenital heart disease and coronary artery atherogenesis. Am J Cardiol 2005;96(2):283–90.

76. Savransky V, Nanayakkara A, Li J, et al. Chronic intermittent hypoxia induces atherosclerosis. Am J Respir Crit Care Med 2007;175(12):1290–7.

77. Sluimer JC, Daemen MJ. Novel concepts in atherogenesis: angiogenesis and hypoxia in atherosclerosis. J Pathol 2009;218(1):7–29.

78. Martinez-Quintana E, Rodriguez-Gonzalez F, Nieto-Lago V, et al. Serum glucose and lipid levels in adult congenital heart disease patients. Metabolism 2010;59(11):1642–8.

79. Hopkins WE. The remarkable right ventricle of patients with Eisenmenger syndrome. Coron Artery Dis 2005;16(1):19–25.

80. Kalogeropoulos AP, Border WL, Georgiopoulou VV, et al. Right ventricular function in adult patients with Eisenmenger physiology: insights from quantitative echocardiography. Echocardiography 2010;27(8): 937–45.

81. Becker-Grunig T, Klose H, Ehlken N, et al. Efficacy of exercise training in pulmonary arterial hypertension associated with congenital heart disease. Int J Cardiol 2013;168(1):375–81.

82. Ammash N, Warnes CA. Cerebrovascular events in adult patients with cyanotic congenital heart disease. J Am Coll Cardiol 1996;28(3):768–72.

83. Broberg CS, Bax BE, Okonko DO, et al. Blood viscosity and its relationship to iron deficiency, symptoms, and exercise capacity in adults with cyanotic congenital heart disease. J Am Coll Cardiol 2006; 48(2):356–65.

84. Tay EL, Peset A, Papaphylactou M, et al. Replacement therapy for iron deficiency improves exercise capacity and quality of life in patients with cyanotic congenital heart disease and/or the Eisenmenger syndrome. Int J Cardiol 2011;151(3):307–12.

85. Broberg CS, Jayaweera AR, Diller GP, et al. Seeking optimal relation between oxygen saturation and hemoglobin concentration in adults with cyanosis from congenital heart disease. Am J Cardiol 2011;107(4):595–9.

86. Wimmer M, Schlemmer M. Long-term hemodynamic effects of nifedipine on congenital heart disease with Eisenmenger's mechanism in children. Cardiovasc Drugs Ther 1992;6(2):183–6.

87. Fernandes SM, Newburger JW, Lang P, et al. Usefulness of epoprostenol therapy in the severely ill adolescent/adult with Eisenmenger physiology. Am J Cardiol 2003;91(5):632–5.

88. Apostolopoulou SC, Manginas A, Cokkinos DV, et al. Long-term oral bosentan treatment in patients with pulmonary arterial hypertension related to congenital heart disease: a 2-year study. Heart 2007;93(3):350–4.

89. Benza RL, Rayburn BK, Tallaj JA, et al. Efficacy of bosentan in a small cohort of adult patients with pulmonary arterial hypertension related to congenital heart disease. Chest 2006;129(4): 1009–15.

90. Christensen DD, McConnell ME, Book WM, et al. Initial experience with bosentan therapy in patients with the Eisenmenger syndrome. Am J Cardiol 2004;94(2):261–3.

91. D'Alto M, Vizza CD, Romeo E, et al. Long term effects of bosentan treatment in adult patients with pulmonary arterial hypertension related to congenital heart disease (Eisenmenger physiology): safety, tolerability, clinical, and haemodynamic effect. Heart 2007;93(5):621–5.

92. Diller GP, Dimopoulos K, Kaya MG, et al. Long-term safety, tolerability and efficacy of bosentan in adults with pulmonary arterial hypertension associated with congenital heart disease. Heart 2007; 93(8):974–6.

93. Gatzoulis MA, Rogers P, Li W, et al. Safety and tolerability of bosentan in adults with Eisenmenger physiology. Int J Cardiol 2005;98(1):147–51.

94. Kotlyar E, Sy R, Keogh AM, et al. Bosentan for the treatment of pulmonary arterial hypertension associated with congenital cardiac disease. Cardiol Young 2006;16(3):268–74.

95. Schulze-Neick I, Gilbert N, Ewert R, et al. Adult patients with congenital heart disease and pulmonary arterial hypertension: first open prospective multicenter study of bosentan therapy. Am Heart J 2005;150(4):716.

96. Sitbon O, Beghetti M, Petit J, et al. Bosentan for the treatment of pulmonary arterial hypertension associated with congenital heart defects. Eur J Clin Invest 2006;36(Suppl 3):25–31.

97. van Loon RL, Hoendermis ES, Duffels MG, et al. Long-term effect of bosentan in adults versus children with pulmonary arterial hypertension associated with systemic-to-pulmonary shunt: does the beneficial effect persist? Am Heart J 2007;154(4): 776–82.

98. Zuckerman WA, Leaderer D, Rowan CA, et al. Ambrisentan for pulmonary arterial hypertension due to congenital heart disease. Am J Cardiol 2011; 107(9):1381–5.

99. Chau EM, Fan KY, Chow WH. Effects of chronic sildenafil in patients with Eisenmenger syndrome

versus idiopathic pulmonary arterial hypertension. Int J Cardiol 2007;120(3):301–5.

100. Lu XL, Xiong CM, Shan GL, et al. Impact of sildenafil therapy on pulmonary arterial hypertension in adults with congenital heart disease. Cardiovasc Ther 2010;28(6):350–5.

101. Tay EL, Papaphylactou M, Diller GP, et al. Quality of life and functional capacity can be improved in patients with Eisenmenger syndrome with oral sildenafil therapy. Int J Cardiol 2011;149(3): 372–6.

102. Zhang ZN, Jiang X, Zhang R, et al. Oral sildenafil treatment for Eisenmenger syndrome: a prospective, open-label, multicentre study. Heart 2011; 97(22):1876–81.

103. Mukhopadhyay S, Nathani S, Yusuf J, et al. Clinical efficacy of phosphodiesterase-5 inhibitor tadalafil in Eisenmenger syndrome–a randomized, placebo-controlled, double-blind crossover study. Congenit Heart Dis 2011;6(5):424–31.

104. Singh TP, Rohit M, Grover A, et al. A randomized, placebo-controlled, double-blind, crossover study to evaluate the efficacy of oral sildenafil therapy in severe pulmonary artery hypertension. Am Heart J 2006;151(4):851.e1–5.

105. Gatzoulis MA, Beghetti M, Galie N, et al. Longer-term bosentan therapy improves functional capacity in Eisenmenger syndrome: results of the BREATHE-5 open-label extension study. Int J Cardiol 2008;127(1):27–32.

106. Galie N, Beghetti M, Gatzoulis MA, et al. Bosentan therapy in patients with Eisenmenger syndrome: a multicenter, double-blind, randomized, placebo-controlled study. Circulation 2006;114(1):48–54.

107. Berger RM, Beghetti M, Galie N, et al. Atrial septal defects versus ventricular septal defects in BREATHE-5, a placebo-controlled study of pulmonary arterial hypertension related to Eisenmenger's syndrome: a subgroup analysis. Int J Cardiol 2010; 144(3):373–8.

108. Diller GP, Alonso-Gonzalez R, Dimopoulos K, et al. Disease targeting therapies in patients with Eisenmenger syndrome: response to treatment and long-term efficiency. Int J Cardiol 2013;167(3): 840–7.

109. Dimopoulos K, Inuzuka R, Goletto S, et al. Improved survival among patients with Eisenmenger syndrome receiving advanced therapy for pulmonary arterial hypertension. Circulation 2010;121(1):20–5.

110. Kempny A, Dimopoulos K, Alonso-Gonzalez R, et al. Six Minute Walk Test Distance and Resting Oxygen Saturation but not Functional Class Predict Outcome in Adult Patients with Eisenmenger Syndrome. Int J Cardiol 2013. [Epub ahead of print].

111. D'Alto M, Romeo E, Argiento P, et al. Bosentan-sildenafil association in patients with congenital heart disease-related pulmonary arterial hypertension and Eisenmenger physiology. Int J Cardiol 2012; 155(3):378–82.

112. Iversen K, Jensen AS, Jensen TV, et al. Combination therapy with bosentan and sildenafil in Eisenmenger syndrome: a randomized, placebo-controlled, double-blinded trial. Eur Heart J 2010;31(9):1124–31.

113. Batista RJ, Santos JL, Takeshita N, et al. Successful reversal of pulmonary hypertension in Eisenmenger complex. Arq Bras Cardiol 1997;68(4): 279–80.

114. Lin MT, Chen YS, Huang SC, et al. Alternative approach for selected severe pulmonary hypertension of congenital heart defect without initial correction–palliative surgical treatment. Int J Cardiol 2011;151(3):313–7.

115. Burkhart HM, Dearani JA, Williams WG, et al. Late results of palliative atrial switch for transposition, ventricular septal defect, and pulmonary vascular obstructive disease. Ann Thorac Surg 2004;77(2): 464–8 [discussion: 468–9].

116. Baruteau AE, Serraf A, Levy M, et al. Potts shunt in children with idiopathic pulmonary arterial hypertension: long-term results. Ann Thorac Surg 2012; 94(3):817–24.

117. Esch JJ, Shah PB, Cockrill BA, et al. Transcatheter Potts shunt creation in patients with severe pulmonary arterial hypertension: initial clinical experience. J Heart Lung Transplant 2013;32(4):381–7.

118. Labombarda F, Maragnes P, Dupont-Chauvet P, et al. Potts anastomosis for children with idiopathic pulmonary hypertension. Pediatr Cardiol 2009; 30(8):1143–5.

119. Gorenflo M, Gu H, Xu Z. Peri-operative pulmonary hypertension in paediatric patients: current strategies in children with congenital heart disease. Cardiology 2010;116(1):10–7.

120. Huang JB, Liu YL, Yu CT, et al. Lung biopsy findings in previously inoperable patients with severe pulmonary hypertension associated with congenital heart disease. Int J Cardiol 2011; 151(1):76–83.

121. Waddell TK, Bennett L, Kennedy R, et al. Heart-lung or lung transplantation for Eisenmenger syndrome. J Heart Lung Transplant 2002;21(7):731–7.

122. Reitz BA, Wallwork JL, Hunt SA, et al. Heart-lung transplantation: successful therapy for patients with pulmonary vascular disease. N Engl J Med 1982;306(10):557–64.

123. Stoica SC, McNeil KD, Perreas K, et al. Heart-lung transplantation for Eisenmenger syndrome: early and long-term results. Ann Thorac Surg 2001; 72(6):1887–91.

Failure of the Fontan Circulation

Marc Gewillig, MD, PhD[a],*, David J. Goldberg, MD[b]

KEYWORDS

- Fontan circulation • Chronic low output • Circulatory failure • Pulmonary vascular resistance

KEY POINTS

- The essence of a Fontan circuit is the creation of the Fontan "neoportal system": this allows for oxygenation at near normal levels, but at the cost of a chronic state of systemic venous congestion and decreased cardiac output.
- The heart, while still the engine of the circuit, cannot compensate for this major flow restriction: the ventricle has lost control of the output and of systemic venous congestion; systolic and diastolic ventricular dysfunction are common and may contribute to overall circulatory failure.
- The abnormal hemodynamics inherent in the Fontan circulation affect organs outside the heart and may lead to liver cirrhosis, protein-losing enteropathy, or plastic bronchitis.
- Failure of the Fontan is progressive; over time there is an insidious increase in both pulmonary vascular resistance and ventricular end-diastolic pressure, which may lead to progressive functional impairment.

THE "FONTAN" CONCEPT

A normal mammalian cardiovascular system consists of a double circuit, pulmonary and systemic, connected in series and powered by a double pump. In the absence of congenital heart disease, the right ventricle pumps to the pulmonary circulation and the left ventricle pumps to the systemic circulation (**Fig. 1A**).

Many complex cardiac malformations are characterized by the existence of only one functional ventricle. This single ventricle has to maintain both the systemic and the pulmonary circulations, which at birth are not connected in series but in parallel (see **Fig. 1B**). Such a circuit has 2 major disadvantages: diminished oxygen saturation of the systemic arterial blood and a chronic volume load to the single ventricle. The chronic ventricular volume load will lead to progressive impairment of

ventricular function and altered pulmonary vasculature, causing a gradual attrition resulting from congestive heart failure and pulmonary hypertension from the third decade, with few survivors beyond the fourth decade.

In 1971, Francis Fontan[1] from Bordeaux, France, reported a new approach to the operative treatment of these malformations, separating the systemic and pulmonary circulations. In a "Fontan circulation" the systemic venous return is connected to the pulmonary arteries without the interposition of a pumping chamber (see **Fig. 1C**). In this construct, residual postcapillary energy is used to push blood through the lungs in a new portal-like system.[2] Advantages of a Fontan circuit include (near) normalization of the arterial oxygen saturation, and abolishment of the chronic volume load on the single ventricle. However, because venous return through the pulmonary vasculature

[a] Leuven University Hospital, Pediatric and Congenital Cardiology, Herestraat 49, Leuven B 3000, Belgium;
[b] Division of Cardiology, The Children's Hospital of Philadelphia, 34th Street and Civic Center Boulevard, Philadelphia, PA 19104, USA
* Corresponding author.
E-mail address: marc.gewillig@uzleuven.be

Heart Failure Clin 10 (2014) 105–116
http://dx.doi.org/10.1016/j.hfc.2013.09.010
1551-7136/14/$ – see front matter © 2014 Elsevier Inc. All rights reserved.

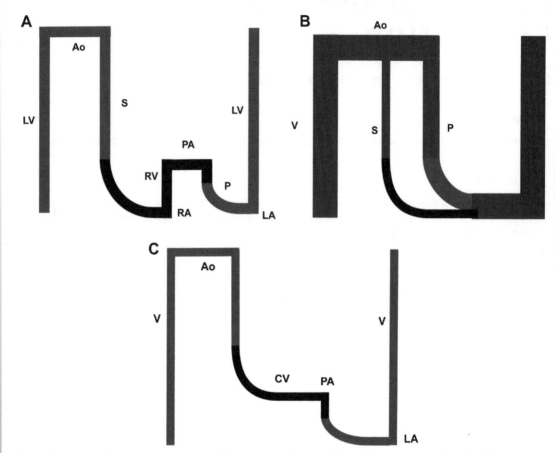

Fig. 1. Normal cardiovascular circulation (*A*), shunted palliation (*B*), and Fontan circulation (*C*). (*A*) Normal circulation. The pulmonary circulation (P) is connected in series with the systemic circulation (S). The right ventricle maintains the right atrial pressure lower than the left atrial pressure, and provides enough energy for the blood to pass through the pulmonary resistance. (*B*) Shunted palliation. The systemic (S) and pulmonary (P) circuits are connected in parallel, with a considerable volume overload to the single ventricle. There is complete admixture of systemic and pulmonary venous blood, causing arterial oxygen desaturation. (*C*) Fontan circuit. The systemic veins (V) are connected to the pulmonary artery, without a subpulmonary ventricle or systemic atrium. The lungs are thereby converted into a neoportal system, which limits flow to the ventricle. In the absence of a fenestration, there is no admixture of systemic and pulmonary venous blood, but the systemic venous pressures are markedly elevated. A fenestration allows the systemic venous blood to bypass the Fontan portal system and limits the damming effect, thereby increasing output and decreasing congestion, but also arterial saturation. Ao, aorta; CV, caval veins; F, fenestration; LA, left atrium; LV, left ventricle; PA, pulmonary artery; RA, right atrium; RV, right ventricle; V, single ventricle. Line thickness reflects output, color reflects oxygen saturation.

is hindered by the pulmonary impedance, this circulation creates a state of chronic hypertension and congestion in the systemic veins, and results in decreased cardiac output, both at rest and during exercise (**Fig. 2**).[3,4] It is these 2 inherent features of the Fontan circulation, elevated systemic venous pressure and chronically low cardiac output, which are the root cause of most of the physiologic impairments, collectively termed Fontan failure.

CARDIAC OUTPUT IN THE FONTAN CIRCULATION

By creating a total cavopulmonary connection, a new portal system is made. A portal system occurs when one capillary bed pools blood into another capillary bed through veins without passing through the heart; for example, the hepatic portal system and the hypophyseal portal system. The Fontan neoportal system dams off and pools the systemic venous blood. As a result, transit of

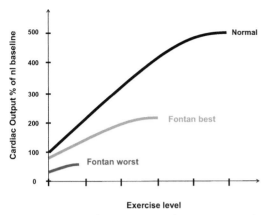

Fig. 2. Exercise and output: normal versus Fontan circulation. A normal subject with a biventricular circuit can increase his output by a factor of 5 (*black line*). In Fontan patients, output is significantly impaired both at rest and during exercise; at best (*green line*), the output is mildly decreased at rest, with moderate capacity to increase flow during moderate exercise. At worst (*red line*), the output is severely reduced at rest and barely augments during minimal exercise.

blood through this neoportal system depends on the pressure gradient from the systemic postcapillary vessels to the pulmonary postcapillary vessels (see **Fig. 1**C). As there is no pump to add energy to the system, small changes in the static resistances and dynamic impedances of the structures within this portal system have a profound impact on the blood flow.

Fontan failure is different from pure systolic or diastolic heart failure in that although the heart itself may function well, the inherent limitations of the Fontan neoportal system determine the degree of circulatory compromise. It is this neoportal system that is the limiting factor of flow, and the underlying cause of venous congestion and diminished cardiac output. The heart, while still the engine of the circuit, cannot compensate for this major flow restriction: the suction required to compensate for the damming effect of the Fontan portal system cannot be generated. The heart therefore no longer controls cardiac output, nor can it alter the degree of systemic venous congestion. In cases where the systemic ventricle functions poorly, the heart can make an already compromised circulation worse. **Fig. 3** illustrates the relationship between output, ventricular contractility, and pulmonary vascular resistance (PVR).

The components that make up the Fontan neoportal system are critically important in the overall function of the Fontan circuit. These components include the venoarterial Fontan connection itself (atriopulmonary in older patients), pulmonary arteries, pulmonary capillary network (including precapillary sphincters), pulmonary veins, and the venoatrial connection. Impairment at any level of this portal system will have profound consequences on the output of the Fontan circuit, much more so than a comparable dysfunction in a 2-ventricle circulation. These impairments

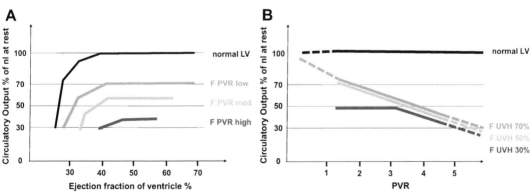

Fig. 3. (*A, B*) Relationship of output at rest, ventricular function, and pulmonary vascular resistance (PVR). (*A*) Modulation by PVR. In a normal subject (*black line*), output at rest is minimally influenced by ventricular function, except when severely depressed. In Fontan patients (*colored lines*), PVR is the primary modulator of cardiac output. As in a 2-ventricle system, systolic performance will only affect output at rest when cardiac function is severely depressed. If ventricular function is not severely depressed, squeezing harder will not result in more output. (*B*) Modulation by ventricular function. In a normal subject (*black line*), cardiac output is not influenced by a mild increase of PVR up to 5 Woods Units. In all Fontan patients (*colored lines*), an increase in PVR is invariably associated with a decrease in cardiac output. If PVR is low, a reasonable output is achieved in patients with normal or moderately depressed ventricular function (*green and yellow lines*). However, severely depressed ventricular function invariably results in low output (*red line*). F, Fontan; LV, left ventricle; PVR, pulmonary vascular resistance; UVH, univentricular heart.

include, but are not limited to, stenosis, hypoplasia, distortion, vasoconstriction, pulmonary vascular disease, loss or exclusion of large or microvessels, turbulence and flow collision, flow mismatch, and obstruction by external compression.

The restriction to cardiac output imposed by the neoportal system can be partially reversed by by-passing the pulmonary vasculature. A Fontan fenestration allows flow to bypass the Fontan neo-portal system, resulting in an increase in cardiac output and a decrease in venous congestion. However, while a fenestration can increase overall output, it does so at the expense of diminished arterial oxygen saturation. Nevertheless, in the setting of a fenestration, the increase in cardiac output can result in an increase in peripheral oxygen delivery even if the saturation is mildly diminished. **Fig. 4** shows the relationship between output, congestion, and arterial saturation in a good and bad (failing) Fontan circuit, and the effect of partial undoing by a fenestration. In a good Fontan circuit, the low-resistance portal system will cause a mild decrease of output with modest increase in systemic venous pressures, making a fenestration unnecessary. In a bad Fontan circuit, inclusion of a high vascular resistance portal system will decrease output and create venous congestion to unacceptable levels; a fenestration will attenuate these changes, but in bad candi-dates with increased PVR an acceptable compro-mise may not be possible.

FUNCTIONAL IMPAIRMENT AFTER THE FONTAN OPERATION

The restriction to cardiac output and the inability to power blood through the pulmonary vasculature results in a circulation whereby the ability to per-form exercise is reduced. Under resting condi-tions, cardiac output in a patient with a Fontan circulation is approximately 70% to 80% of what would be normal for age or body surface area. During exercise, the limitations of the Fontan cir-cuit are substantially magnified such that the small differences in cardiac output at rest become much larger differences in cardiac output during activity (see **Fig. 2**). At peak exercise, a well-trained athlete with a normal heart can increase blood flow through the lungs by up to 5-fold. This increased flow is accomplished through a substantial in-crease in right ventricular systolic pressure (up to 70 mm Hg![5]) as well as flow acceleration coupled with a decrease in PVR. In a patient with Fontan physiology, there is no physiologic mechanism to allow for a similar increase in cardiac output: the maximal mean venous pressure rarely reaches 30 mm Hg, there is no blood acceleration, and the reactivity of PVR is attenuated or absent.[6] In combination, these limitations result in a dimin-ished ability to augment cardiac output in res-ponse to increased metabolic demand, and therefore limit the ability of a patient with a Fontan to perform exercise.

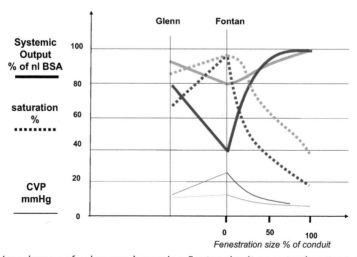

Fig. 4. Effect of various degrees of pulmonary bypass in a Fontan circuit on systemic output, saturation, and sys-temic venous congestion. A "good Fontan" with low neoportal resistance (*green lines*) has an output (*thick solid lines*) of about 80% of normal for body surface area (BSA), with a high saturation (*dotted lines*) and a mildly elevated central venous pressure (CVP) (*thin lines*). The "bad Fontan" with a high portal resistance has an output with a similar saturation, but with a very low to unacceptable output despite a high CVP. Partial bypassing of the Fontan portal system by a fenestration invariably increases systemic output and decreases systemic congestion, but in the "bad Fontan" this occurs at an unacceptable degree of cyanosis.

Through childhood and until puberty, the mean maximal exercise capacity for patients with a Fontan circulation is in the range of 65% predicted for gender and age.[7] The situation worsens as patients pass through puberty and their body composition changes while the efficiency of the Fontan circuit diminishes. Whereas good Fontan patients may remain stable for many years, poor Fontan patients suffer an accelerated increase of PVR and increasing filling pressures of the ventricle as a result of chronic preload deprivation with disuse hypofunction. Longitudinal studies of late adolescents and young adults demonstrate this point well; as patients progress to late adolescence and early adulthood, exercise capacity tends to continue to decline by about 2.6% predicted per year.[8]

The impact of the functional impairment of the Fontan patient may only limit activities at first, but at an advanced stage is predictive of the need for hospitalization and, possibly, death and/or the need for transplant. In many forms of congenital heart disease, an exercise capacity of 45% to 50% predicted appears to be the cutoff for the development of symptoms of heart failure.[9] In the Fontan physiology, assuming a starting point of 65% predicted for age at the onset of puberty and a decline of 2.6% per year thereafter, the cutoff of 45% predicted can be expected to be reached at the end of the second decade of life. Not surprisingly, this is fairly close to what is actually reported. Diller and colleagues[10] followed 321 patients with various Fontan connections for a median of 21 months. The mean age of patients at the onset of the study was 21 years, with a maximal predicted oxygen consumption of 52%. Not surprisingly, during the follow-up period 41% of patients required hospitalization for heart failure and 9% of patients either died or underwent heart transplantation.

Although the exercise data and the rate of functional decline suggest significant impairment by the end of the second decade, there are several reasons why adults with a Fontan circuit in the current era do not reflect where the current cohort of patients will be in several decades. Many of the original candidates for a Fontan operation, the current adult cohort, were suboptimal for this type of surgery from a hemodynamic standpoint, with many significant residual lesions and sequelae related to the original cardiac malformation and palliative procedures. A shunt procedure performed during the period from the 1960s to the 1980s was evaluated based on the goal of the long-term relief of cyanosis: "the pinker the better." Often a second aortopulmonary shunt was created to augment pulmonary blood flow after the first shunt was deemed inadequate. The idea that these shunts could induce pulmonary vascular disease, ventricular overgrowth, hypertrophy and dysfunction, or pulmonary artery distortion was not—as it is now—a principal preoccupation of the surgeon. At present, the success of a shunt is evaluated by obtaining acceptable relief of cyanosis without significant volume overload to the ventricle, and by the induction of adequate pulmonary growth without causing changes to PVR. In addition, in the modern palliation the systemic to pulmonary shunt is designed to last 4 to 6 months, enough time to allow vascular resistance to drop such that a partial cavopulmonary connection can safely be created. **Fig. 5** illustrates the different loading conditions of the single ventricle at the various stages of palliation, highlighting the differences in management before the 1990s (typically 2 aortopulmonary shunts before full Fontan) and after (typically 1 shunt, then partial and later complete Fontan).

THE HEART AND PULMONARY VASCULATURE IN THE FONTAN CIRCULATION
The Heart

In the Fontan construct, the heart is exposed to several stressors that can result in altered structure and impaired function. Chronic preload deprivation and increased systemic vascular resistance create a milieu that favors development of both systolic and diastolic dysfunction. Although the heart is not the primary determinant of cardiac output after the Fontan, alterations in cardiac function can result in functional impairments beyond what might be expected from the Fontan construct itself, and so cannot be overlooked.

Over the long term, systolic dysfunction of the single ventricle results from both decreased preload and the chronic impact of pumping against increased resistance. The effects of chronic deprivation are significantly aggravated by the ventricle being overgrown by the time it reaches the Fontan state.[4] This combination leads to a situation whereby the optimal point for contractility on the Frank-Starling preload-contractility curve cannot be achieved and the heart appears both under-filled and hypertrophied; an "overgrown pump."[11] In addition to the factors related to the limitations of the Fontan physiology, the single ventricle may also exhibit systolic dysfunction as a result of the malformation itself (right vs left ventricle, fiber disarray), or as a result of overgrowth and damage by the volume or pressure overload state that was present early in the palliative course.

Diastolic function after the Fontan is also typically abnormal, and the impairment is progressive. The unloading of the ventricle at the time of the

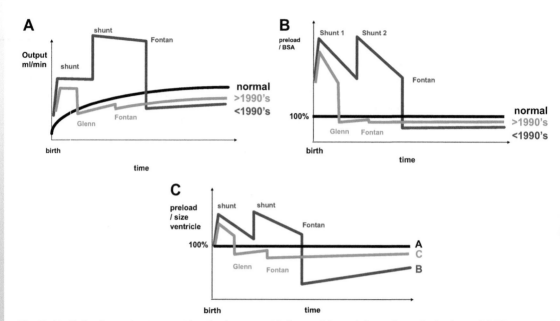

Fig. 5. (*A–C*) Cardiac output versus time in the normal left ventricle and the univentricular heart (UVH) managed before and after the 1990s. Each graph tells the same story but expressed with a different reference frame: in absolute value (*A*), related to BSA (*B*), and related to ventricular size (*C*). (*A*) Cardiac output expressed as absolute value: The black line shows output of a normal ventricle, which increases proportional to growth. At birth the volume load to the UVH is about 250% to 300% of that of a normal left ventricle. Before the 1990s, a neonatal and infant large shunt is created with significant increase in output (*red line*); the shunts are abolished at the time of the Fontan operation, and the Fontan portal dam reduces preload even further. After the 1990s, a small neonatal shunt is created for a short time, and the ventricle is progressively unloaded at both the Glenn and the Fontan operation (*green line*). (*B*) Cardiac output related to BSA. Black line: output of normal remains at 100% for body surface area (BSA). This representation assumes only dilation and stretch without any overgrowth of the ventricle. The patient with a UVH is born with a large ventricle (volume load of 250% of normal for BSA). Before the 1990s (*red line*), the preload to the ventricle is augmented shortly after birth by a shunt procedure to ±350% of normal for BSA. The patient slowly outgrows his shunt, thereby gradually reducing the volume overload. A second shunt is created, augmenting the volume overload again. As this patient again outgrows his shunt, a Fontan circuit is made, reducing the volume load to less than 80%. After the 1990s (*green line*), a small neonatal shunt is created for a short time; the patient slowly outgrows his shunt, and the ventricle is progressively unloaded at both the Glenn and Fontan operation (*green line*). (*C*) Cardiac output related to ventricular size. This representation assumes adapted overgrowth of the ventricle at every stage in the function of chronic preload, A: output of normal remains at 100% for ventricular size. The patient with a UVH is born with an appropriate ventricle for volume load (100% of normal for ventricular size). Before the 1990s (*B, red line*), the preload to the ventricle is augmented shortly after birth by a shunt procedure to ±150%. The patient slowly outgrows his shunt and adapts his ventricle, thereby gradually reducing the volume overload to ±100% for its size. A second shunt is created, augmenting the volume overload again to 150%. As this patient again outgrows his shunt, a Fontan circuit is made, reducing the volume load to 25% of its "due" preload. After the 1990s (*C, green line*), a small neonatal shunt is created for a short time; the patient slowly outgrows his shunt, and the ventricle is progressively unloaded at both the Glenn and Fontan operation in much milder steps, avoiding acute unloading and severe deprivation.

Fontan procedure results in less recoil, impaired compliance, and decreased suction in the acute phase.[12] Owing to persistent preload deprivation, the pressure-volume curve may show "reversed creep," with an upward shift and increasing filling pressures (**Fig. 6**). The ventricle may now enter a vicious cycle whereby the chronic low preload results in remodeling, reduced compliance with increasing diastolic pressures, poor ventricular filling, and, eventually, progressively declining cardiac output. This phenomenon of progressive "disuse hypofunction" occurs at a chronic preload of less than 70% of the preload expected for ventricular size.[13]

The response of the heart to the stressors associated with the Fontan operation appears to be heterogeneous. In some patients the heart can appear fairly normal for many years, and function

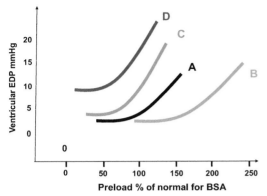

Fig. 6. Ventricular end-diastolic pressure (EDP) in various phases of ventricle. A, normal ventricle; B, shunted ventricle with chronic volume overload leading to enhanced compliance; C, Fontan ventricle after acute phase, with mild preload deprivation of the overgrown ventricle; D, Fontan ventricle with low output as a result of severe chronic preload deprivation, leading to elevated filling pressures.

may be relatively well preserved, whereas in other patients the ventricle appears thickly trabeculated and "overgrown" starting at, or even before, the time of Fontan surgery. The variability may be related in part to native anatomy or myocardial disarray from conformation changes resulting from the palliative surgeries preceding the Fontan, but there may also be a genetic heterogeneity in the response of an individual to the stressors associated with single-ventricle physiology. Polymorphisms in the renin-angiotensin-aldosterone system have been shown to have measurable impact on ventricular hypertrophy and on the response of the myocardium to treatment with angiotensin-converting enzyme inhibitors.[14] It may be that these and other unmeasured genetic variants are in part responsible for the variable response of the heart to the Fontan circulation. However, even for those in whom the genetic pre-programming is favorable, the basic physiology of the Fontan will invariably lead to some element of progressive systolic and diastolic dysfunction.

The Pulmonary Vasculature

Abnormal growth and development of the pulmonary vasculature are a hallmark of single-ventricle congenital heart disease. Decreased flow to the pulmonary arterial tree may begin during fetal life, depending on the specific lesion, and will certainly exist by necessity after the first stage of palliation during partial or complete cavopulmonary connection (**Fig. 7**). As a result, hypoplasia of the pulmonary vascular bed is common. Stenosis resulting from abnormal connections, ductal constriction, or surgical scarring can further

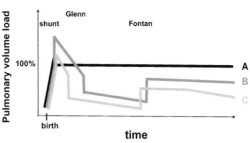

Fig. 7. Pulmonary volume load (and outcome) of Fontan since the 1990s. In the normal circulation, pulmonary blood flow increases at birth and remains at 100% of normal for BSA (A, black line). In a univentricular heart, a phase of significant pulmonary overflow exists immediately after birth until a shunt or band is placed to limit blood flow. With adequate pulmonary growth (B, green line), pulmonary blood flow is reduced to about 50% of normal for BSA after the superior cavopulmonary connection (stage 2 palliation). Pulmonary flow is then increased by completion of the total cavopulmonary connection (the Fontan operation). If flow to the lungs is too low after the initial palliation, this may result in inadequate growth (C, orange line). The cyanosis from low pulmonary blood flow may lead to early referral for superior cavopulmonary connection, which may further reduce flow and growth. When the Fontan circuit is created, the Fontan portal system will have a high impedance, resulting in a poor Fontan circulation irrespective of the ventricular function, with low cardiac output and a progressive functional impairment.

compromise the normal pulmonary architecture. The loss of pulsatile flow after cavopulmonary connection complicates the matter further by affecting the usual vasoreactivity of the pulmonary bed. Ideally the lung vessels should be slightly oversized with low resistance. However, more frequently the abnormal development may result in relative hypoplasia of the large vessels coupled with endothelial dysfunction. The chronic low-flow conditions will induce an overall state of pulmonary (and systemic) vasoconstriction, bringing the whole circuit into a negative spiral. Failing Fontans typically have a high PVR, although this is often reversible after transplantation (higher output of pulsatile flow).[15] The low-flow hemodynamic condition of the Fontan may also cause microthrombi, which further increase PVR.

SECONDARY COMPLICATIONS OF THE FONTAN CIRCULATION
Liver Fibrosis/Cirrhosis

The liver is in a particularly precarious state following the Fontan operation, as it is wedged between the capillary bed of the organs of the abdominal viscera and the capillary bed of the lungs. This placement results in substantially diminished perfusion of the liver from decreased portal flow, in addition the burden imposed by the chronic elevation in the pressure in the central veins of the liver.[16]

In recent years, the impact of abnormal flow patterns on the liver has become more evident. A large and growing number of imaging and histologic studies have demonstrated significant fibrosis and even frank cirrhosis in patients with the Fontan circulation.[17,18] In some cases this has led to the need for heart/liver transplant as end-stage therapy following Fontan failure, whereas in other cases changes to the liver parenchyma have resulted in malignant transformation of the hepatocytes and the development of hepatocellular carcinoma.[19]

The timing of the onset of the pathologic changes in the liver is variable. Reviews of autopsies performed in patients with Fontan failure demonstrate fibrotic changes even in fairly young patients.[20] However, there does also seem to be an element of time associated with liver changes, such that those who have lived with Fontan physiology for a longer duration seem to have more substantial disease.[21] This aspect suggests that changes in liver architecture may occur early in those with a complicated early course, while the Fontan physiology itself may result in slowly progressive changes on top of the burden imposed by the early years of multiple surgeries, congestion, and chronic hypoxemia.

Protein-Losing Enteropathy

In a circulation characterized by low cardiac output and high venous pressure, the gastrointestinal tract is at a particularly high risk for poor perfusion as the autoregulatory systems attempt to maintain perfusion to other vital organs. Poor perfusion and dilated lymphatic vessels, perhaps in combination with inflammation and a genetic predisposition, are thought to be responsible for the development of protein-losing enteropathy (PLE).[22] In support of this notion, investigators have described an increase in vascular resistance in children with Fontan physiology, even in those without PLE. In children with PLE this elevation in vascular resistance has been more pronounced, and results in a substantial decrease in both systolic and diastolic blood flow.

Although PLE can occur at any time after the Fontan, there appear to be 2 particular peaks in the onset of disease. The first peak occurs in the early years after the Fontan operation, and can occur in patients who seem otherwise reasonably well. In this group, treatment with oral controlled-release budesonide appears to result in some improvement in symptoms, with a normalization in protein levels after an induction period of several months.[23] The second peak in the onset of PLE is in late adolescence or early adulthood, and may occur more frequently in patients with more severely impaired hemodynamics. This group does not seem to be as responsive to steroids, suggesting that inflammation may not play as much of a role in the pathogenesis.[24] In this group, chronic dilation of the lymphatic system, as a result of the underlying hemodynamic abnormalities, likely plays a more pronounced role.

It is not yet clear why some patients develop PLE while others with similar hemodynamics are spared. However, the difficulty in predicting which patients will develop PLE points to the possibility of a prominent genetic predisposition. Recently, a diminished expression of glycosaminoglycan in the enterocytes of children with PLE has been suggested (Rychik J, unpublished data, 2013). This protein is essential for maintaining the integrity of the gut epithelium, and the underexpression may be a significant contributor to the pathophysiology of the disease. An altered expression of glycosaminoglycan would suggest either that those who develop PLE have a baseline deficiency in this protein, or that the inflammation and hemodynamic abnormalities of the Fontan operation result in altered expression.

While much remains to be understood about the development and pathophysiology of PLE in the Fontan population, it is clear that the development of this illness results in chronic debilitation and early death. Although new approaches to medical therapies have improved outcomes over the last 2 decades, there is still no definitive cure. Early cardiac transplantation has been used in some cases and does seem to be effective at eliminating the stimulus for the disease, but transplantation in this population is a high-risk endeavor with its own constellation of morbidities and a limited life span of graft.[25]

Plastic Bronchitis

In rare cases, the accumulation of proteinaceous material in the airways of patients with Fontan physiology may result in the formation of "casts" associated with plastic bronchitis. These casts can lead to acute obstruction of the airway, resulting in acute respiratory distress or airway compromise. The underlying pathophysiology of plastic bronchitis remains poorly understood, although abnormal connections between the lymphatics in the mediastinum and the airways are thought to contribute. Inhaled tissue plasminogen activator has been described as a medical treatment option to control the formation of plastic casts, likely by dissolving or breaking up the protein formations.[26] A case report describing the resolution of plastic bronchitis following thoracic duct ligation suggests that limiting lymphatic flow may also result in symptomatic improvement.[27] However, in severe intractable cases of plastic bronchitis, fenestration and cardiac transplantation have also been reported to result in resolution of symptoms.[28–30]

TREATMENT OF CIRCULATORY FAILURE IN FONTAN CIRCULATION

In "classical cardiology" with primary myocardial disease such as ischemic heart disease or cardiomyopathy, ventricular function is most frequently the limiting factor of cardiac output; typically ventricular preload is abundant. Most cardiac algorithms and treatment strategies have focused on augmenting systolic performance. However, in some conditions the systemic ventricle is not the limiting factor but rather the preload of that ventricle: obstructed inflow after Mustard repair, primary pulmonary hypertension, constrictive pericarditis, supravalvular and valvular mitral stenosis, and the Fontan circuit.

The circulatory problem in a Fontan circuit is primarily created by the damming effect of the Fontan neoportal system and the subsequent limit on cardiac preload. As such, strategies aimed at maximizing the efficiency of this portal system may be more effective than "traditional" heart-failure therapies. Such modulation may consist of increasing the pressure before the dam (systemic venous pressure), lowering the height (resistance of Fontan neoportal system) of the dam, enhancing the runoff after the dam (ventricular suction), or bypassing the dam (fenestration).

Elevated Systemic Venous Pressure (Increasing Pressure Before the Dam)

An acute increase of systemic venous pressure, as is achieved during exercise (up to 30 mm Hg), can temporarily increase output.[31] However, such an elevation cannot be maintained for a long time. A chronic elevation of venous pressures higher than 18 to 20 mm Hg, as in patients with a high-resistance Fontan portal circuit, will result in unacceptable side effects such as vascular congestion, edema, ascites, and lymphatic failure. Diuretics can partially control these complications of congestion, but may further increase the problems of low output. General aerobic fitness may play a role in the transient ability to increase central venous pressure, but even then the venous pressure cannot approximate the change in driving pressure that can be achieved by a subpulmonary ventricle.

Impedance and Pulmonary Vascular Resistance (Lowering the Height of the Dam)

In the current era, the surgical technique used to create a total cavopulmonary connection is usually satisfactory, with minimal focal stenoses, reduced turbulence, and flow of the inferior caval vein (with the "hepatic factor") to both lungs.[32,33] Previous connections, including valved pathways and atrial-ventricular-pulmonary connections, are now considered outdated or even obsolete. For those who received older-style Fontan operations, conversion to cavopulmonary connection should be considered when the patient becomes symptomatic, or even prophylactically, to limit any energy loss in the Fontan portal system[34,35] and to avoid recurrent atrial arrhythmias. Nevertheless, in the setting of elevated Fontan pressure or reduced physical capacity, care should be taken to ensure that focal areas of stenosis, hypoplasia, distortion, or abundant collateral flow are addressed when possible.

The total cross-sectional area of the pulmonary vascular bed is an important factor for Fontan efficiency, but one that is hard to modulate in the absence of a subpulmonary ventricle following Fontan. The first palliative procedure is probably the most important and crucial intervention in the development of the pulmonary vasculature in a patient with single-ventricle physiology (see **Fig. 7**). It is during these early days that pulmonary arterial growth is most likely. However, the goal of providing sufficient pulmonary blood flow must be balanced with the concern of creating increased vascular resistance.

In the last few years, the pulmonary vasculature itself has emerged as a therapeutic target to improve output. In the Fontan circuit, PVR is generally mildly elevated at baseline but, in the absence of pulsatile flow, it does not decrease normally with increased cardiac output. Advances in the treatment options for primary pulmonary hypertension suggest that the pulmonary resistance might also be considered as a potential target of medication intervention in the Fontan circulation. Several agents have been reported (oxygen at altitude, sildenafil, bosentan, inhaled iloprost), although the short-term improvements as a result of these agents have been modest.[36–39] Longer-term studies with pulmonary vasodilators are needed to understand whether these agents can affect the long-term outcomes of patients after Fontan, and alter what is characteristically a slow, downward slope of exercise capacity and cardiovascular functionality.

Ventricular Suction (Enhancing Runoff After the Dam)

The contraction of the ventricle itself has a role in helping blood flow through the pulmonary vascular bed. As the atrioventricular annulus contracts toward the apex of the heart, a vacuum is created to "pull" blood into the pulmonary atrium. The total contribution of this "suction" is hard to quantify, but is clearly lost in the settings of atrioventricular dyssynchrony or significantly elevated atrial pressure. In the Fontan circulation, the systemic ventricle functions in a preload-deprived state. In this state, ventricular contractility is limited (as dictated by the Frank-Starling curve), further limiting the contribution of ventricular suction.

Fenestration (Bypassing the Dam)

One sure way to improve cardiac output in the Fontan is to create a bypass around the congested pulmonary circuit in the form of a small fenestration. This concept was originally reported as a means to help with the physiologic adjustment in the perioperative state following the Fontan surgery itself.[40] After the institution of the fenestration, the incidence of prolonged pleural effusions and long hospital stays decreased significantly. In addition, a limited bypass of the Fontan portal system also results in chronic improvement of congestion and circulatory output in the Fontan circuit. The downside to a fenestration is decreased arterial oxygen saturation. Nevertheless, the improved output may result in better overall oxygen delivery, and will also help to alleviate the congestion felt in upstream organs, particularly the liver.

Whereas a fenestration at the time of Fontan is well tolerated and may be viable for years or decades after surgery, the creation of a fenestration in later years in a patient who has not had one is not as well tolerated. These patients are referred for fenestration creation because of the failure of their Fontan circuit, often characterized by elevated PVR and a high transpulmonary gradient. In this setting, achieving the proper balance in the creation of a fenestration is difficult, and may not be possible. A small fenestration will not allow the degree of decompression necessary to alleviate symptoms, and a larger fenestration might alleviate congestion and augment cardiac output, but in so doing will result in an unacceptable level of cyanosis (see **Fig. 4**). Nevertheless, fenestration creation may have a role in a failing Fontan as a bridge to heart transplantation.

Heart Rate, Contractility, and Afterload

In a ventricle with preload reserve, an increase of heart rate within the normal physiologic range will result in increased output. In a Fontan circuit with no ventricular preload reserve, an increase in heart rate will result in a proportional decrease of stroke volume, and subsequently no change in output.[41] In excessive bradycardia, pacing with a heart rate in physiologic range will increase output and decrease congestion.[42] However, excessive tachycardia may actually result in a decrease in cardiac output related to the inability to augment diastolic filling.

Because systolic performance is not generally the primary issue in the Fontan circulation, the role of inotropic agents is often limited. These agents can make the Fontan ventricle squeeze harder, but will not result in clinically significant more output. Such a response is typical for a preload-deprived ventricle. There may be a role for inotropes in the Fontan patient with significant ventricular dysfunction that is not due to chronic underloading, but in general the role of these agents is somewhat limited.

The afterload faced by the systemic ventricle may have a role in the structural characteristics of the ventricle, and thus some thought should be given to the use of an afterload-reducing agent. Any patient who is in a chronic state of low cardiac output will invariably generate an increased systemic vascular resistance to maintain blood pressure. In a failing but normally connected biventricular circulation with a hypocontractile ventricle and preload reserve, a decrease of afterload results in an increase in output, which will counter the tendency for hypotension, thus resulting in a good clinical response. However, in a Fontan patient a substantial decrease of afterload without preload reserve will not result in an increase in output, but may be detrimental by causing hypotension. Whether there is a role for low-dose afterload reduction in attempting to modulate ventricular diastolic function remains as yet unknown. In the only randomized trial of enalapril after Fontan, no beneficial effect was seen.[43] However, the time course in this trial was 10 weeks; it may be that the benefit of afterload-reducing agents lies in the chronic impact on diastolic function rather than the short-term impact on systemic resistance.

MECHANICAL SUPPORT AND HEART TRANSPLANTATION

Mechanical support for the failing single ventricle is still in its infancy. The usual ventricular assist devices are designed to aid a failing systemic ventricle. In the failing Fontan circulation, the problem is typically not systolic performance, but rather failure of the physiology itself related to the neoportal system and chronic preload deprivation. In this setting the interposition of a subpulmonary assist device is required, and this has been reported in one instance as a bridge to transplantation.[44] In a second case, a total artificial heart was used to bridge a patient with a failing Fontan circulation to transplantation.[45] The surgery to place a subpulmonary assist device or a total artificial heart is extensive, and requires the takedown of the Fontan construct itself.

In many cases of Fontan failure, heart transplantation is likely to be the final outcome. Heart transplantation in the Fontan cohort is constitutes a higher risk than in those without congenital heart disease, and may be even higher in those with Fontan failure but preserved ventricular function.[46]

SUMMARY

The Fontan construct has allowed for the survival of countless children born with congenital heart disease. However, this palliation creates a form of man-made heart failure characterized by a neoportal system that leads to chronic preload deprivation, resulting in low cardiac output and systemic venous congestion. Careful attention to pulmonary blood flow and pulmonary arterial growth in the initial stages of Fontan palliation are crucial, as are the technical details of the geometry of the Fontan connections. Avoiding overload of the systemic ventricle is important, while excessive protection from volume overload may result in pulmonary artery hypoplasia. Nevertheless, even in a "perfect" Fontan, it can be difficult to predict how durable this man-made form of heart failure will be over the longer term.

Overall treatment options for circulatory failure of a Fontan circuit are disappointing; avoidance of problems is most important, because once the Fontan circuit is created it "runs on auto-pilot," and allows little modulation. However, trials are under way to evaluate the potential benefits of modulators of PVR and to determine whether aerobic training may help to forestall the insidious onset of circulatory failure. At the same time, new support devices are coming to the market that may help to bridge those patients with a failing Fontan to cardiac transplantation.

REFERENCES

1. Fontan F, Baudet E. Surgical repair of tricuspid atresia. Thorax 1971;26:240–8.
2. Gewillig M. The Fontan circulation. Heart 2005;91:839–46.
3. Gewillig M, Brown SC, Eyskens B, et al. The Fontan circulation: who controls cardiac output? Interact Cardiovasc Thorac Surg 2010;10:428–33.
4. Gewillig M, Kalis N. Pathophysiological aspects after cavopulmonary anastomosis. Thorac Cardiovasc Surg 2000;48:336–41.
5. La Gerche A, Gewillig M. What limits cardiac performance during exercise in normal subjects and in healthy Fontan patients? Int J Pediatr 2010;2010. pii:791291.
6. Van de Bruaene A, La Gerche A, Claessen G, et al. Sildanafil improves exercise hemodynamics in Fontan patients [abstract]. Cardiol Young 2013;23:S54.
7. Paridon SM, Mitchell PD, Colan SD, et al. A cross-sectional study of exercise performance during the first 2 decades of life after the Fontan operation. J Am Coll Cardiol 2008;52:99–107.
8. Giardini A, Hager A, Pace Napoleone C, et al. Natural history of exercise capacity after the Fontan operation: a longitudinal study. Ann Thorac Surg 2008;85:818–21.
9. Diller GP, Dimopoulos K, Okonko D, et al. Exercise intolerance in adult congenital heart disease: comparative severity, correlates, and prognostic implication. Circulation 2005;112:828–35.
10. Diller GP, Giardini A, Dimopoulos K, et al. Predictors of morbidity and mortality in contemporary Fontan patients: results from a multicenter study including cardiopulmonary exercise testing in 321 patients. Eur Heart J 2010;31:3073–83.
11. Gewillig MH, Lundstrom UR, Deanfield JE, et al. Impact of Fontan operation on left ventricular size and contractility in tricuspid atresia. Circulation 1990;81:118–27.
12. Gewillig M, Daenen W, Aubert A, et al. Abolishment of chronic volume overload. Implications for diastolic function of the systemic ventricle immediately after Fontan repair. Circulation 1992;86:II93–9.
13. Silverstein DM, Hansen DP, Ojiambo HP, et al. Left ventricular function in severe pure mitral stenosis as seen at the Kenyatta National Hospital. Am Heart J 1980;99:727–33.
14. Mital S, Chung WK, Colan SD, et al. Renin-angiotensin-aldosterone genotype influences ventricular remodeling in infants with single ventricle. Circulation 2011;123:2353–62.
15. Mitchell MB, Campbell DN, Ivy D, et al. Evidence of pulmonary vascular disease after heart transplantation for Fontan circulation failure. J Thorac Cardiovasc Surg 2004;128:693–702.
16. Rychik J, Veldtman G, Rand E, et al. The precarious state of the liver after a Fontan operation: summary of a multidisciplinary symposium. Pediatr Cardiol 2012;33:1001–12.

17. Bulut OP, Romero R, Mahle WT, et al. Magnetic resonance imaging identifies unsuspected liver abnormalities in patients after the Fontan procedure. J Pediatr 2013;163:201–6.

18. Wu FM, Ukomadu C, Odze RD, et al. Liver disease in the patient with Fontan circulation. Congenit Heart Dis 2011;6:190–201.

19. Asrani S, Warnes C, Kamath P. Hepatocellular carcinoma after the Fontan procedure. N Engl J Med 2013;368:1756–7.

20. Schwartz MC, Sullivan LM, Glatz AC, et al. Portal and sinusoidal fibrosis are common on liver biopsy after Fontan surgery. Pediatr Cardiol 2013;34:135–42.

21. Friedrich-Rust M, Koch C, Rentzsch A, et al. Noninvasive assessment of liver fibrosis in patients with Fontan circulation using transient elastography and biochemical fibrosis markers. J Thorac Cardiovasc Surg 2008;135:560–7.

22. Rychik J. Protein-losing enteropathy after Fontan operation. Congenit Heart Dis 2007;2:288–300.

23. Thacker D, Patel A, Dodds K, et al. Use of oral budesonide in the management of protein-losing enteropathy after the Fontan operation. Ann Thorac Surg 2010;89:837–42.

24. John AS, Driscoll DJ, Warnes CA, et al. The use of oral budesonide in adolescents and adults with protein-losing enteropathy after the Fontan operation. Ann Thorac Surg 2011;92:1451–6.

25. Griffiths ER, Kaza AK, Wyler von Ballmoos MC, et al. Evaluating failing Fontans for heart transplantation: predictors of death. Ann Thorac Surg 2009;88: 558–63 [discussion: 563–4].

26. Heath L, Ling S, Racz J, et al. Prospective, longitudinal study of plastic bronchitis cast pathology and responsiveness to tissue plasminogen activator. Pediatr Cardiol 2011;32:1182–9.

27. Shah SS, Drinkwater DC, Christian KG. Plastic bronchitis: is thoracic duct ligation a real surgical option? Ann Thorac Surg 2006;81:2281–3.

28. Chaudhari M, Stumper O. Plastic bronchitis after Fontan operation: treatment with stent fenestration of the Fontan circuit. Heart 2004;90:801.

29. ElMallah MK, Prabhakaran S, Chesrown SE. Plastic bronchitis: resolution after heart transplantation. Pediatr Pulmonol 2011;46:824–5.

30. Wilson J, Russell J, Williams W, et al. Fenestration of the Fontan circuit as treatment for plastic bronchitis. Pediatr Cardiol 2005;26:717–9.

31. Shachar GB, Fuhrman BP, Wang Y, et al. Rest and exercise hemodynamics after the Fontan procedure. Circulation 1982;65:1043–8.

32. de Leval MR, Kilner P, Gewillig M, et al. Total cavopulmonary connection: a logical alternative to atriopulmonary connection for complex Fontan operations. Experimental studies and early clinical experience. J Thorac Cardiovasc Surg 1988;96:682–95.

33. Van Haesdonck JM, Mertens L, Sizaire R, et al. Comparison by computerized numeric modeling of energy losses in different Fontan connections. Circulation 1995;92:II322–6.

34. Conte S, Gewillig M, Eyskens B, et al. Management of late complications after classic Fontan procedure by conversion to total cavopulmonary connection. Cardiovasc Surg 1999;7:651–5.

35. Mavroudis C, Deal BJ, Backer CL, et al. The favorable impact of arrhythmia surgery on total cavopulmonary artery Fontan conversion. Seminars in thoracic and cardiovascular surgery. Semin Thorac Cardiovasc Surg Pediatr Card Surg Annu 1999;2: 143–56.

36. Darst JR, Vezmar M, McCrindle BW, et al. Living at an altitude adversely affects exercise capacity in Fontan patients. Cardiol Young 2010;20: 593–601.

37. Goldberg DJ, French B, McBride MG, et al. Impact of oral sildenafil on exercise performance in children and young adults after the Fontan operation: a randomized, double-blind, placebo-controlled, crossover trial. Circulation 2011;123:1185–93.

38. Ovaert C, Thijs D, Dewolf D, et al. The effect of bosentan in patients with a failing Fontan circulation. Cardiol Young 2009;19:331–9.

39. Rhodes J, Ubeda-Tikkanen A, Clair M, et al. Effect of inhaled iloprost on the exercise function of Fontan patients: a demonstration of concept. Int J Cardiol 2013;168(3):2435–40.

40. Bridges ND, Lock JE, Castaneda AR. Baffle fenestration with subsequent transcatheter closure. Modification of the Fontan operation for patients at increased risk. Circulation 1990;82:1681–9.

41. Barber G, Di Sessa T, Child JS, et al. Hemodynamic responses to isolated increments in heart rate by atrial pacing after a Fontan procedure. Am Heart J 1988;115:837–41.

42. Cohen MI, Rhodes LA, Wernovsky G, et al. Atrial pacing: an alternative treatment for protein-losing enteropathy after the Fontan operation. J Thorac Cardiovasc Surg 2001;121:582–3.

43. Kouatli AA, Garcia JA, Zellers TM, et al. Enalapril does not enhance exercise capacity in patients after Fontan procedure. Circulation 1997;96: 1507–12.

44. Pretre R, Haussler A, Bettex D, et al. Right-sided univentricular cardiac assistance in a failing Fontan circulation. Ann Thorac Surg 2008;86:1018–20.

45. Rossano J, Goldberg D, Fuller S, et al. Successful use of the total artificial heart in the failing Fontan circulation. Ann Thorac Surg, in press.

46. Seddio F, Gorislavets N, Iacovoni A, et al. Is heart transplantation for complex congenital heart disease a good option? A 25-year single centre experience. Eur J Cardiothorac Surg 2013;43:605–11 [discussion: 611].

Pregnancy in Women with Heart Disease
Risk Assessment and Management of Heart Failure

Jasmine Grewal, MD, FRCPC[a],*,
Candice K. Silversides, MD, FRCPC[b,c],
Jack M. Colman, MD, FRCPC[b,c]

KEYWORDS

- Pregnancy • Heart failure • Congenital heart disease • Cardiomyopathy

KEY POINTS

- Heart disease, present in 0.5% to 3% of pregnant women, is an important cause of morbidity and the leading cause of death among pregnant women in the developed world.
- Certain heart conditions are associated with an increased risk of heart failure during pregnancy or the postpartum period; for these conditions, management during pregnancy benefits from multidisciplinary care at a center with expertise in pregnancy and heart disease.
- This review focuses on cardiac risks and management strategies for women with acquired and congenital heart disease at increased risk of heart failure.

INTRODUCTION

Between 0.5% and 3.0% of women have a form of heart disease (HD) either known before or diagnosed during pregnancy.[1] HD is the leading cause of death among pregnant women in the developed world.[1] For women with preexisting HD, the hemodynamic stress of pregnancy can result in cardiac complications, including heart failure (HF). Some heart conditions are associated with a higher risk of developing HF during pregnancy or in the postpartum period, especially complex congenital HD (CHD), significant valve disease, and cardiomyopathy. Many women are aware of their heart condition before pregnancy, but in others the hemodynamic stress of pregnancy can unmask a previously quiescent lesion that manifests as clinical HF. Moreover, conditions that develop de novo during pregnancy such as peripartum cardiomyopathy or preeclampsia may cause HF. This review focuses on: (1) physiologic changes of pregnancy that contribute to the risk of HF, (2) diagnosing HF in pregnancy, (3) risk assessment for women with HD, (4) general management strategies, and (5) HF risk in and management for select high-risk cardiac lesions.

Disclosures: None.
[a] University of British Columbia Cardiac Obstetrics Clinic and Pacific Adult Congenital Heart Clinic, Division of Cardiology, St. Paul's Hospital, University of British Columbia, Room 344-1081, Burrard Street, Vancouver, British Columbia V6Z 1Y6, Canada; [b] University of Toronto Program in Pregnancy and Heart Disease, Obstetric Medicine Program, Division of Cardiology, Mount Sinai Hospital, 600 University Avenue, Room 1603, Toronto, ON M5G 1X5, Canada; [c] Toronto Congenital Cardiac Centre for Adults, Peter Munk Cardiac Centre, University Health Network, 5 North, 585 University Avenue, Toronto, ON M5G 2N2, Canada
* Corresponding author.
E-mail address: jasmine.grewal@vch.ca

Heart Failure Clin 10 (2014) 117–129
http://dx.doi.org/10.1016/j.hfc.2013.09.014
1551-7136/14/$ – see front matter Crown Copyright © 2014 Published by Elsevier Inc. All rights reserved.

CARDIOVASCULAR CHANGES DURING NORMAL PREGNANCY THAT CONTRIBUTE TO THE RISK OF HEART FAILURE

Underlying or evolving HD may lead to adverse pregnancy outcomes by affecting the ability of the cardiovascular system to adapt to hemodynamic changes of pregnancy. During pregnancy, systemic vascular resistance decreases while cardiac output and blood volume increase (**Fig. 1**). The initial decrease in systemic vascular resistance is thought to be due to circulating estrogen, vasodilator peptides, nitric oxide, and other factors.[2,3] Mean arterial pressure declines beginning in the first trimester, largely due to a decline in diastolic blood pressure. Blood pressure reaches a nadir at around 20 weeks gestational age before returning to normal or supranormal levels by 38 weeks' gestation.[4,5] Blood volume increases by 40% to 50%, primarily because of increased plasma volume, with a lesser increase in red cell mass.[5,6] This disparity contributes to the physiologic anemia of pregnancy. Heart rate increases by 10 to 20 beats per minute, peaking early in the third trimester. These increases in stroke volume and heart rate lead to an increase in cardiac output, which peaks during the second trimester

at 25% to 50% above nongravid levels and then remains stable throughout the third trimester.[4,7–11]

In the absence of analgesia, labor induces a 30% increase in cardiac output above the end-of-pregnancy level, which is due to increased heart rate and stroke volume occurring predominantly in relation to uterine contractions.[12] In the second-stage of labor, bearing down further increases cardiac output. These cardiovascular stresses may be poorly tolerated, leading to HF especially in women with lesions such as cardiomyopathy or left-sided heart obstruction. Effective anesthesia/analgesia during labor can blunt the increase in blood pressure and cardiac output, mitigating their adverse effects. During the third stage of labor the placenta is delivered and the uterus contracts, further increasing intravascular volume. However, blood loss associated with delivery, averaging 500 mL for vaginal deliveries, mitigates this. During the first 2 postpartum weeks cardiac output decreases substantially, and reaches nonpregnant levels by 24 weeks postpartum.[13] Despite the return toward normal hemodynamics, women remain at risk for HF during this period. Women with peripartum cardiomyopathy are particularly vulnerable.

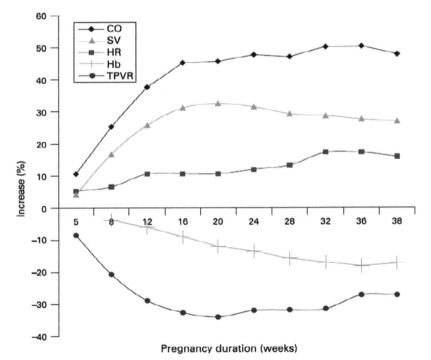

Fig. 1. Cardiovascular changes during normal pregnancy. CO, changes in cardiac output; Hb, hemoglobin concentration; HR, heart rate; SV, stroke volume; TPVR, total peripheral vascular resistance. (*From* Karamermer Y, Roos-Hesselink JW. Pregnancy and adult congenital heart disease. Expert Rev Cardiovasc Ther 2007;5(5):859–69; with permission.)

CHALLENGES OF DIAGNOSING HEART FAILURE IN PREGNANCY

The cardinal cardiac symptoms of dyspnea, tachypnea, orthopnea, fatigue, and decreased exercise tolerance are not uncommon during a normal healthy pregnancy, and thus are not specific for HF even in a woman with underlying HD. Moreover, physical findings during a normal pregnancy overlap with findings of HF and/or the underlying heart condition. These possibly normal findings include mild distension of jugular veins, a displaced apex, a parasternal lift, increased intensity of the first heart sound, prominent pulmonary component of the second heart sound, third heart sound, early peaking systolic ejection murmur, and pedal edema. A physician needs to recognize these signs and symptoms that in some cases are markers of abnormality and in other cases are normal findings. The distinction is important, as it may trigger changes in management on the one hand, or allow welcome reassurance on the other. In cases where HF is suspected, additional investigations (**Box 1**) may confirm or refute the diagnosis, demonstrate worsening of a preexisting condition, and/or define a previously undiagnosed condition. It is often helpful to perform such tests at baseline and repeat them serially to look for changes.

Box 1
Investigations that aid in the diagnosis and management of heart failure in pregnancy: normal findings, special considerations, and utility

Electrocardiogram

- Normal pregnancy findings include: sinus tachycardia, postpartum transient sinus bradycardia, left-axis deviation, nonspecific ST-T abnormalities.
- Atrial and ventricular extrasystoles are often seen in a normal healthy pregnancy.[60] New arrhythmias may be seen in relation to heart failure.

Exercise Testing

- Preconception testing can clarify exercise capacity, assess blood pressure response to exercise, and identify exercise-induced arrhythmias.
- Prognostic value: an abnormal chronotropic response to exercise has been associated with adverse outcomes in pregnancy.[61]
- A submaximal stress echocardiogram can be performed safely during pregnancy when indicated.

Echocardiogram

- Normal pregnancy findings include: small increase in dimensions of all cardiac chambers, small increase in left ventricular mass, increased regurgitation across the mitral and tricuspid valves (increase of up to one grade is normal).[62] Systolic function normally does not change.
- Changes in systolic function, valve function, or severity of pulmonary hypertension may be observed in women who develop heart failure.

Cardiac Magnetic Resonance Imaging

- Can be used during pregnancy if indicated, ideally after the first trimester.
- Gadolinium should be avoided because teratogenic effects of high doses have been demonstrated in animal studies.[63]

Diagnostic Tests Using Ionizing Radiation

- These tests include: diagnostic radiography, computed tomography, cardiac catheterization, and nuclear imaging.
- Ionizing radiation should generally be avoided in pregnancy, but can be considered if critical to management and the information cannot be otherwise obtained.

Brain Natriuretic Peptide

- Elevated brain natriuretic peptide (BNP) levels are found in women with clinical heart failure; however, BNP can also be elevated in pregnant women with heart disease who do not develop heart failure during pregnancy.
- A normal BNP level has been shown to have a high negative predictive value for excluding cardiac complications during pregnancy.[64]

MATERNAL GLOBAL RISK ASSESSMENT

HF and arrhythmias are the most common adverse maternal cardiac events during pregnancy in women with HD.[14,15] Other adverse events include stroke, endocarditis, and, rarely, death. Risk stratification allows women to make informed pregnancy choices and to plan safe pregnancy care. In addition to the general risk estimates described in this section, lesion-specific risks should be considered when known, so that issues unique to the lesion can be taken into account. Some high-risk lesions are known to be underrepresented in the study populations from which global risk scores were derived. Therefore, pregnancy risk in such patients is not accurately predicted by global risk scores.

A commonly used pregnancy risk score was based on 2 studies of pregnancy outcomes in 851 Canadian women with HD (252 in a retrospective study and 599 in a multicenter prospective observational study).[15,16] Seventy-four percent of the patients in the prospective study had congenital HD. In the multicenter prospective study, a risk score (CARPREG score) was derived that predicted risk for adverse maternal cardiac events during pregnancy independent of specific underlying cardiac diagnosis, based on prepregnancy maternal characteristics (**Fig. 2**).[15] In this study, 13% of pregnancies were complicated by an adverse maternal cardiac event, half of which were HF.[15]

A subsequent retrospective study in a CHD population by Khairy and colleagues[14] suggested that the addition of subpulmonary ventricular systolic dysfunction and/or severe pulmonary regurgitation to the CARPREG risk score improves maternal cardiac risk assessment. Twenty-five percent of pregnancies were complicated by an adverse maternal cardiac event, of which 67% were HF.

The ZAHARA investigators proposed a weighted scoring system for women with CHD, and incorporated several additional variables into their risk prediction model (**Table 1**).[17] Of 1302 pregnancies, 8% were complicated by an adverse maternal cardiac event, of which 20% were HF; arrhythmias comprised the majority of adverse events.

MANAGEMENT STRATEGIES
Multidisciplinary Team

A woman of childbearing age with HD contemplating pregnancy or already pregnant should be referred to a cardiologist with expertise in pregnancy and HD for at least one visit, to review risks and counsel the patient and health care providers on the approach to further management. Such women require special attention focusing on the issues outlined in **Box 2**. Based on lesion complexity, residual disease, functional class, pregnancy risk, and logistical considerations, a woman should be stratified to 1 of the following 3 care pathways.

1. Exclusive care by an expert multidisciplinary team at a center with expertise in pregnancy and HD (**Fig. 3**)

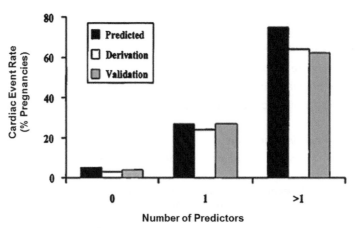

Fig. 2. CARPREG risk score. Frequency of adverse maternal cardiac events, as predicted by the CARPREG risk index, and observed in derivation and validation groups, expressed as a function of the number of predictors. Predictors, taken to be of equal weight, are: (1) poor functional status (New York Heart Association functional class >II) or cyanosis, (2) history of cardiac events before pregnancy (arrhythmia, stroke, or heart failure), (3) left heart obstruction, and (4) systemic ventricular systolic dysfunction (ejection fraction <40%). (*From* Siu SC, Sermer M, Colman JM, et al. Prospective multicenter study of pregnancy outcomes in women with heart disease. Circulation 2001;104(5):520; with permission.)

Table 1
ZAHARA weighted risk score of cardiac complications

Variable	Points
Prior arrhythmias	1.5
NYHA >II	0.75
Left heart obstruction (aortic valve peak gradient >50 mm Hg)	2.5
Cardiac medications prepregnancy	1.5
Moderate to severe systemic AV valve regurgitation	0.75
Moderate to severe pulmonary valve regurgitation	0.75
Mechanical valve prosthesis	4.5
Cyanotic heart disease	1.0

Risk score for cardiac complications during completed (>20 weeks of gestation) pregnancies in women with congenital HD. Translation of total points to risk%: 0 points = 2.9%; 0.5–1.5 points = 7.5%; 1.51–2.5 points = 17.5%; 2.51–3.5 points = 43.1%; >3.5 points = 70%.
Abbreviations: AV, atrioventricular; NYHA, New York Heart Association functional class.

2. Shared care including regular review by a cardiologist with expertise in pregnancy and HD and local obstetric care
3. Local obstetric care, with regular cardiology follow-up not required during pregnancy after initial review by cardiologist with expertise in pregnancy and HD

Antenatal Care

Chronic heart failure
Chronic HF during pregnancy should be managed according to standard guidelines,[18,19] taking into account potential adverse effects of medications on the developing fetus. Angiotensin-converting enzyme inhibitors, angiotensin receptor blockers, and renin inhibitors are contraindicated because of fetotoxicity.[20,21] If afterload reduction is indicated, hydralazine with or without nitrates can be used instead, although the evidence supporting this approach in pregnancy is limited. When β-blocker therapy is indicated, β1-selective drugs are preferred. The largest experience in pregnancy is with metoprolol. Atenolol should not be used because in comparison with other β-blockers a higher risk of babies of low birth weight has been reported.[22] Anticoagulation is recommended in some women with significant left ventricular left ventricular systolic dysfunction, intracardiac thrombus, history of thromboembolism, or atrial fibrillation. Low molecular weight heparin is often used, but vitamin K antagonists are also

Box 2
General approach to the care of pregnant women at risk for heart failure

All women with heart disease considering pregnancy or already pregnant should be given special attention with focus on the following:

- Ascertain anatomic, physiologic, and electrical features of the condition and functional status of the woman.
- Consider need for potential interventions in future independent of pregnancy, and at a preconception evaluation, consider whether such interventions would improve the pregnancy outcome.
- Ensure that the woman understands her condition.
- Estimate the risk of an adverse maternal cardiac, obstetric, or neonatal event using a combination of general and lesion-specific maternal cardiac and obstetric risk factors.
- Share the risk assessment with the woman, ensure that she understands the risks, and clarify her tolerance of those risks.
- Discuss important issues around maternal health and life expectancy that would affect the ability to raise a child.
- Assess risk of recurrence of heart disease in the offspring and, when indicated, offer genetics consultation, genetic testing, fetal echocardiography, and postpartum clinical and echocardiographic assessment of the infant.
- Provide recommendations from the cardiac standpoint with regard to the need for high-risk versus standard obstetric consultation and/or ongoing care, further cardiac monitoring, and investigations during pregnancy, and care and delivery at a high-risk center versus a local hospital.
- Discuss future pregnancies.
- Discuss the need for and type of contraception with women not yet pregnant.
- Plan for postpartum contraception in women currently pregnant.

appropriate between weeks 14 and 36. Full-dose low molecular weight heparin requires confirmation of dosing using anti-Xa levels; dosing by weight alone may not be appropriate in pregnancy.[23] The involvement of a hematologist is helpful in this scenario. Management of anticoagulation for mechanical valves is especially fraught, and should be the topic of intensive counseling both before and during pregnancy.

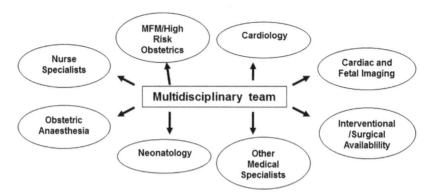

Fig. 3. A model of expert multidisciplinary care for pregnant women at high risk for heart failure. MFM, maternal-fetal medicine.

Acute heart failure

Precipitating causes of acute decompensation should be sought, and chronic HF therapy maintained. Diuretics should be used to treat pulmonary congestion, using caution to avoid overdiuresis, which may have an adverse impact on placental blood flow.[24] Furosemide is the most frequently used diuretic in pregnancy. Spironolactone is associated with antiandrogenic effects in the first trimester, and should be avoided.[25] Safety data for eplerenone are lacking. If intravenous vasodilators are considered, intravenous nitroglycerin is favored because nitroprusside and nesiritide have potential fetal toxicities. If inotropic drugs are required, dopamine, dobutamine, and milrinone can be used, recognizing that their impact on the fetus has not been adequately studied. If severe left ventricular systolic dysfunction develops, the woman should be transferred urgently to a facility where intra-aortic balloon counterpulsation, ventricular assist devices, and transplant consult teams are available.

Labor and Delivery

Women deemed to be at moderate to high risk of morbidity and/or mortality should be managed and delivered at a center with expertise in pregnancy and HD. Multidisciplinary care should be provided (see **Fig. 3**) and detailed plans for labor and delivery developed in advance, documented, and distributed. In most instances, women can be monitored noninvasively. For women with clinical HF at the time of delivery, invasive blood-pressure monitoring may be useful. Pulmonary artery catheters are very rarely indicated.[26] Epidural anesthesia established early in labor minimizes pain and prevents excess catecholamine surges that can lead to hemodynamic lability and HF in women at moderate to high risk. Intravenous fluids should be given judiciously. In the event of

hemodynamic instability or refractory HF, an urgent delivery irrespective of gestational age may be necessary. Delivery should be planned incorporating input from obstetrics, obstetric anesthesia, and cardiology. In the absence of an obstetric indication for a cesarean delivery, the authors generally advocate vaginal delivery, which can be performed safely in most women with HD.[26,27]

Postpartum

After delivery, additional standard therapies for HF can be initiated or resumed. Most β-blockers are safe during breast feeding, as is angiotensin-converting enzyme inhibitor therapy, with benazepril, captopril, and enalapril preferred because of minimal excretion into breast milk.[28] Anticoagulation in the immediate postdelivery phase must be restarted cautiously, once bleeding has stopped and after discussion with the obstetrician.

LESION-SPECIFIC RISK ASSESSMENT AND PRINCIPLES OF MANAGEMENT

Many different heart conditions can result in HF during pregnancy (**Box 3**), some of which require specific management. Pregnancy is increasing in frequency among women with CHD, and HF is an important cardiac complication (**Fig. 4**).[29] Analysis of the Nationwide Inpatient Survey of women undergoing delivery in the United States from 1998 to 2007 demonstrated a 35% increase in annual deliveries in women with CHD, compared with an increase of 21% in the general population.[30] In this section some additional issues unique to lesion-specific HF risk and management are reviewed.

Cardiomyopathy

Approaches to assessment, risk stratification, and management of cardiomyopathies most commonly seen in pregnancy are outlined in **Box 4**. In general,

Box 3
Causes of heart failure during pregnancy

Cardiac Causes

Cardiomyopathy

- Dilated cardiomyopathy
- Peripartum cardiomyopathy
- Hypertrophic cardiomyopathy
- Tachycardia-induced cardiomyopathy
- Hypertensive cardiomyopathy
- Ischemic cardiomyopathy
- Chemotherapy-induced cardiomyopathy
- Other rare causes

Congenital

- Complete transposition of the great arteries: atrial switch operation
- Congenitally corrected transposition of the great arteries
- Tetralogy of Fallot
- Pulmonary atresia
- Single-ventricle hearts including those with Fontan operation
- Left ventricular outflow tract obstruction
- Eisenmenger syndrome

Valvular[a]

- Aortic stenosis
- Mitral stenosis
- Regurgitant lesions

Noncardiac Causes

- Preeclampsia
- Hyperthyroidism
- Anemia
- Pulmonary hypertension

[a] Valvular lesions may be due to congenital as well as acquired heart disease.

the risk of deterioration is highest late in pregnancy or postpartum.

In pregnant women with dilated cardiomyopathy, the risk of adverse cardiac events, specifically HF, is considerable. Prepregnancy characteristics can identify women at the highest risk (**Fig. 5**).[31] Cardiac complications are significantly more common in pregnant than in nonpregnant women with dilated cardiomyopathy. During a 16-month follow-up period, an approximately 6-fold increase in complications has been found.[31]

Peripartum cardiomyopathy is a disorder of unclear etiology, in which HF typically develops in the last month of pregnancy or within 5 months of delivery.[32] However, data suggest that women presenting earlier during gestation may be a part of the peripartum cardiomyopathy spectrum, although only a small percentage present before 36 weeks of gestation.[33] By contrast, women with underlying HD may present with HF in the second trimester, coincident with an increase in hemodynamic burden. Subsequent pregnancies in a woman with peripartum cardiomyopathy carry a recurrence risk of 30% to 50%, so counseling for future pregnancies is important even if the left ventricular ejection fraction has recovered.[24,34]

Transposition of the Great Arteries

In complete transposition of the great arteries following an atrial switch procedure (Mustard or Senning operation), and in congenitally corrected transposition of the great arteries, the right ventricle supports the systemic circulation. Systolic dysfunction of the subaortic right ventricle is common, raising concern about the ability of this ventricle to respond adequately to the increased cardiac work of pregnancy.[35,36] HF developing late in pregnancy or postpartum has been reported in 5% to 15% of women with atrial switch operations.[35,37,38] Lower rates of HF, between 1% and 5%, have been described in congenitally corrected transposition.[39,40] However, a description of subaortic ventricular function is not available in many of these studies. Women with severe subaortic right ventricular dysfunction are thought, based on limited data, to be at high risk for complications and should be cautioned against pregnancy. The role of routine HF therapy, including β-blockers and angiotensin-converting enzyme inhibitors, is unclear in patients with a subaortic right ventricle. If used, β-blockers need to be administered cautiously for fear of exacerbating bradyarrhythmias. It has been reported that pregnancy is associated with an increase in subaortic ventricular dimensions in 30% and a decrease in systolic function in 25% of pregnant women with complete transposition treated with atrial switch surgery.[41] Another study, incorporating a nonpregnant control group comparison, suggests that pregnancy, and not merely time, is associated with more deterioration in subaortic right ventricular function and reduction in functional class than in women who do not undergo pregnancy.[42]

Tetralogy of Fallot

Women with repaired tetralogy of Fallot usually tolerate pregnancy well. However, right ventricular

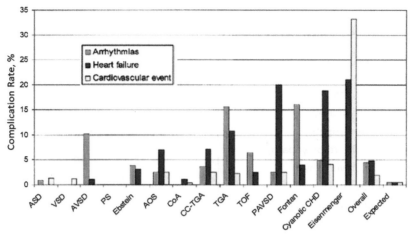

Fig. 4. Rates of the most important complications encountered during pregnancy in women with congenital heart disease. The rightmost columns depict the expected rates in healthy women. AOS, aortic stenosis; ASD, atrial septal defect; AVSD, atrioventricular septal defects; CC-TGA, congenital corrected transposition of the great arteries; CHD, congenital heart disease; CoA, aortic coarctation; Ebstein, Ebstein anomaly; Eisenmenger, Eisenmenger syndrome; Fontan, patients after Fontan repair; PAVSD, pulmonary atresia with ventricular septal defects; PS, pulmonary valve stenosis; TGA, complete transposition of the great arteries; TOF, tetralogy of Fallot; VSD, ventricular septal defect. (*From* Drenthen W, Pieper PG, Roos-Hesselink JW, et al. Outcome of pregnancy in women with congenital heart disease. J Am Coll Cardiol 2007;49(24):2306; with permission.)

dysfunction and/or moderate to severe pulmonary regurgitation are risk factors for adverse events.[14] The most frequent cardiovascular events are arrhythmias, but HF occurs in 1% to 2%, associated with either severe pulmonary regurgitation or left ventricular dysfunction.[43,44] It has been suggested that women with tetralogy of Fallot who have completed a pregnancy have a trend to accelerated rate of adverse right ventricular remodeling, manifested as increased end-diastolic volume on magnetic resonance imaging.[45]

Fontan Circulation

Few data are available on the HF risk in this population. A review of 52 women (60 live births) found that the most common cardiac event was supraventricular arrhythmia.[46] There were 7 reported cases of HF in this review. Deterioration in New York Heart Association (NYHA) functional class without overt HF has also been reported.[47,48] Despite limited data, women with significantly depressed ventricular function and/or severe atrioventricular valve regurgitation are considered to be at high risk of HF, and pregnancy should be discouraged. The long-term impact of pregnancy on a woman with a univentricular heart is unknown.

Eisenmenger Syndrome

Eisenmenger patients have a right to left shunt as a consequence of severe pulmonary hypertension. A high maternal mortality of between 20% and 50% is associated with pregnancy in Eisenmenger

patients, with the highest risk occurring in the peripartum and early postpartum period.[49,50] HF, thromboembolism, and arrhythmias complicate approximately 30% of pregnancies. If pregnancy occurs, the extreme risk should be reviewed and termination offered, recognizing that the risk of termination is also considerable. During ongoing pregnancy, restriction of physical activity and supplemental oxygen are recommended. Right-sided HF may occur, but diuretics need to be used carefully to avoid hemoconcentration and intravascular volume depletion. Hypovolemia can lead to increased right to left shunting, reduced cardiac output, and refractory hypoxemia. Volume overload should also be avoided, as it cannot be accommodated by the compromised pulmonary vascular bed and may result in HF and an increased right to left shunt. Iron deficiency is common and should be treated, as it may precipitate HF. The authors advocate a planned elective admission for vaginal delivery with an assisted second stage of labor. Blood pressure must be monitored closely, as decreases in blood pressure can be especially dangerous for a woman with Eisenmenger syndrome. Oxytocic drugs induce vasodilation and arterial hypotension, and should be avoided or used very cautiously, avoiding bolus injection.

Aortic Stenosis

In women of childbearing age, the main cause of aortic stenosis is congenital bicuspid aortic valve.

Box 4
Cardiomyopathy in pregnancy: risk assessment and management

Idiopathic dilated cardiomyopathy

- If first presentation is during pregnancy, it is difficult to differentiate from peripartum cardiomyopathy.
- When first presentation is during pregnancy, a family history of dilated cardiomyopathy favors idiopathic over peripartum cardiomyopathy.

Maternal Risk:

- Baseline EF <40% and/or NYHA III/IV are predictors of adverse maternal cardiac events. Such women should be followed closely at a center with expertise in pregnancy and heart disease.[31]
- LVEF <20% is associated with high maternal mortality. Pregnancy should be discouraged.
- Caution should be exercised in any woman with a diagnosis of dilated cardiomyopathy, even with milder depression of EF.

Peripartum cardiomyopathy

- Predisposing factors: multiparity, multiple gestation, family history, ethnicity, smoking, diabetes, hypertension, preeclampsia, advanced or adolescent maternal age, β-sympathomimetic tocolytic therapy, cocaine abuse.[24,65]
- Diagnostic criteria: documented LVEF <45% or fractional shortening <30% by echocardiography, absence of an identifiable cause of HF, typical timing of presentation.[32]
- Genetic and cultural factors affect incidence between 1:300 and 1:4000 pregnancies.[24,65]
- Initial presentation can range from mild symptoms to intractable HF, arrhythmias, and/or thromboembolism leading to rapid death.

Maternal Risk:

- Mortality ranges from 0% to 9% in the white North American population and up to 15% in African Americans.[33,66]
- Recovery usually occurs within 6 months, so therapies such as a biventricular pacemaker or ventricular assist device should be delayed if possible, in anticipation of possible recovery.[33,67] Further pregnancies should be discouraged if LVEF has not recovered.
- Even with LVEF >40% there is a risk of progressive HF symptoms and recurrent left ventricular dysfunction.[24,34]

Management:

- Prophylactic low molecular weight heparin is appropriate because of the risk of thromboembolism. If thromboembolism has been documented, full-dose anticoagulation is indicated.[23]

Hypertrophic Cardiomyopathy

- Unexplained left ventricular hypertrophy associated with nondilated ventricular chambers.

Maternal Risk:

- Asymptomatic women with hypertrophic cardiomyopathy usually tolerate pregnancy well.
- Women who are symptomatic prepregnancy or have a high outflow-tract gradient demonstrate an increased risk of maternal complications including HF. Such women should be followed at a center with expertise in pregnancy and heart disease.[68,69]
- Common complications include HF as a result of diastolic dysfunction, severe left ventricular outflow tract obstruction, and arrhythmias.

Management:

- β-Blocker therapy should be considered in women with symptoms, with more than mild left ventricular outflow tract obstruction, with maximal wall thickness >15 mm, to secure rate control for atrial arrhythmias and/or to suppress ventricular arrhythmias.[70]
- Women already on β-blockers should continue using them.
- Atrial fibrillation is often poorly tolerated, and early cardioversion should be considered.

- Epidural anesthesia should be used with caution in women with severe left ventricular outflow tract obstruction, as it can increase the severity of obstruction by provoking systemic vasodilatation and hypotension.
- Intravenous fluid administration prevents hypovolemia-induced exacerbation of left ventricular outflow tract obstruction, but must be balanced against the impact of diastolic dysfunction, whereby high filling pressures may provoke HF.
- Oxytocin may cause hypotension and tachycardia, especially when administered as bolus injection. It should only be given as a slow infusion.

Abbreviations: EF, ejection fraction; HF, heart failure; LVEF, left ventricular ejection fraction; NYHA, New York Heart Association functional class.

Although maternal deaths are rare (<1% in contemporary case series), HF and arrhythmias occur in 10% to 44% of pregnancies.[51–54] HF occurs in approximately 10% of pregnant women with severe AS.[55] Women with moderate or severe asymptomatic AS during pregnancy are also at high risk of requiring cardiac interventions late after pregnancy in comparison with controls.[56] Women with symptomatic severe aortic stenosis should have valve replacement before pregnancy. Preconception intervention in a woman with asymptomatic severe aortic stenosis is more difficult; decision making may be assisted by an exercise test to assess exercise capacity, arrhythmia development, and blood-pressure response to exercise.[54] When women with aortic stenosis develop HF, judicious diuresis is important to avoid hypotension. An echocardiogram should be performed to assess for worsening ventricular systolic function. Pregnant women with severe aortic stenosis and NYHA functional class III/IV symptoms despite medical therapy should be considered for percutaneous aortic valvuloplasty during pregnancy if valve morphology is appropriate. If this is not an option, surgical valve replacement may be considered, taking into account the substantial attendant fetal risk.[57]

Mitral Stenosis

Most women of childbearing age with mitral stenosis have rheumatic HD. Less commonly, mitral stenosis is due to a congenital cardiac lesion such as cor triatriatum or parachute mitral valve. HF can occur among pregnant women with moderate to severe mitral stenosis even if previously asymptomatic.[52,53,58] Increased cardiac output and especially uncontrolled tachycardia, which shortens the diastolic left atrial emptying time, are the main responsible factors. The onset of atrial fibrillation is a common precipitant of overt HF, and is even more likely if mitral stenosis was previously unrecognized and prophylactic therapy (usually β-blocker) to control the heart rate had not been established in advance. A woman with severe mitral stenosis should be counseled against pregnancy, even if asymptomatic, until an intervention can be performed. Ideally this should be a percutaneous mitral valvuloplasty,[23] which is often feasible in rheumatic mitral stenosis but is unlikely to be effective in congenital mitral stenosis. If symptoms or pulmonary hypertension (pulmonary systolic pressure ≥50 mm Hg by echocardiography) develop during pregnancy, activity should be restricted and aggressive control of heart rate pursued, usually by using β-blockers.[59] Diuretic therapy can be given when HF persists despite rate control.[59] Open mitral valvuloplasty or mitral valve replacement surgery may be considered if all other measures have failed. Vaginal delivery is appropriate in women with

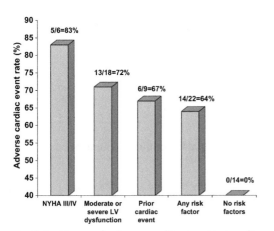

Fig. 5. Incidence of adverse cardiac events according to maternal risk factors in women with a dilated cardiomyopathy. The first 3 risk categories are not mutually exclusive. Any risk factor refers to the presence of any 1 of the 3 risk factors (moderate or severe LV dysfunction, NYHA functional class III or IV, previous cardiac events). LV, left ventricular; NYHA, New York Heart Association functional class. (*From* Grewal J, Siu SC, Ross HJ, et al. Pregnancy outcomes in women with dilated cardiomyopathy. J Am Coll Cardiol 2009;55:49; with permission.)

mitral stenosis in NYHA functional class I/II with no evidence of pulmonary hypertension. Cesarean delivery has been advocated in women with moderate to severe mitral stenosis and in NYHA III/IV or with pulmonary hypertension,[23] although the authors generally favor vaginal delivery even in such patients.[26,27]

REFERENCES

1. de Swiet M. Maternal mortality: confidential enquiries into maternal deaths in the United Kingdom. Am J Obstet Gynecol 2000;182(4):760–6.

2. Stevenson JC, Macdonald DW, Warren RC, et al. Increased concentration of circulating calcitonin gene related peptide during normal human pregnancy. Br Med J (Clin Res Ed) 1986;293(6558): 1329–30.

3. Williams DJ, Vallance PJ, Neild GH, et al. Nitric oxide-mediated vasodilation in human pregnancy. Am J Physiol 1997;272(2 Pt 2):H748–52.

4. Easterling TR, Benedetti TJ, Schmucker BC, et al. Maternal hemodynamics in normal and preeclamptic pregnancies: a longitudinal study. Obstet Gynecol 1990;76(6):1061–9.

5. Pritchard JA. Changes in the blood volume during pregnancy and delivery. Anesthesiology 1965;26: 393–9.

6. Hunter S, Robson SC. Adaptation of the maternal heart in pregnancy. Br Heart J 1992;68(6): 540–3.

7. Gilson GJ, Mosher MD, Conrad KP. Systemic hemodynamics and oxygen transport during pregnancy in chronically instrumented, conscious rats. Am J Physiol 1992;263(6 Pt 2):H1911–8.

8. Gilson GJ, Samaan S, Crawford MH, et al. Changes in hemodynamics, ventricular remodeling, and ventricular contractility during normal pregnancy: a longitudinal study. Obstet Gynecol 1997;89(6):957–62.

9. Hennessy TG, MacDonald D, Hennessy MS, et al. Serial changes in cardiac output during normal pregnancy: a Doppler ultrasound study. Eur J Obstet Gynecol Reprod Biol 1996;70(2):117–22.

10. Karamermer Y, Roos-Hesselink JW. Pregnancy and adult congenital heart disease. Expert Rev Cardiovasc Ther 2007;5(5):859–69.

11. Robson SC, Hunter S, Boys RJ, et al. Serial study of factors influencing changes in cardiac output during human pregnancy. Am J Physiol 1989;256(4 Pt 2): H1060–5.

12. Hendricks CH, Quilligan EJ. Cardiac output during labor. Am J Obstet Gynecol 1956;71(5):953–72.

13. Robson SC, Hunter S, Moore M, et al. Haemodynamic changes during the puerperium: a Doppler and M-mode echocardiographic study. Br J Obstet Gynaecol 1987;94(11):1028–39.

14. Khairy P, Ouyang DW, Fernandes SM, et al. Pregnancy outcomes in women with congenital heart disease. Circulation 2006;113(4):517–24.

15. Siu SC, Sermer M, Colman JM, et al. Prospective multicenter study of pregnancy outcomes in women with heart disease. Circulation 2001;104(5):515–21.

16. Siu SC, Sermer M, Harrison DA, et al. Risk and predictors for pregnancy-related complications in women with heart disease. Circulation 1997;96(9): 2789–94.

17. Drenthen W, Boersma E, Balci A, et al. Predictors of pregnancy complications in women with congenital heart disease. Eur Heart J 2010;31(17):2124–32.

18. Jessup M, Abraham WT, Casey DE, et al. 2009 focused update: ACCF/AHA guidelines for the diagnosis and management of heart failure in adults: a report of the American College of Cardiology Foundation/American Heart Association Task Force on Practice Guidelines: developed in collaboration with the International Society for Heart and Lung Transplantation. Circulation 2009;119(14): 1977–2016.

19. McKelvie RS, Moe GW, Ezekowitz JA, et al. The 2012 Canadian Cardiovascular Society heart failure management guidelines update: focus on acute and chronic heart failure. Can J Cardiol 2013;29(2):168–81.

20. Cooper WO, Hernandez-Diaz S, Arbogast PG, et al. Major congenital malformations after first-trimester exposure to ACE inhibitors. N Engl J Med 2006;354(23):2443–51.

21. Schaefer C. Angiotensin II-receptor-antagonists: further evidence of fetotoxicity but not teratogenicity. Birth Defects Res A Clin Mol Teratol 2003; 67(8):591–4.

22. Lydakis C, Lip GY, Beevers M, et al. Atenolol and fetal growth in pregnancies complicated by hypertension. Am J Hypertens 1999;12(6):541–7.

23. Regitz-Zagrosek V, Blomstrom Lundqvist C, Borghi C, et al. ESC Guidelines on the management of cardiovascular diseases during pregnancy: the Task Force on the Management of Cardiovascular Diseases during Pregnancy of the European Society of Cardiology (ESC). Eur Heart J 2011;32(24):3147–97.

24. Sliwa K, Fett J, Elkayam U. Peripartum cardiomyopathy. Lancet 2006;368(9536):687–93.

25. Mirshahi M, Ayani E, Nicolas C, et al. The blockade of mineralocorticoid hormone signaling provokes dramatic teratogenesis in cultured rat embryos. Int J Toxicol 2002;21(3):191–9.

26. Robertson JE, Silversides CK, Mah ML, et al. A contemporary approach to the obstetric management of women with heart disease. J Obstet Gynaecol Can 2012;34(9):812–9.

27. Goldszmidt E, Macarthur A, Silversides C, et al. Anesthetic management of a consecutive cohort

of women with heart disease for labor and delivery. Int J Obstet Anesth 2010;19(3):266–72.

28. Beardmore KS, Morris JM, Gallery ED. Excretion of antihypertensive medication into human breast milk: a systematic review. Hypertens Pregnancy 2002;21(1):85–95.

29. Drenthen W, Pieper PG, Roos-Hesselink JW, et al. Outcome of pregnancy in women with congenital heart disease: a literature review. J Am Coll Cardiol 2007;49(24):2303–11.

30. Opotowsky AR, Siddiqi OK, D'Souza B, et al. Maternal cardiovascular events during childbirth among women with congenital heart disease. Heart 2012;98(2):145–51.

31. Grewal J, Siu SC, Ross HJ, et al. Pregnancy outcomes in women with dilated cardiomyopathy. J Am Coll Cardiol 2009;55(1):45–52.

32. Pearson GD, Veille JC, Rahimtoola S, et al. Peripartum cardiomyopathy: National Heart, Lung, and Blood Institute and Office of Rare Diseases (National Institutes of Health) workshop recommendations and review. JAMA 2000;283(9): 1183–8.

33. Elkayam U, Akhter MW, Singh H, et al. Pregnancy-associated cardiomyopathy: clinical characteristics and a comparison between early and late presentation. Circulation 2005;111(16): 2050–5.

34. Habli M, O'Brien T, Nowack E, et al. Peripartum cardiomyopathy: prognostic factors for long-term maternal outcome. Am J Obstet Gynecol 2008; 199(4):415.e1–5.

35. Dos L, Teruel L, Ferreira IJ, et al. Late outcome of Senning and Mustard procedures for correction of transposition of the great arteries. Heart 2005; 91(5):652–6.

36. Graham TP Jr, Bernard YD, Mellen BG, et al. Long-term outcome in congenitally corrected transposition of the great arteries: a multi-institutional study. J Am Coll Cardiol 2000;36(1):255–61.

37. Drenthen W, Pieper PG, Ploeg M, et al. Risk of complications during pregnancy after Senning or Mustard (atrial) repair of complete transposition of the great arteries. Eur Heart J 2005;26(23): 2588–95.

38. Canobbio MM, Morris CD, Graham TP, et al. Pregnancy outcomes after atrial repair for transposition of the great arteries. Am J Cardiol 2006; 98(5):668–72.

39. Connolly HM, Grogan M, Warnes CA. Pregnancy among women with congenitally corrected transposition of great arteries. J Am Coll Cardiol 1999; 33(6):1692–5.

40. Therrien J, Barnes I, Somerville J. Outcome of pregnancy in patients with congenitally corrected transposition of the great arteries. Am J Cardiol 1999;84(7):820–4.

41. Guedes A, Mercier LA, Leduc L, et al. Impact of pregnancy on the systemic right ventricle after a Mustard operation for transposition of the great arteries. J Am Coll Cardiol 2004;44(2):433–7.

42. Bowater SE, Selman TJ, Hudsmith LE, et al. Long-term outcome following pregnancy in women with a systemic right ventricle: is the deterioration due to pregnancy or a consequence of time? Congenit Heart Dis 2013;8(4):302–7.

43. Balci A, Drenthen W, Mulder BJ, et al. Pregnancy in women with corrected tetralogy of Fallot: occurrence and predictors of adverse events. Am Heart J 2011;161(2):307–13.

44. Veldtman GR, Connolly HM, Grogan M, et al. Outcomes of pregnancy in women with tetralogy of Fallot. J Am Coll Cardiol 2004;44(1):174–80.

45. Egidy Assenza G, Cassater D, Landzberg M, et al. The effects of pregnancy on right ventricular remodeling in women with repaired tetralogy of Fallot. Int J Cardiol 2013;168(3):1847–52.

46. Le Gloan L, Mercier LA, Dore A, et al. Pregnancy in women with Fontan physiology. Expert Rev Cardiovasc Ther 2011;9(12):1547–56.

47. Drenthen W, Pieper PG, Roos-Hesselink JW, et al. Pregnancy and delivery in women after Fontan palliation. Heart 2006;92(9):1290–4.

48. Canobbio MM, Mair DD, van der Velde M, et al. Pregnancy outcomes after the Fontan repair. J Am Coll Cardiol 1996;28(3):763–7.

49. Presbitero P, Somerville J, Stone S, et al. Pregnancy in cyanotic congenital heart disease. Outcome of mother and fetus. Circulation 1994; 89(6):2673–6.

50. Weiss BM, Zemp L, Seifert B, et al. Outcome of pulmonary vascular disease in pregnancy: a systematic overview from 1978 through 1996. J Am Coll Cardiol 1998;31(7):1650–7.

51. Balint OH, Siu SC, Mason J, et al. Cardiac outcomes after pregnancy in women with congenital heart disease. Heart 2010;96(20):1656–61.

52. Lesniak-Sobelga A, Tracz W, KostKiewicz M, et al. Clinical and echocardiographic assessment of pregnant women with valvular heart diseases— maternal and fetal outcome. Int J Cardiol 2004; 94(1):15–23.

53. Hameed A, Karaalp IS, Tummala PP, et al. The effect of valvular heart disease on maternal and fetal outcome of pregnancy. J Am Coll Cardiol 2001;37(3):893–9.

54. Silversides CK, Colman JM, Sermer M, et al. Early and intermediate-term outcomes of pregnancy with congenital aortic stenosis. Am J Cardiol 2003;91(11):1386–9.

55. Yap SC, Drenthen W, Pieper PG, et al. Risk of complications during pregnancy in women with congenital aortic stenosis. Int J Cardiol 2008; 126(2):240–6.

56. Tzemos N, Silversides CK, Colman JM, et al. Late cardiac outcomes after pregnancy in women with congenital aortic stenosis. Am Heart J 2009; 157(3):474–80.

57. Barth WH Jr. Cardiac surgery in pregnancy. Clin Obstet Gynecol 2009;52(4):630–46.

58. Silversides CK, Colman JM, Sermer M, et al. Cardiac risk in pregnant women with rheumatic mitral stenosis. Am J Cardiol 2003;91(11):1382–5.

59. Elkayam U, Bitar F. Valvular heart disease and pregnancy part I: native valves. J Am Coll Cardiol 2005;46(2):223–30.

60. Gowda RM, Khan IA, Mehta NJ, et al. Cardiac arrhythmias in pregnancy: clinical and therapeutic considerations. Int J Cardiol 2003;88(2–3):129–33.

61. Lui GK, Silversides CK, Khairy P, et al. Heart rate response during exercise and pregnancy outcome in women with congenital heart disease. Circulation 2011;123(3):242–8.

62. Campos O, Andrade JL, Bocanegra J, et al. Physiologic multivalvular regurgitation during pregnancy: a longitudinal Doppler echocardiographic study. Int J Cardiol 1993;40(3):265–72.

63. Okuda Y, Sagami F, Tirone P, et al. Reproductive and developmental toxicity study of gadobenate dimeglumine formulation (E7155) (3)—study of embryo-fetal toxicity in rabbits by intravenous administration. J Toxicol Sci 1999;24(Suppl 1): 79–87.

64. Tanous D, Siu SC, Mason J, et al. B-type natriuretic peptide in pregnant women with heart disease. J Am Coll Cardiol 2010;56(15):1247–53.

65. Sliwa K, Hilfiker-Kleiner D, Petrie MC, et al. Current state of knowledge on aetiology, diagnosis, management, and therapy of peripartum cardiomyopathy: a position statement from the Heart Failure Association of the European Society of Cardiology Working Group on peripartum cardiomyopathy. Eur J Heart Fail 2010;12(8):767–78.

66. Sliwa K, Forster O, Libhaber E, et al. Peripartum cardiomyopathy: inflammatory markers as predictors of outcome in 100 prospectively studied patients. Eur Heart J 2006;27(4):441–6.

67. Lampert MB, Weinert L, Hibbard J, et al. Contractile reserve in patients with peripartum cardiomyopathy and recovered left ventricular function. Am J Obstet Gynecol 1997;176(1 Pt 1): 189–95.

68. Autore C, Conte MR, Piccininno M, et al. Risk associated with pregnancy in hypertrophic cardiomyopathy. J Am Coll Cardiol 2002;40(10): 1864–9.

69. Thaman R, Varnava A, Hamid MS, et al. Pregnancy related complications in women with hypertrophic cardiomyopathy. Heart 2003;89(7): 752–6.

70. Spirito P, Autore C. Management of hypertrophic cardiomyopathy. BMJ 2006;332(7552):1251–5.

The Tricuspid Valve in Adult Congenital Heart Disease

Jonathan Ginns, MD[a],*, Naser Ammash, MD[b],
Pierre-Luc Bernier, MD, MPH, FRCSC[a]

KEYWORDS

- Tricuspid valve • ACHD • Functional tricuspid regurgitation • Annuloplasty • Ebstein anomaly
- ASD • VSD

KEY POINTS

- Tricuspid valve disease is a common finding primarily and secondarily in congenital heart disease and tends to be underestimated in its clinical significance.
- The clinical assessment of tricuspid valve disease is subtle but critically important to management.
- Echocardiographic and magnetic resonance imaging assessment of tricuspid valve disease is essential to assess cause, severity, and management options.
- Surgical management of tricuspid valve disease is complex and evolving and can involve multiple repair techniques, or valve replacement.
- More attention in terms of research needs to be focused on the management of tricuspid valve disease in adult congenital heart disease.

 Videos of valve repair accompany this article at http://www.heartfailure.theclinics.com/

INTRODUCTION

Tricuspid valve disease is a frequent primary and secondary issue in adult congenital heart disease (ACHD), although its incidence has not been well defined.[1] In the past, tricuspid valve disease has been underappreciated in its importance, although this seems to be changing.[2–5] It has received less attention in terms of research or guidelines. Guidelines for surgical management of tricuspid disease are less aggressive and more subjective than those of other valves.[6] Indications for surgical intervention, and methods of approach and repair, are not uniform across institutions.

These issues also apply to acquired tricuspid disease. However, over the past decade significant progress has been made in establishing the importance of tricuspid valve disease, predominantly tricuspid regurgitation (TR), to patient outcomes in acquired heart disease.[7] In addition, rational approaches to methods of repair have been formed and relative agreement on modes of replacement has been developed. Nevertheless, tricuspid valve repair remains underused in this population.

Rigorous understanding of the contribution of this important lesion to symptoms, morbidity, and mortality is not well established in the ACHD population. Much understanding in this area comes from acquired heart disease. Imaging of tricuspid valve disease is complex and multimodality imaging is often required.[8] It is up to the ACHD community to perform more rigorous and extensive studies to define the extent of the problem and its contribution to disease in this population. Clinical assessment, pathologic entities,

Disclosures: None.
[a] Columbia University Medical Center, New York, NY 10032, USA; [b] Mayo Clinic, Rochester, MN 55905, USA
* Corresponding author.
E-mail address: jng2125@columbia.edu

Heart Failure Clin 10 (2014) 131–153
http://dx.doi.org/10.1016/j.hfc.2013.09.019
1551-7136/14/$ – see front matter © 2014 Elsevier Inc. All rights reserved.

investigations, management (both nonsurgical and surgical) are addressed in this article.

EMBRYOLOGY, ANATOMY, AND RELATIONSHIPS OF THE TRICUSPID VALVE
Embryology

The tricuspid valve forms after the division of the primitive atrioventricular (AV) canal (the connection between the primitive atrium and primitive ventricle) into 2 parts with the ingrowth and fusion of the anterior and posterior endocardial cushions (**Box 1**). As the ventricle enlarges, the tricuspid leaflet tissue delaminates from the wall of the ventricle, along with chordal and papillary muscle apparatus. The endocardial cushions contribute to the formation of the valve, particularly the septal leaflet. In various congenital heart conditions this process occurs abnormally. For example, in the endocardial cushion defects, there is abnormal or no fusion of the anterior and posterior cushions, giving rise to atrial and ventricular septal defects (VSDs) but also abnormal formation of the AV valve tissue. In Ebstein anomaly, delamination of the tricuspid valve from the right ventricle (RV) is abnormal, giving rise to the classic findings of septal and posterior leaflet fusion to the ventricular wall and abnormal excessive chordal attachments.

Anatomy

The tricuspid valve has several distinctive anatomic features (**Box 2**).[9,10] It has 3 leaflets: anterior, posterior, and septal. The anterior leaflet is the largest of these three and usually occupies about 40% of the circumference of the annulus (**Figs. 1** and **2**). The tricuspid valve annulus is displaced more toward the apex than in the mitral valve. The annulus is saddle shaped (highest anteriorly and posteriorly) and slightly ovoid. There are 2 major papillary muscles (anterior and posterior) providing attachment to the anterior and posterior

---

Box 1
Embryology of the tricuspid valve

- Tricuspid valve forms when the primitive common AV valve is divided by anterior and posterior endocardial cushions
- Delaminates from the endomyocardium of the right ventricle (RV)
- Failure of the endocardial cushions to fuse causes AV canal defects
- Failure of delamination from the RV causes Ebstein anomaly

Box 2
Anatomy and relationships of the tricuspid valve

- Tricuspid valve annulus more apically displaced than mitral annulus
- Tricuspid valve has 3 leaflets: anterior (the largest), posterior, and septal
- Two major papillary muscles (anterior and posterior) that arise from the RV free wall, but commonly there are septal chordal attachments (unlike the mitral valve)
- Annulus is saddle shaped (highest points are anterior and posterior)
- The triangle of Koch is immediately above the septal leaflet, with the AV node at its apex, vulnerable to surgery in this area

---

leaflets and the posterior and septal leaflets respectively. There are also septal chordal connections via the muscle of Lancisi (unlike the mitral valve), which provide additional support to the anterior and septal leaflets in the region of the anteroseptal commissure and are vulnerable to injury during surgery that involves the septum, such as patch closure of VSD.

Relationships

Several important anatomic structures are closely related to the tricuspid valve. The right atrium (RA) in patients with normal situs and D-looping of the ventricles is immediately above the tricuspid valve. The triangle of Koch sits superiorly to the septal leaflet. This anatomic triangle is made up of the coronary sinus ostium at its base, the tendon of Todaro (which is the anterior continuation of the eustachian valve), and the septal leaflet of the tricuspid valve. At its apex lies the AV node, which is susceptible to damage during surgery (**Fig. 3**). Anterior to this structure lies the central fibrous body, penetrated by the His bundle, and further anterior lies the membranous septum. The mitral annulus is leftward of the tricuspid annulus. The aortic valve lies in the space between the two AV valves anteriorly.

CLINICAL ASSESSMENT
History

History in the patient with tricuspid valve disease can be vague (**Box 3**). It is uncommon for patients with significant tricuspid valve disease to complain of shortness of breath. Much more commonly patients with tricuspid disease describe lack of energy and poor exercise capacity as fatigue and

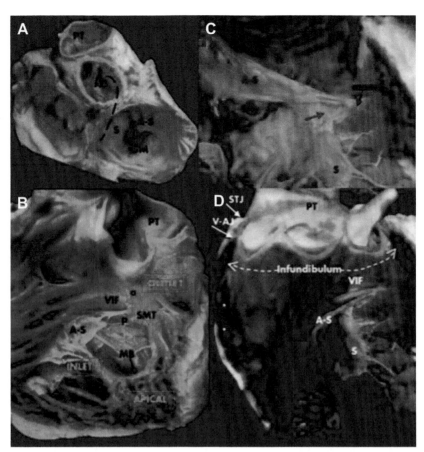

Fig. 1. (*A*) This dissection of the cardiac base shows the central location of the aortic valve, wedged between the mitral and tricuspid valves, and behind the pulmonary valve. The broken line marks the curved ventricular septum. The leaflets of the tricuspid valve are designated septal (S), anterosuperior (A-S), and mural (M). (*B*) The septal aspect of the RV is displayed to show the septomarginal trabeculation (SMT) with its anterior (a) and posterior (p) arms embracing the ventriculoinfundibular fold (VIF). The moderator band (MB) crosses the ventricular cavity as a distinct bundle. (*C*) The commissure between anterosuperior and septal leaflets is supported by the medial papillary muscle (mpm). This heart lacks formation of leaflet tissue in the region of the membranous septum (*arrow*). (*D*) This dissection of the outflow tract shows the muscular infundibulum supporting the pulmonary valve. Septoparietal trabeculations (*asterisks*) are flat. The semilunar leaflets have been removed to reveal the hinge lines crossing the ventriculoarterial junction (V-AJ) and rising to the sinotubular junction (STJ). (*From* Ho SY, Nihoyannopoulos P. Anatomy, echocardiography, and normal right ventricular dimensions. Heart 2006;92:i2–13; with permission.)

running out of energy. Patients with tricuspid valve disease commonly present late in the course of their disease because of this issue. One of the chief difficulties in patients with ACHD is that they often have other lesions that can contribute to exercise intolerance, including other valve disease, ventricular dysfunction, single-ventricle physiology, right-to-left shunting causing hypoxemia, bradycardia/pacemaker requirement, and noncardiac causes of limitation, such as restrictive lung disease, obesity, and general debility and deconditioning.

Other findings of significant tricuspid valve disease include poor appetite, nausea, and abdominal fullness caused by liver and intestinal venous distension and later ascites. Massive weight gain is common because salt and water retention can occur slowly and can pass unnoticed by the patient. As disease progresses and long-standing anorexia leads to malnutrition, weight loss can occur as muscle and fat is gradually shed because of inadequate caloric intake and lack of activity. Abdominal swelling is common in young patients. Patients often falsely ascribe the increased abdominal girth to dietary excess. Leg swelling and edema occur, but seem to be less frequent findings in young patients than in older patients, unless there is concomitant venous

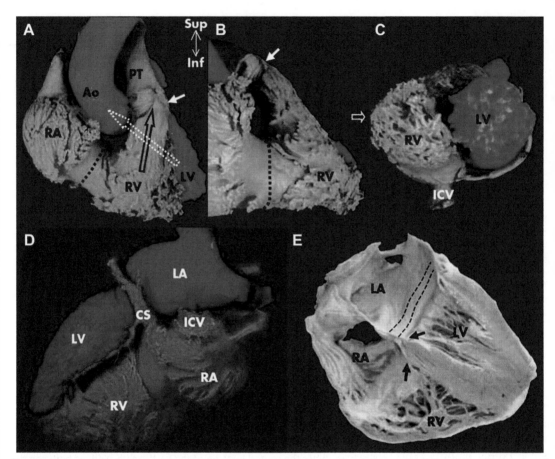

Fig. 2. An endocast of a normal heart, with right heart chambers colored blue and left heart chambers colored red, viewed from different perspectives to display the spatial relationships between cardiac chambers. (*A*) Viewed from the anterior aspect, the crossover arrangement between left (*dotted arrow*) and right ventricular (*open arrow*) outflow tracts is apparent. The pulmonary valve (*solid arrow*) is situated superiorly. (*B*) This view from right and anterior shows the triangular shape of the RV delimited by the tricuspid (*dotted line*) and pulmonary (*arrow*) valves. (*C*) Viewed from the apex, the RV is crescentic, wrapping round the left ventricle. The open arrow marks the acute margin. The coronary sinus is related to the inferior wall of the left atrium. (*D*) This view from the diaphragmatic aspect shows the course of the coronary sinus and the cardiac crux. (*E*) This 4-chamber section through a heart shows the offset arrangement of the hinge lines of the tricuspid and mitral valves (*arrows*) with the tricuspid valve attached closer to the cardiac apex than the mitral valve. The broken lines trace the course of the coronary sinus passing along the inferior aspect of the left atrium. Ao, aorta; CS, coronary sinus; ICV, inferior caval vein; LA, left atrium; LV, left ventricle; PT, pulmonary trunk; RA, right atrium. (*From* Ho SY, Nihoyannopoulos P. Anatomy, echocardiography, and normal right ventricular dimensions. Heart 2006;92:i2–13; with permission.)

disease of the lower limbs (as is common in patients with ACHD who have frequently had injury to lower limb venous structures caused by prior cardiac catheterization).

Palpitations can occur; mostly caused by supraventricular arrhythmias. The commonest arrhythmic complication of significant tricuspid disease is atrial flutter, or, in Ebstein anomaly, atrioventricular reciprocating tachycardia (AVRT) caused by Wolff-Parkinson-White syndrome, which occurs in approximately 25%. It is common for atrial arrhythmias to occur silently, and patients just present with worsening signs of right heart

failure caused by the loss of atrial kick, followed by sustained increase in filling pressures. Chest pain is uncommon in tricuspid disease.

Examination

Clinical examination findings again tend to be subtle in tricuspid valve disease, and are listed later (**Box 4**).

General

If present, cachexia can be masked by massive fluid overload. After appropriate diuresis, the dry

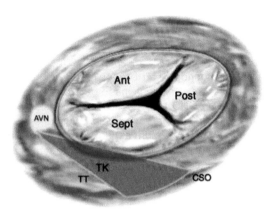

Fig. 3. Surgical anatomy of the tricuspid valve: the triangle of Koch (TK) is indicated by the orange area. Ant, anterior; AVN, AV node; CSO, coronary sinus orifice; Post, posterior; Sept, septal; TT, tendon of Todaro. (*From* Taramasso M, Vanermen H, Maisano F, et al. The growing clinical importance of secondary tricuspid regurgitation. J Am Coll Cardiol 2012;59(8):703–10; with permission.)

weight is often surprisingly low and suggests significant malnutrition.

Vitals

There can be weight loss or weight gain, depending on the volume status. Blood pressure can be low. Heart rate can be fast and/or irregular because of atrial arrhythmia. Cyanosis is a common finding, caused by VQ mismatch or right-to-left shunting across the atrial septum that tends to worsen with exercise.

Face

Plethora caused by chronic cyanosis and central cyanosis of the tongue can sometimes be appreciated.

Neck

Increase of the jugular venous pressure (JVP) is common, but may not occur in some instances

---

Box 3
History

- Fatigue, reduced exercise tolerance
- Shortness of breath uncommon
- Poor appetite, nausea, weight gain or loss (depending on volume status/diuretic use)
- Abdominal fullness
- Leg swelling
- Palpitations frequently caused by supraventricular arrhythmias

---

Box 4
Examination

- Cachexia, edema, anasarca
- Cyanosis with right to left atrial-level shunt or VQ mismatch
- Increased jugular venous pressure, especially prominent v waves
- RV heave if the RV is dilated or hypertrophied
- Pansystolic murmur at lower left sternal border that worsens with inspiration
- Systolic clicks in Ebstein anomaly
- Abdominal fullness
- Liver enlargement and pulsatility
- Lower limb edema

---

such as in Ebstein anomaly caused by a large capacitant chamber of the RA plus the atrialized portion of the RV or when the patient has been well diuresed. Prominent a waves can occur if there is right ventricular noncompliance or tricuspid stenosis. Large v waves frequently occur in the presence of severe TR.

Precordium

Right ventricular heave may be present. Apex beat can be displaced if there is additional dilatation of the left ventricle.

Lungs

Lung examination tends to be clear until pleural effusions occur (a late finding).

Heart sounds

S1 may be soft or absent in severe TR. There may be a prominent P2 when there is pulmonary hypertension. S2 may occur late (widely split S2) with right bundle branch block, which is commonly present in patients with previous right-sided cardiac surgery. Right ventricular S3 may be present if there is RV dysfunction. Systolic clicks can occur in systole in Ebstein anomaly caused by sudden straightening of abnormal chordal attachments. Murmur caused by TR tends to be of medium pitch, pansystolic, and loudest at the lower left sternal border. It is louder with inspiration. The murmur is the sound generated between the fast-moving layers of the TR jet and the relatively motionless blood in the right atrial chamber. In some cases of severe TR there may be no murmur because of the laminar flow of a very severe, broad jet of TR. A diastolic rumble over the tricuspid region may be present because of tricuspid stenosis or high flow when there is massive TR. In the systemic RV the sound of TR often takes on a high pitch or whistling quality because of higher pressures.

Abdomen

The abdomen is often full, lacking its usual scaphoid appearance in young patients, because of passive congestion of abdominal viscera. This condition may be noted as a general firmness of the abdomen. The liver may be enlarged and/or pulsatile. The presence of liver pulsatility is a helpful sign of severe TR. The spleen may be palpable. There may be ascites present, but this can be difficult to detect when mild.

Lower limbs

Edema may be appreciated. Chronic venous changes are not usually caused by TR itself, but often accompany and contribute to leg swelling when the patient has a history of venous injury from cardiac catheterization in childhood or prior venous thrombosis.

KEY PATHOLOGIC ENTITIES CAUSING TRICUSPID DISEASE IN ACHD
Functional TR

Functional TR is defined as TR that is secondary to changes in the RV or distortion of tricuspid leaflets, annulus, or chords that is not caused by a primary disorder of the tricuspid valve (Video 1). Much of the understanding of the pathogenesis of functional TR is taken from acquired left-sided heart disease in adult patients, in whom it is a common problem[11] and usually caused by RV dysfunction induced by left-sided heart disease with pulmonary hypertension.[6]

Functional TR carries a significant adverse prognosis in acquired heart disease.[11,12] Whether this adverse prognosis can be applied in congenital heart disease (CHD) remains to be proved. Functional TR in CHD may occur in many lesions in which there is abnormal preload or afterload affecting the RV, such as atrial septal defect (ASD), anomalous pulmonary venous return, pulmonary regurgitation, pulmonary hypertension, and in the failing systemic RV.[7]

Functional TR occurs because of reduced leaflet coaptation for 3 reasons[13]:

- Annular dilatation that occurs predominantly laterally and posteriorly (**Fig. 4**). Annular dilatation has been strongly correlated with degree of TR (**Fig. 5**)
- Annular deformation: the tricuspid annulus loses its usual saddle shape becomes flatter and more circular, which leads to leaflets coapting abnormally because of alteration in their spatial relationships and change in orientation of the chordal apparatus and papillary musculature (**Fig. 6**)
- With RV dilatation, chordal apparatus and papillary muscles are displaced laterally, causing tethering of the tricuspid leaflets and worsening coaptation (**Fig. 7**)[14]

The size and location of the tricuspid annulus can be abnormal in CHD, which complicates the disorder and assessment in this situation, and the tricuspid leaflets often have intrinsic disorders.

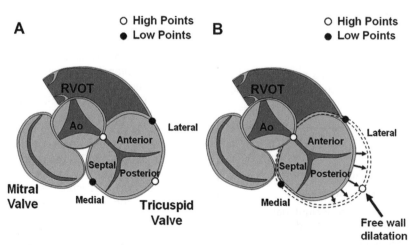

Fig. 4. (*A*) tricuspid valve viewed from the atrium. The valve relative to anatomic structures is displayed, showing the location of high and low points. (*B*) Dilatation along the free wall aspect of the tricuspid valve with functional TR (*dashed lines*). RVOT, RV outflow tract. (*From* Ton-Nu TT, Levine RA, Handschumacher MD, et al. Geometric determinants of functional tricuspid regurgitation: insights from 3-dimensional echocardiography. Circulation 2006;114(2):143–9; with permission.)

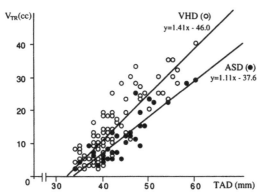

Fig. 5. Correlation of regurgitant volume per beat (VTR) and tricuspid annular dimension at end-diastole. There is a significant correlation between preoperative TAD and volume of tricuspid regurgitation in the VHD group ($r = 0.87$) and the ASD group ($r = 0.88$). However, the slope of the correlation line is steeper for the valvular heart disease group than for the ASD group. (*From* Sugimoto T, Okada M, Ozaki N, et al. Long-term evaluation of treatment for functional tricuspid regurgitation with regurgitant volume: characteristic differences based on primary cardiac lesion. J Thorac Cardiovasc Surg 1999;117(3):463–71; with permission.)

The development of functional TR is self-reinforcing because worsening TR begets further annular and RV dilation and further worsening of TR. Previously functional TR was thought to spontaneously improve following treatment of the primary lesion in acquired heart disease.[15] In the last decade multiple studies have shown this premise to be false, with many series showing later onset of TR or persistence of TR where a valve disorder was not addressed at the primary surgery.[16]

ASD

ASD can lead to long-term volume overload of the RV. When this overload causes annular dilatation or dysfunction, secondary TR can ensue

(Video 2). In a study by Toyono and colleagues,[17] 32 of 180 patients undergoing ASD closure had moderate or greater TR before closure (device or surgical). Fifty percent of patients with moderate or worse TR before ASD closure had residual TR after the procedure. The presence of pulmonary hypertension before ASD closure was a marker for predicting residual TR after secundum ASD closure in this cohort. In those who underwent concomitant tricuspid valve repair, preoperative RV systolic function, sphericity, and pulmonary artery systolic pressure (PASP) were predictors of residual TR.[18] However, Yalonetsky and Lorber[19] showed significant improvement in TR following device closure in all patients in a series of 46 patients.

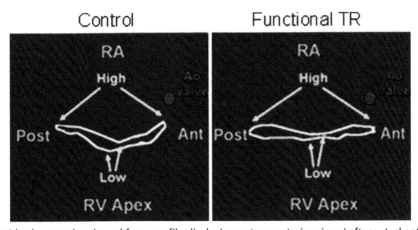

Fig. 6. Tricuspid valve annulus viewed from profile displaying anteroposterior view. Left: control patient (normal tricuspid valve) with 2 high points located anteroposteriorly. Right: patient with functional TR. The annulus has become flatter with no distinct high point. (*From* Hung J. The pathogenesis of functional tricuspid regurgitation. Semin Thorac Cardiovasc Surg 2010;22(1):76–8; with permission.)

A

B

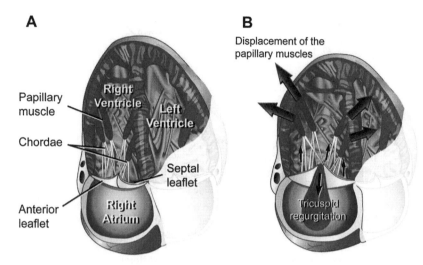

Fig. 7. (A) Normal tricuspid valve. (B) Functional TR: enlargement of the RV results in displacement of the papillary muscles and tethering of the tricuspid leaflets. In addition there is dilatation of the tricuspid annulus. (*From* Mascherbauer J, Maurer G. The forgotten valve: lessons to be learned in tricuspid regurgitation. Eur Heart J 2010;31:2841–3; with permission.)

VSD

In perimembranous VSD, the defect is frequently partially closed by aneurysmal tissue of the septal leaflet of the tricuspid valve, which infrequently causes deformity of this leaflet and chordae supplying the anteroseptal commissure, giving rise to reduced leaflet coaptation and secondarily TR (Video 3). The septal leaflet of the tricuspid valve has attachments to the septum and these can be damaged during VSD repair, leading to significant TR. During repair of VSD, there is rarely injury to the tricuspid with resultant significant TR. In a study by Mongeon and colleagues,[20] 46 adults patients undergoing VSD closure, 6% had severe preoperative TR, 24% required tricuspid repair during surgery, and 13% had moderate or worse TR at late follow-up.

AV Canal Defect

The right-sided AV valve can occasionally be left with varying degrees of stenosis and regurgitation after repair, which likely depends preoperative anatomy (Video 4). The right AV valve is composed of a portion of the inferior and superior bridging leaflet, and the right anterior, right lateral, and right posterior leaflet. The multiple clefts in this situation can give rise to TR. In addition, depending on the size of the common AV valve orifice and the location of the septal patch, an element of tricuspid stenosis can be seen, although this is uncommon. Dodge-Khatami and colleagues[21] reported a 6.6% incidence of significant right AV valve disease at

follow-up of a series of 76 patient undergoing repair for complete AV canal defect.

Ebstein Anomaly

During embryologic development, the tricuspid valve fails to delaminate from the RV in this lesion (Videos 5 and 6). The septal leaflet and posterior leaflet are the most affected.[22] In addition to the failure of delamination, the atrialized portion of the RV fails to develop normal musculature and is myopathic. The functional RV can be small. The leaflets are abnormal, often leading to poor leaflet coaptation and leading to varying severities of TR. SVT caused by AV bypass tracts are sometimes associated.

Tricuspid Valve Dysplasia

Tricuspid valve dysplasia can occur primarily or concomitantly with other lesions (Video 7). It shares some features with Ebstein anomaly but lacks the apical displacement of the septal and posterior leaflets of the tricuspid valve. If abnormally tethered, fenestrated leaflets can lead to severe TR and occasionally tricuspid stenosis.

Tricuspid Atresia/Hypoplasia

In tricuspid atresia, the tricuspid valve fails to form out of the primitive AV canal (Videos 8 and 9). This lesion is frequently treated with the Fontan operation. In a small number of patients in whom there was an adequate RV some form of operation to restore continuity between the RA and the RV, such as the Bjork modification Fontan and homograft RA-RV conduit, may have been performed. These patients have varying degrees of stenosis and regurgitation through the connection between the RA and RV and frequently require surgical or catheter-based repair.[23]

Repaired Tetralogy of Fallot/Pulmonary Stenosis

Patients with repaired tetralogy of Fallot (TOF) and pulmonary stenosis are commonly left with severe pulmonary regurgitation (Video 10). This pulmonary regurgitation can lead to RV dilatation and dysfunction over time. Secondary TR can result from this. Kogon and colleagues[24] showed than in 35 patients undergoing pulmonary valve replacement for repaired TOF or PS with preoperative moderate or worse TR, degree of postoperative TR was similar between those who did (16 of 35) and those who did not (19 of 35) undergo tricuspid valve repair.

Pulmonary Atresia with Intact Ventricluar Septum

The tricuspid valve forms abnormally in pulmonary atresia with intact ventricluar septum (PA-IVS). The tricuspid annulus is frequently hypoplastic (Video 11). Often abnormal attachments and tethering occur. As part of biventricular repair, significant pulmonary incompetence often results (66.7% in series by Hoashi[25]). This condition can lead to dilation of the hypoplastic RV to accommodate the increased volume. The tricuspid valve that is hypoplastic then becomes tethered, analogously to a dilated ventricle in pulmonary regurgitation caused by PS or TOF. This abnormal tethering leads to central TR, which is moderate or worse in 44.4%.[25] In a series of 13 patients by Bautista-Hernandez and colleagues,[26] 85% had moderate or worse TR and 69% required concomitant tricuspid valve repair when undergoing PVR for severe PI at a median age of 15.5 years, which was a higher rate than a matched cohort of patients with TOF undergoing PVR (only 8% requiring concomitant tricuspid valve repair).

Systemic RV in Congenitally Corrected Transposition of the Great Arteries, D Transposition of the Great Arteries After Mustard/Senning and Hypoplastic Left Heart Syndrome

The physiology of TR in these lesions is different from those discussed earlier because as it represents disease of the systemic AV valve, with physiology akin to mitral regurgitation (Videos 12 and 13). These patients may present with shortness of breath, pulmonary hypertension, or right heart failure symptoms caused by subpulmonic left ventricular (LV) failure.

TR can occur in CCTGA, in which dysplasia of the tricuspid valve (sharing some features with Ebstein anomaly) is a common finding.[27] Tricuspid valve replacement is recommended in this situation if significant AV valve regurgitation is appreciated,[28] and may prevent deterioration in systemic RV function over time.[29] In contrast with this, TR in D-TGA after Mustard or Senning operation is often secondary.[30] Akin to functional mitral regurgitation, tricuspid valve replacement is not advised if there is significant dysfunction of the systemic RV.[28] Aggressive medical therapy and early referral of consideration of cardiac transplantation or mechanical support are essential.

In hypoplastic left heart syndrome the systemic RV may be affected by significant TR. TR is a risk factor for mortality in these patients. Up to 25% of patients after Norwood operation require surgery for TR. The tricuspid valve may be regurgitant in these patients because of systemic RV dysfunction or intrinsic abnormalities of the tricuspid valve, including dysplasia, prolapse, and increased/decreased number of leaflets.[31,32]

Pulmonary Hypertension

Pulmonary hypertension by itself does not usually cause TR, but, when RV dilatation and dysfunction develop, secondary TR can result (Videos 14 and 15). This condition seems to have the usual causes, as discussed earlier, with annular dilatation and deformation and, as RV dysfunction develops, tethering of the tricuspid valve leaflets. Resolution of pulmonary hypertension after thromboendarterectomy in chronic pulmonary thromboembolic disease tends to reduce severity of TR.[33,34]

Pacemakers and Implantable Cardioverter-Defibrillator

Heart block and ventricular arrhythmias in adults with CHD often necessitate placement of permanent pacemakers and implantable cardioverter-defibrillators (ICDs) (Video 16). The ventricular lead often causes the tricuspid valve to function abnormally, leading to significant TR, which can be caused by leaflet perforation, laceration, or scarring/adhesion to the lead (**Fig. 8**). One report noted that 17.8% of patients with mild TR at baseline developed moderate-severe TR after pacemaker or ICD lead placement.[35] The lead usually lies in the anteroposterior or posteroseptal commissure. Significant TR is more likely to happen with ICD leads (presumably because of

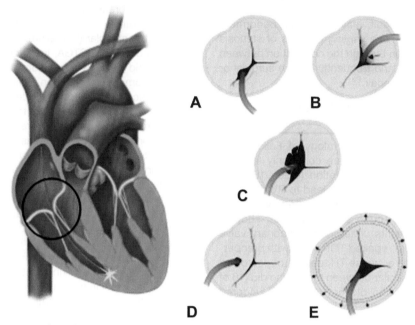

Fig. 8. Mechanisms of mechanical TR in the setting of permanent pacemaker or implantable cardioverter-defibrillator leads. (A) Valve obstruction caused by lead placed between leaflets. (B) Lead adherence caused by fibrosis and scar formation to valve causing incomplete closure. (C) Lead entrapment in the tricuspid valve apparatus. (D) Valve perforation or laceration. (E) Annular dilatation. (*From* Al-Bawardy R, Krishnaswamy K, Bhargava M, et al. Tricuspid regurgitation in patients with pacemakers and implantable cardiac defibrillators: a comprehensive review. Clin Cardiol 2013;36(5):249–54; with permission.)

their bulk) and may occur even when no regurgitation existed before lead placement. If the lead is removed, residual TR may persist, caused by annular dilatation or leaflet damage.[36–39]

INVESTIGATIONS
Transthoracic Echocardiography

Subcostal views are particularly useful to assess venous flow in the inferior vena cava (IVC), hepatic veins, and sometimes to see the tricuspid valve when poorly imaged from other views. Assessment of the IVC diameter and whether there is inspiratory collapse supplements the clinical findings of the jugular venous assessment. When there is systolic reversal in the hepatic venous flow, this suggests severe TR.

Apical views show the anterior leaflet and septal leaflet on typical 4-chamber views. Assessment in this view includes measurement of the tricuspid annulus, motion, thickening, location of septal attachment, assessment of severity of TR, assessment based on effective regurgitant orifice, vena contracta width, and size of jet area in RA. In addition, this view is useful for assessment of any gradient across the tricuspid valve in cases of tricuspid stenosis or hypoplasia.

Assessment of right atrial size and assessment of right ventricular size and function in this view should be routine.

Parasternal views generally allow the best assessment (because the echo window has the shortest distance to the valve in this location) of the tricuspid valve morphology, motion and abnormalities of leaflet positions, size, thickening, prolapsed, and fenestrations. The long axis (parasternal long axis [PLAX] and parasternal short axis [PSAX]) views allow assessment of the anterior leaflet, septal leaflet, and posterior leaflets individually. Annular dimension is often greatest in the PLAX view because the annulus typically dilates greatest posteriorly. Assessment of TR is supplemented in these views and often the cause of regurgitation is better assessed here. In cases where the apical views do not allow adequate assessment of TR severity (such as in the presence of bioprosthetic tricuspid valve or pacemaker leads), the parasternal views should be relied on to better assess the severity of any TR present. PSAX views also allow assessment of RV size and function over the entire ventricle and allow better assessment of regional variation (such as in RV outflow tract/scar/patch in TOF). Right parasternal views can also be used to supplement, particularly in cases of abnormal cardiac position, and can allow closer assessment of the interatrial septum and superior vena cava and IVC.

Three-dimensional transthoracic echocardiogram

Three-dimensional transthoracic echocardiogram (3D TTE) may enable improved identification of individual leaflets and regurgitant jets; improved ability to quantify RV size and function; identification of chordal ruptures, papillary muscles, and flail leaflets; and measurement of tenting volume. 3D TTE may be particularly useful in pacemaker-related TR to assess the lead location.

Transesophageal echocardiogram

Transesophageal echocardiogram (TEE) can be helpful when suboptimal imaging of the tricuspid valve is obtained on TTE. Sedation and volume reduction with fasting can change the severity of TR significantly, and TEE should be not relied on wholly when discrepant to the TTE. Perioperative TEE is susceptible to the same pitfalls when TR is frequently underestimated in the presence of lower-than-usual blood flows, vasodilating anesthetic agents, and unpredictable fluid shifts.[8]

Cardiac MRI

Cardiac MRI has become the gold standard in assessment of right ventricular volumes and function. Assessment of right ventricular size and function is notoriously difficult by echocardiography, especially in the context of abnormal body habitus, complex anatomy, or poor acoustic penetration. This modality also allows reliable serial imaging to assess changes in right ventricular size and volume to follow tricuspid valve disease over time. Assessment of TR severity can be attempted by MRI, although it can be subject to pitfalls. Other limitations include susceptibility to artifact, the necessity of a cooperative patient, and the presence of arrhythmias, and many patients in these groups have pacemakers or ICDs, which currently are a contraindication to cardiac MRI at most institutions. Cardiac computed tomography can be used as an alternative, with newer techniques leading to reduced radiation dose.

Cardiac catheterization

Cardiac catheterization can be useful in the assessment of tricuspid valve disease in which assessment of hemodynamics is suboptimal by echo and clinical examination. Underestimation of central venous pressure can occur clinically. Right ventriculography may be useful if echo imaging is suboptimal, and arrhythmias do not allow adequate assessment by cardiac MRI.

MANAGEMENT
Management Strategies are Presented in Outline Form, Reflecting Data-driven and Experience-driven Care Guidelines

Overall approach

- Appreciate tricuspid valve disease severity and assess its impact
- Determine the underlying cause
- Manage any contributing factors, such as volume overload, arrhythmia, pulmonary hypertension, left-sided heart disease, myopathic disease, concomitant valvular disease, infection
- Surgical therapy by appropriately trained and experienced surgeon if appropriate on tricuspid valve and/or any other concomitant valve/disease process, using technique appropriate to the disease
- Cardiologists should be cognizant of various repair techniques, their durability, the types of valve replacement available, and percutaneous options available to guide therapy

Nonsurgical

- Diuretics to control volume status. This strategy generally improves edema, shortness of breath caused by pleural effusions, abdominal swelling, and ascites if present. Volume control should not be seen as an end in itself.
- Loop diuretics are first-line agents. The addition of a powerful thiazide diuretic can sometimes be warranted, although care must be taken to avoid hypokalemia in this setting. Addition of spironolactone can be especially helpful if there is an element of hepatic dysfunction. Renal function and daily weight should be recorded.
- Antiarrhythmics and AV nodal blocking agents should be considered if appropriate to control supraventricular arrhythmias.
- Inotropic support can be appropriate when right ventricular dysfunction has led to low-output state. The long-term use of inotropes is controversial, except in the setting of awaiting cardiac transplantation. Short-term use may also be helpful to optimize the patient before undergoing high-risk surgery involving the tricuspid valve.
- When pulmonary hypertension caused by pulmonary vascular disease is present, the addition of oral, inhaled, or parenteral pulmonary vasodilators is appropriate. These vasodilators reduce RV afterload, and therefore tend to improve RV compliance and secondary TR when present.

- Consideration of electrophysiology study and ablation when supraventricular arrhythmias are present. In general, right-sided atrial flutter can be addressed with greater than 90% success rate. Ablation is typically safe; this procedure can safely be undertaken even in patients with precarious hemodynamics.
- Catheter-based intervention to the tricuspid valve, in particular valve-in-valve replacement, is increasingly considered when bioprosthetic valve dysfunction is present, as is transcatheter closure of paravalvular leaks.[40–42]

Surgery

Indications for tricuspid surgery

The American College of Cardiology (ACC)–American Heart Association (AHA) ACHD care guidelines mention the tricuspid valve when addressing certain indications (**Box 5**).

The guidelines mention surgery on the tricuspid valve in the context of other lesion repair, or as an indication for other lesion repair. In addition, they address tricuspid valve disease in Ebstein anomaly and in the systemic RV. However, other isolated tricuspid disease is not specifically addressed, for which concomitant surgery is not

---

Box 5
ACHD guidelines

In ASD/VSD repair TR should be addressed if significant

In TOF with severe PI, moderate or severe TR is a class IIa indication for PVR (significant TR in this setting should be addressed with either repair or replacement depending on valve morphology) (level of evidence, C)

In D-TGA after atrial baffle repair with moderate-severe systemic AV valve regurgitation and preserved RV function, surgery is a class I indication (level of evidence, B)

In D-TGA/VSD/PS after Rastelli repair with severe conduit regurgitation, more than moderate TR is a class I indication for conduit replacement (level of evidence, C)

Unrepaired CCTGA with any severe AV valve regurgitation or evidence of moderate or progressive systemic AV valve regurgitation is considered a class I indication for surgery (level of evidence, B)

In Ebstein anomaly class I indications for surgery include:

    Symptoms or deteriorating exercise capacity (level of evidence, B)

    Cyanosis (oxygen saturation less than 90%) (level of evidence, B)

    Paradoxic embolism (level of evidence, B)

    Progressive cardiomegaly on chest radiograph (level of evidence, B)

    Progressive RV dilatation or reduction of RV systolic function (level of evidence, B)

In Ebstein anomaly following prior surgery, surgical rerepair or replacement of the tricuspid valve is recommended for the following class I indications:

    Symptoms, deteriorating exercise capacity, or New York Heart Association functional class III or IV (level of evidence, B)

    Severe TR after repair with progressive RV dilatation, reduction of RV systolic function, or appearance/progression of atrial and/or ventricular arrhythmias (level of evidence, B)

    Bioprosthetic tricuspid valve dysfunction with significant mixed regurgitation and stenosis (level of evidence, B)

    Predominant bioprosthetic valve stenosis (mean gradient greater than 12–15 mm Hg) (level of evidence, B)

    Operation can be considered earlier with lesser degrees of bioprosthetic stenosis with symptoms or decreased exercise tolerance (level of evidence, B)

Adapted from Warnes CA, Williams RG, Bashore TM, et al. ACC/AHA 2008 guidelines for the management of adults with congenital heart disease: a report of the American College of Cardiology/American Heart Association Task Force on Practice Guidelines (Writing Committee to Develop Guidelines on the Management of Adults With Congenital Heart Disease). Developed in Collaboration With the American Society of Echocardiography, Heart Rhythm Society, International Society for Adult Congenital Heart Disease, Society for Cardiovascular Angiography and Interventions, and Society of Thoracic Surgeons. J Am Coll Cardiol 2008;52(23):e143–263; with permission.

required and clinicians must look to adult guidelines for guidance (**Box 6**).

These guidelines apply to the adult patient with acquired heart disease in whom functional TR is the most common lesion. Some experts have suggested other indications for intervention, including prophylactic repair at a particular level of annular dilatation because this may more accurately represent tricuspid disease than degree of TR. Possible indications for prophylactic repair in the context of concomitant cardiac surgery when the degree of TR is less than severe include:

- Echo/surgical indications: annulus greater than 40 mm or 21 mm/m^2 from the apical 4-chamber view
- Intraoperative finding of annular dimensions greater than 70 mm from anteroseptal commissure to posteroseptal commissure[4]

The current guidelines may lead to late intervention when patients have become medically refractory. The high mortality of tricuspid surgery may indicate that late surgery tends to be the norm. Caution is needed in extending these guidelines to the patient with ACHD for the following reasons:

- Patients affected by most common left-sided lesions are older than typical patients with ACHD, and the long-term effect of severe volume load on the RV is greater over the lifetime, especially in active young patients
- The high mortality for tricuspid valve surgery in these adults likely affects the aggressiveness of these guidelines; however, it is likely that many patients previously operated on for this lesion mostly had late-stage disease
- Tricuspid valve repair is preferred in many situations, but it is common for at least moderate TR to remain after repair

SURGICAL APPROACH TO TRICUSPID DISEASE
General

To understand tricuspid disease, the ACHD cardiologist needs a good appreciation of the types of surgeries, their risks, and potential long-term outcomes. In ACHD, variability in disorders of the tricuspid valve is the norm, and frequently an additional component of functional tricuspid valve regurgitation is present. In addition, the RV is frequently abnormal because of malformation or previous surgery. The outcomes

---

Box 6
Applicable ACC-AHA care guidelines for adults with tricuspid valve disease

Class I

Tricuspid valve repair is beneficial for severe TR in patients with mitral valve disease requiring MV surgery (level of evidence, B)

Class IIa

1. Tricuspid valve replacement or annuloplasty is reasonable for severe primary TR when symptomatic (level of evidence, C)

2. Tricuspid valve replacement is reasonable for severe TR secondary to diseased/abnormal tricuspid valve leaflets not amenable to annuloplasty or repair (level of evidence, C)

Class IIb

Tricuspid annuloplasty may be considered for less-than-severe TR in patients undergoing MV surgery when there is pulmonary hypertension or tricuspid annular dilatation (level of evidence, C)

Class III

1. Tricuspid valve replacement or annuloplasty is not indicated in asymptomatic patients with TR whose pulmonary artery systolic pressure is less than 60 mm Hg in the presence of a normal MV (level of evidence, C)

2. Tricuspid valve replacement or annuloplasty is not indicated in patients with mild primary TR (level of evidence, C)

Adapted from Bonow RO, Carabello BA, Chatterjee K, et al. 2008 focused update incorporated into the ACC/AHA 2006 guidelines for the management of patients with valvular heart disease: a report of the American College of Cardiology/American Heart Association Task Force on Practice Guidelines (Writing Committee to Revise the 1998 Guidelines for the Management of Patients with Valvular Heart Disease). Endorsed by the Society of Cardiovascular Anesthesiologists, Society for Cardiovascular Angiography and Interventions, and Society of Thoracic Surgeons. J Am Coll Cardiol 2008;52(13):e1–142; with permission.

for the various procedures are not well documented in this population, although this is an area of active research.

Repair is appropriate in many circumstances, but can be difficult to achieve. The type of repair should be tailored to the underlying disorder. Patients may have recurrent TR when only the primary disorder is treated, even when significant TR is not present before surgery (especially when significant annular dilatation, RV dilatation/dysfunction, pulmonary hypertension, or leaflet tethering are present).

TECHNIQUES OF TRICUSPID VALVE REPAIR
Annuloplasty Techniques

Correction of annular dilatation, which is one of the key anatomic deformities that lead to significant TR in functional tricuspid valve disease, can be achieved with a variety of methods of annuloplasty (**Table 1**). Techniques to reduce annular dimensions include suture-based techniques, as well as the use of band and ring annuloplasties.

Suture-based techniques include the Kay (**Fig. 9**) and De Vega annuloplasty (**Fig. 10**). These annuloplasties are quickly performed and have low cost, low risk of complication, and moderate durability. The De Vega annuloplasty involves a more extensive suture line than the Kay annuloplasty and is thought to be more effective.

Annuloplasty rings provide a more rigid support (**Figs. 11** and **12**). They can be partial or full. Partial annuloplasty rings have the advantage of leaving an area over the septal leaflet (the danger zone) around the location of the AV node free of sutures to avoid AV block. However, full annuloplasty rings can be sewn into the septal leaflet to avoid suturing directly into the annulus in the location of the AV node, or sutures can be omitted in this area.

Experience in the population of patients with acquired tricuspid valve disease has shown superiority for ring annuloplasty techniques rather than suture techniques alone. There is a slightly higher incidence of postoperative AV block and a slightly longer bypass/cross-clamp time required.

Residual significant TR is associated with poorer outcomes, although this may relate to underlying, more severe, disorders. However, reoperation for TR carries high mortality. Annuloplasty can worsen tethering, because of pulling chords/papillary muscles in an even more oblique angle (therefore clinicians should consider replacement when annuloplasty alone is not going to be successful).

One disadvantage of annuloplasty rings in patients with CHD is that they were designed for patients with a normal adult annulus. However, many patients with CHD have abnormal annuli, unlike anything seen in acquired heart disease, in which the ring may prove to be the wrong shape or size. In addition, the introduction of a foreign body with the potential for scar formation and later difficulty with repeat surgery is a concern. Therefore many congenital heart surgeons continue to use suture-based techniques primarily. The difference in outcomes seen between the two techniques has yet to be shown in this population.

Other Repair Techniques

- Commissural or cleft closure for areas of commissural/cleft leak (**Fig. 13**)

Table 1
Comparison of selected annuloplasty approaches for functional TR

	Bicuspidization/ Kay	De Vega	Flexible Band	Rigid Ring
Simplicity	Yes	Yes	No	No
Added time (min)	<5	<10	10–20	15–20
Reproducibility	Low	Moderate	High	Very high
Annular stabilization	Posterior	Anterior/ posterior	Anterior/ posterior	Septal/anterior/ posterior
Risk of heart block	None	Minimal	Minimal	Low
Residual TR	High	Moderate	Low	Low
Recurrent TR	High	Moderate	Low	Low
Cost	Cheap	Cheap	Expensive	Expensive

This assumes techniques are applied by general cardiac surgeons without specific expertise in either repair technique.
Adapted from Chikwe J, Anyanwu AC. Surgical strategies for functional tricuspid regurgitation. Semin Thorac Cardiovasc Surg 2010;22(1):90–6; with permission.

A

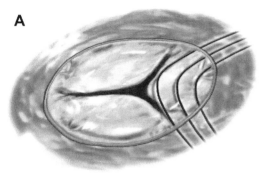

B

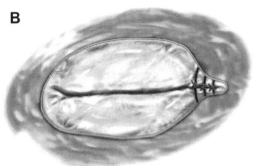

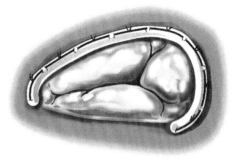

Fig. 11. A measured plication of the annulus adjacent to the anterior and posterior leaflets is achieved and the conduction system is not jeopardized. (*From* McCarthy JF, Cosgrove DM. Tricuspid valve repair with the Cosgrove-Edwards Annuloplasty System. Ann Thorac Surg 1997;64(1):267–8; with permission.)

- Cusp augmentation: autologous pericardium or the use of prosthetic materials has been used to increase the length of the anterior leaflet or other leaflets in order to increase the degree of coaptation (**Fig. 14**)
- Clover technique (**Fig. 15**)

Tricuspid Valve Replacement

When satisfactory repair cannot be achieved, tricuspid valve replacement is appropriate. In acquired heart disease, tricuspid valve replacement may carry mortality of up to 20%[43]; higher than repair, with a hazard ratio greater than 5:1,[44–46] although this may reflect more severe disorders in patients who underwent tricuspid replacement who were not repairable (there is no randomized trial comparing repair with replacement). Currently most patients are referred for bioprosthetic tricuspid valve replacement given the significant risk of thrombosis associated with a mechanical valve in this position (**Table 2**).[45,46]

SPECIAL SITUATIONS
Ebstein Anomaly

Given the unusual anatomy in Ebstein disorder, specific techniques have been designed to achieve repair in this condition. Continual progress is being made in techniques of repair, indicating that further refinement over time is likely to occur. Some of the techniques involved in repair in other conditions can and need to be applied to Ebstein anomaly. Guiding principles in these repairs are to reduce TR, reduce annular dimension if appropriate, and to restore the tricuspid valve to the normal annular plane, thus increasing the size of

Fig. 9. Kay repair technique. (*A*) Tricuspid valve bicuspidization is accomplished by plicating the annulus along the posterior leaflet. (*B*) The sutures are tied, obliterating the posterior leaflet and creating a bicuspid valve. (*From* Taramasso M, Vanermen H, Maisano F, et al. The growing clinical importance of secondary tricuspid regurgitation. J Am Coll Cardiol 2012;59(8):703–10; with permission.)

- Leaflet repair: perforations/fenestrations can be repaired with direct suturing or a patch of autologous or glutaraldehyde-treated pericardium

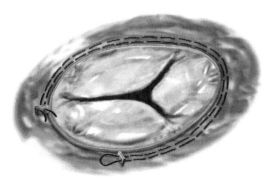

Fig. 10. De Vega repair: a single suture is placed around the tricuspid annulus, avoiding the area of the AV node. The suture is tied, completing the annuloplasty. (*From* Taramasso M, Vanermen V, Maisano F, et al. The growing clinical importance of secondary tricuspid regurgitation. J Am Coll Cardiol 2012;59(8):703–10; with permission.)

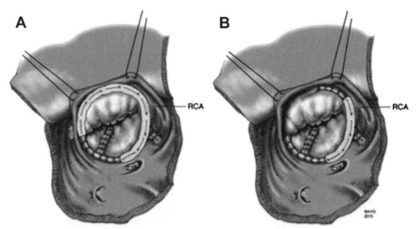

Fig. 12. (*A*) The tricuspid annulus is usually dilated and a flexible annuloplasty ring is used beginning at the anteroseptal commissure and extending clockwise and anchored into the coronary sinus. (*B*) In young patients, an eccentric ring from the anteroinferior to inferoseptal commissures can be used because this is the annular site most vulnerable to dilation. The band serves to decrease the stress on the repair and support the reconstructed cone. RCA, right coronary artery one-quarter right coronary artery. (*From* Dearani JA, Said SM, Burkhart HM, et al. Strategies for tricuspid re-repair in Ebstein malformation using the cone technique. Ann Thorac Surg 2013;96:202–10; with permission.)

the function RV and eliminating the atrialized portion of the RV, with (it is hoped) improved compliance and overall systolic function. Another key issue is whether to close any ASD that is present at the same time, particularly if there was

evidence of right-to-left shunting before surgery, either at rest or with exercise. However, elimination of the pop-off mechanism (especially in adults with reduced ventricular compliance) may lead to reduced cardiac output both acutely and chronically and may even worsen exercise capacity though this is uncommon if adequate repair is achieved.

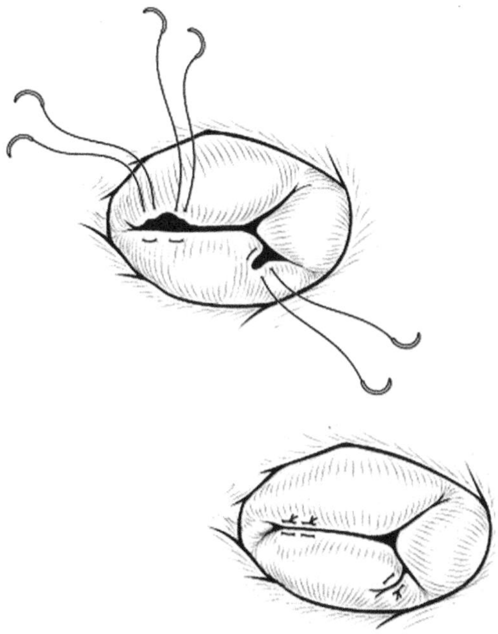

TYPES OF REPAIR

Table 3 shows the historical evolution of Ebstein repair. These 3 techniques have, over time, been the most popular among congenital heart surgeons, although the second and third are currently most performed. Elements of each technique can vary from patient to patient (because each patient with Ebstein anomaly is different). Other techniques of repair, as mentioned earlier, may also be necessary, such as closure of commissures, fenestrations, cusp augmentation, and annuloplasty (whether ring or suture based) as appropriate (**Figs. 16–21**).

Systemic RV

Late onset of TR is generally secondary in D-TGA, but may be a primary issue in CCTGA. In general, replacement is preferred rather than repair of structurally abnormal valves in CCTGA to reduce the risk of reoperation. PA banding to reestablish the crescent shape of the RV was advocated in the past, but experience with this procedure in adults has generally been disappointing, with

Fig. 13. Partial commissure closure and leaflet cleft repair. (*From* Ohye RG, Gomez CA, Goldberg CS, et al. Tricuspid valve repair in hypoplastic left heart syndrome. J Thorac Cardiovasc Surg 2004;127(2):465–72; with permission.)

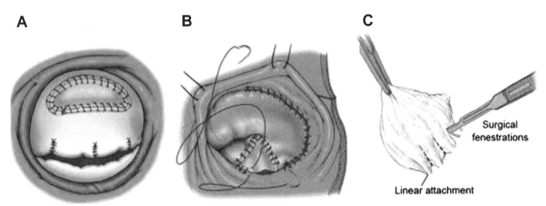

Fig. 14. (*A*) The tricuspid valve anterior leaflet augmentation can be performed using CorMatrix membrane or an autologous pericardial patch to increase the leaflet height and improve coaptation. Multiple small plications along the annular free edge of the leaflet can also be performed to increase the leaflet height. (*B*) A triangular patch may be used to augment the reconstructed cone to increase the diameter of the neotricuspid valve and help avoid tricuspid valve stenosis. (*C*) In a linear attachment (ie, absent chordae with adherence of the leading edge to the endocardium), multiple vertical fenestrations are made into the linear attachment to create a new leading edge. (*From* Dearani JA, Said SM, Burkhart HM, et al. Strategies for tricuspid re-repair in Ebstein malformation using the cone technique. Ann Thorac Surg 2013;96:202–10; with permission.)

frequent induction of LV failure, because it does not seem possible to train the LV in adulthood.

AV Canal Defect

There are often clefts (between a portion of the superior and inferior bridging leaflets) that require primary closure. Associated annular dilatation may require annuloplasty. Valve replacement is rarely required.

Pacemaker Leads

Pacemaker leads may need to be extracted. As an alternative, the leads can be placed in the base of a commissure and edge-to-edge repair and/or annuloplasty can be performed inside the lead.

Conversion to epicardial pacemaker may be necessary. In tricuspid valve replacement, the lead needs to be placed around the prosthesis. Placing a pacemaker lead across a bioprosthetic valve is generally avoided if possible.

Combined Arrhythmia Surgery

The addition of right atrial maze, or single ablation line across the cavotricuspid isthmus, can be appropriate if EPS/ablation has been unsuccessful, although prior mapping of the arrhythmia in the EP laboratory is more likely to lead to a successful operation because ablation lines can be directed. Caveats are that electrical success cannot be determined in the operating room

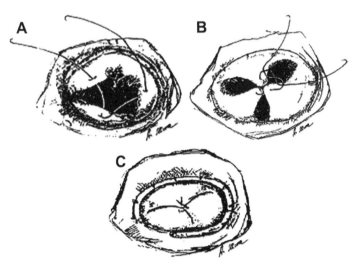

Fig. 15. Surgical steps of the clover technique. (*From* Alfieri O, De Bonis M, Lapenna E, et al. The "clover technique" as a novel approach for correction of post-traumatic tricuspid regurgitation. J Thorac Cardiovasc Surg 2003; 126(1):75–9; with permission.)

Table 2
Bioprosthetic versus mechanical prosthesis

	Bioprosthetic	Mechanical
Pros	No requirement for anticoagulation Probably suitable for percutaneous valve-in-valve replacement	Durable
Cons	Failure rates leading to re-replacement	Need for systemic anticoagulation with INR 2.5–3.5 Significant risk of valve thrombosis

Abbreviation: INR, International Normalized Ratio.

Adapted from van Slooten YJ, Freling HG, van Melle JP, et al. Long-term tricuspid valve prosthesis-related complications in patients with congenital heart disease. Eur J Cardiothorac Surg 2013. [Epub ahead of print], with permission; and Garatti A, Nano G, Bruschi G, et al. Twenty-five year outcomes of tricuspid valve replacement comparing mechanical and biologic prostheses. Ann Thorac Surg 2012;93(4):1146–53, with permission.

and watchful waiting for months afterward is necessary. The recurrence of arrhythmias is not insignificant and can lead to further EP procedures being required. In addition, it is difficult to determine whether the operation reduces risk of thromboembolism, and if ongoing systemic anticoagulation is appropriate, particularly when uncertainty of arrhythmia recurrence exists and there are other risk factors for stroke.[50]

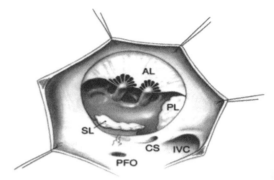

Fig. 16. Surgeon's view of the RV through the tricuspid valve in Ebstein anomaly. AL, anterior leaflet; CS, coronary sinus; PL, posterior leaflet; PFO, patent foramen ovale; SL, septal leaflet. (*From* Dearani JA, Danielson GK. Tricuspid valve repair for Ebstein's anomaly. Operat Tech Thorac Cardiovasc Surg 2003;8(4):188–92; with permission.)

POSTOPERATIVE MANAGEMENT

Shock is a common postoperative problem, especially in Ebstein anomaly, for which preoperative RV dysfunction is worsened with a period of cardioplegic arrest. Consideration to performing tricuspid surgery on the beating heart if the tricuspid valve disease is the primary problem, or, if simple annuloplasty is required concomitantly, tricuspid surgery can be performed during rewarming after the main procedure is completed.

Inotropes, pulmonary vasodilators, and generous fluid loading are used to keep RA

Table 3
Types of Ebstein repair

	Danielson (Figs. 16 and 17)	Carpentier	Cone (Figs. 18–21)
Date of first description	1979	1988	2007
Primary nature of repair	Anterior leaflet and chordal apparatus directly sutured to coapt with septum and annulus	Anterior leaflet mobilized by detaching from annulus and rotating clockwise	All 3 leaflets mobilized by detaching anterior leaflet and surgically delaminating other leaflets if possible
Annulus	Functionally remains displaced apically	Restored to anatomic annulus	Restored to anatomic annulus
Leaflets used in repair	Anterior leaflet to create monocuspid valve	Anterior leaflet to create monocuspid valve	All 3 leaflets
Annuloplasty	Yes	Variable; some use vertical plication of the atrialized RV to reduce annulus	Yes
Other elements	Sebening stitch to appose anterior leaflet to septum	Horizontal or vertical plication	Surgical delamination of septal leaflet to use in repair

Adapted from Refs.[47–49]

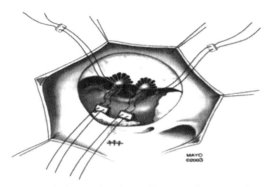

Fig. 17. The base of each papillary muscle is moved toward the ventricular septum at the appropriate level with horizontal mattress sutures backed with felt pledgets. (*From* Dearani JA, Danielson GK. Tricuspid valve repair for Ebstein's anomaly. Operat Tech Thorac Cardiovasc Surg 2003;8(4):188–92; with permission.)

pressures higher (analogy with management of RV infarction is valuable for adult cardiologist). Strict pulmonary care, early extubation, and consideration of use of inhaled pulmonary vasodilator therapy are applied to avoid increases in PVR.

One and one-half ventricle repair is sometimes used by creating a bidirectional Glenn shunt to offload if the RV is felt to be inadequate although this is controversial.

COMPLICATIONS

The risk of AV block is modest and related to the close relationship between the septal annulus and the AV node and His bundle. AV block is variably reversible; it is important to give adequate time for recovery of AV conduction after surgery (especially

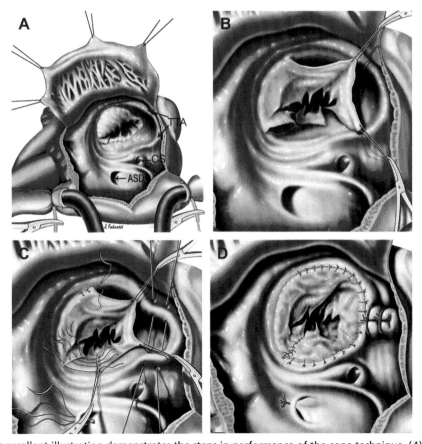

Fig. 18. This excellent illustration demonstrates the steps in performance of the cone technique. (*A*) Opened RA showing displacement of the tricuspid valve. (*B*) Detached part of the anterior and posterior leaflet forming a single piece. (*C*) Clockwise rotation of the posterior leaflet edge to be sutured to the anterior leaflet septal edge and plication of the true tricuspid annulus. (*D*) Complete valve attachment to the true tricuspid annulus and valved closure of the ASD. TTA, true tricuspid annulus. (*From* da Silva JP, Baumgratz JF, da Fonseca L, et al. The cone reconstruction of the tricuspid valve in Ebstein's anomaly. J Thorac Cardiovasc Surg 2007;133(1):215–23; with permission.)

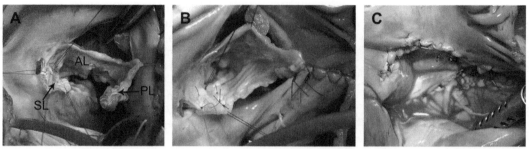

Fig. 19. This figure demonstrates the intraoperative appearances of the sequence seen in the **Fig. 18**. Surgical sequence of tricuspid valve cone repair with incorporation of the septal leaflet. (*A*) Detached septal and posterior leaflets and part of the anterior leaflet of the tricuspid valve. (*From* da Silva JP, Baumgratz JF, da Fonseca L, et al. The cone reconstruction of the tricuspid valve in Ebstein's anomaly. J Thorac Cardiovasc Surg 2007;133(1):215–23; with permission.)

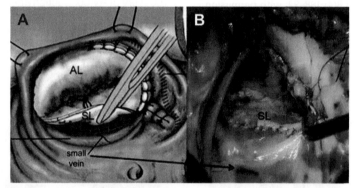

Fig. 20. This figure demonstrates the technique described by Dearani et al to avoid the conduction system during reattachment of the septal leaflet in the cone type of repair. The septal leaflet is reattached to the ventricular side of the conduction tissue (*dashed arrow*), which is usually marked by a small vein and the white membranous septum. (*B*) The completed cone repair. (*From* Dearani JA, Said SM, Burkhart HM, et al. Strategies for tricuspid re-repair in Ebstein malformation using the cone technique. Ann Thorac Surg 2013;96(1):202–21; with permission.)

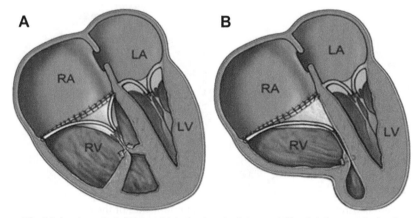

Fig. 21. The modified Sebening stitch (*A*) in which the head of the mobilized right ventricular free wall papillary muscle is approximated to the corresponding smaller head of a septal papillary muscle (as opposed to approximation to the ventricular septum in the original Sebening stitch). (*B*) It is important to avoid dimpling of the right ventricular free wall because this indicates excessive tension. (*From* Dearani JA, Said SM, Burkhart HM, et al. Strategies for tricuspid re-repair in Ebstein malformation using the cone technique. Ann Thorac Surg 2013;96:202–10; with permission.)

if the development of AV block is delayed and not immediate) before placing a pacemaker, especially if tricuspid replacement is used, and consideration of epicardial placement should be given, particularly if resolution of tricuspid disorder was the primary aim of the surgery.

SUMMARY

Tricuspid valve disease is a significant primary and secondary problem in CHD. It is frequently under-recognized, and its hemodynamic effects are under-appreciated, leading to missed opportunities to address this lesion before irreversible ventricular dysfunction or end-organ damage has occurred. ACHD clinicians need to be aware of this silent disease and approach it with as much respect as they have for any other valvular heart lesion. Despite there being so many techniques (or perhaps because there are), clinicians need to work hard to find better ways to address tricuspid valve disease, whether that is medically, percutaneously, or surgically, or likely a combination of these things to improve outcomes. Further research on describing the frequency, severity, and outcomes of tricuspid valve disease in the ACHD population; better ways to quantitatively define the timing of intervention in TR; and the defining role of earlier/more aggressive surgical or interventional approaches are eagerly anticipated.

SUPPLEMENTARY DATA

Supplementary data related to this article can be found at http://dx.doi.org/10.1016/j.hfc.2013.09.019.

REFERENCES

1. Said SM, Burkhart HM, Dearani JA. Surgical management of congenital (non-Ebstein) tricuspid valve regurgitation. Semin Thorac Cardiovasc Surg Pediatr Card Surg Annu 2012;15(1):46–60.
2. Bruce CJ, Connolly HM. Right-sided valve disease deserves a little more respect. Circulation 2009; 119(20):2726–34.
3. Colombo T, Russo C, Ciliberto GR, et al. Tricuspid regurgitation secondary to mitral valve disease: tricuspid annulus function as guide to tricuspid valve repair. Cardiovasc Surg 2001;9(4):369–77.
4. Dreyfus GD, Corbi PJ, Chan KM, et al. Secondary tricuspid regurgitation or dilatation: which should be the criteria for surgical repair? Ann Thorac Surg 2005;79(1):127–32.
5. Tager R, Skudicky D, Mueller U, et al. Long-term follow-up of rheumatic patients undergoing left-sided valve replacement with tricuspid annuloplasty–validity of preoperative echocardiographic criteria in the decision to perform tricuspid annuloplasty. Am J Cardiol 1998;81(8):1013–6.
6. Bonow RO, Carabello BA, Chatterjee K, et al. 2008 focused update incorporated into the ACC/AHA 2006 guidelines for the management of patients with valvular heart disease: a report of the American College of Cardiology/American Heart Association Task Force on Practice Guidelines (Writing Committee to Revise the 1998 Guidelines for the Management of Patients with Valvular Heart Disease). Endorsed by the Society of Cardiovascular Anesthesiologists, Society for Cardiovascular Angiography and Interventions, and Society of Thoracic Surgeons. J Am Coll Cardiol 2008;52(13):e1–142.
7. Hung J. The pathogenesis of functional tricuspid regurgitation. Semin Thorac Cardiovasc Surg 2010;22(1):76–8.
8. Davlouros PA, Niwa K, Webb G, et al. The right ventricle in congenital heart disease. Heart 2006; 92(Suppl 1):i27–38.
9. Rogers JH, Bolling SF. The tricuspid valve: current perspective and evolving management of tricuspid regurgitation. Circulation 2009;119(20): 2718–25.
10. Ho SY, Nihoyannopoulos P. Anatomy, echocardiography, and normal right ventricular dimensions. Heart 2006;92(Suppl 1):i2–13.
11. Koelling TM, Aaronson KD, Cody RJ, et al. Prognostic significance of mitral regurgitation and tricuspid regurgitation in patients with left ventricular systolic dysfunction. Am Heart J 2002;144(3): 524–9.
12. Sagie A, Schwammenthal E, Newell JB, et al. Significant tricuspid regurgitation is a marker for adverse outcome in patients undergoing percutaneous balloon mitral valvuloplasty. J Am Coll Cardiol 1994;24(3):696–702.
13. Ton-Nu TT, Levine RA, Handschumacher MD, et al. Geometric determinants of functional tricuspid regurgitation: insights from 3-dimensional echocardiography. Circulation 2006;114(2):143–9.
14. Spinner EM, Shannon P, Buice D, et al. In vitro characterization of the mechanisms responsible for functional tricuspid regurgitation. Circulation 2011;124(8):920–9.
15. Braunwald NS, Ross J Jr, Morrow AG. Conservative management of tricuspid regurgitation in patients undergoing mitral valve replacement. Circulation 1967;35(Suppl 4):I63–9.
16. Matsuyama K, Matsumoto M, Sugita T, et al. Predictors of residual tricuspid regurgitation after mitral valve surgery. Ann Thorac Surg 2003;75(6): 1826–8.
17. Toyono M, Krasuski RA, Pettersson GB, et al. Persistent tricuspid regurgitation and its predictor in adults after percutaneous and isolated

surgical closure of secundum atrial septal defect. Am J Cardiol 2009;104(6):856–61.

18. Toyono M, Fukuda S, Gillinov AM, et al. Different determinants of residual tricuspid regurgitation after tricuspid annuloplasty: comparison of atrial septal defect and mitral valve prolapse. J Am Soc Echocardiogr 2009;22(8):899–903.

19. Yalonetsky S, Lorber A. Comparative changes of pulmonary artery pressure values and tricuspid valve regurgitation following transcatheter atrial septal defect closure in adults and the elderly. Congenit Heart Dis 2009;4(1):17–20.

20. Mongeon FP, Burkhart HM, Ammash NM, et al. Indications and outcomes of surgical closure of ventricular septal defect in adults. JACC Cardiovasc Interv 2010;3(3):290–7.

21. Dodge-Khatami A, Herger S, Rousson V, et al. Outcomes and reoperations after total correction of complete atrio-ventricular septal defect. Eur J Cardiothorac Surg 2008;34(4):745–50.

22. Attenhofer Jost CH, Connolly HM, Dearani JA, et al. Ebstein's anomaly. Circulation 2007;115(2):277–85.

23. Eicken A, Fratz S, Hager A, et al. Transcutaneous melody valve implantation in "tricuspid position" after a Fontan Bjork (RA-RV homograft) operation results in biventricular circulation. Int J Cardiol 2010;142(3):e45–7.

24. Kogon B, Patel M, Leong T, et al. Management of moderate functional tricuspid valve regurgitation at the time of pulmonary valve replacement: is concomitant tricuspid valve repair necessary? Pediatr Cardiol 2010;31(6):843–8.

25. Hoashi T, Kagisaki K, Kitano M, et al. Late clinical features of patients with pulmonary atresia or critical pulmonary stenosis with intact ventricular septum after biventricular repair. Ann Thorac Surg 2012;94(3):833–41 [discussion: 841].

26. Bautista-Hernandez V, Hasan BS, Harrild DM, et al. Late pulmonary valve replacement in patients with pulmonary atresia and intact ventricular septum: a case-matched study. Ann Thorac Surg 2011;91(2):555–60.

27. Graham TP Jr, Bernard YD, Mellen BG, et al. Long-term outcome in congenitally corrected transposition of the great arteries: a multi-institutional study. J Am Coll Cardiol 2000;36(1):255–61.

28. Warnes CA, Williams RG, Bashore TM, et al. ACC/AHA 2008 guidelines for the management of adults with congenital heart disease: a report of the American College of Cardiology/American Heart Association Task Force on Practice Guidelines (Writing Committee to Develop Guidelines on the Management of Adults With Congenital Heart Disease). Developed in Collaboration With the American Society of Echocardiography, Heart Rhythm Society, International Society for Adult Congenital Heart Disease, Society for Cardiovascular Angiography and Interventions, and Society of Thoracic Surgeons. J Am Coll Cardiol 2008;52(23):e143–263.

29. Mongeon FP, Connolly HM, Dearani JA, et al. Congenitally corrected transposition of the great arteries ventricular function at the time of systemic atrioventricular valve replacement predicts long-term ventricular function. J Am Coll Cardiol 2011; 57(20):2008–17.

30. Warnes CA. Transposition of the great arteries. Circulation 2006;114(24):2699–709.

31. Ugaki S, Khoo NS, Ross DB, et al. Tricuspid valve repair improves early right ventricular and tricuspid valve remodeling in patients with hypoplastic left heart syndrome. J Thorac Cardiovasc Surg 2013; 145(2):446–50.

32. Tsang VT, Raja SG. Tricuspid valve repair in single ventricle: timing and techniques. Semin Thorac Cardiovasc Surg Pediatr Card Surg Annu 2012; 15(1):61–8.

33. Sadeghi HM, Kimura BJ, Raisinghani A, et al. Does lowering pulmonary arterial pressure eliminate severe functional tricuspid regurgitation? Insights from pulmonary thromboendarterectomy. J Am Coll Cardiol 2004;44(1):126–32.

34. Menzel T, Kramm T, Wagner S, et al. Improvement of tricuspid regurgitation after pulmonary thromboendarterectomy. Ann Thorac Surg 2002;73(3): 756–61.

35. Kim JB, Spevack DM, Tunick PA, et al. The effect of transvenous pacemaker and implantable cardioverter defibrillator lead placement on tricuspid valve function: an observational study. J Am Soc Echocardiogr 2008;21(3):284–7.

36. Al-Bawardy R, Krishnaswamy A, Bhargava M, et al. Tricuspid regurgitation in patients with pacemakers and implantable cardiac defibrillators: a comprehensive review. Clin Cardiol 2013;36(5):249–54.

37. Nazmul MN, Cha YM, Lin G, et al. Percutaneous pacemaker or implantable cardioverter-defibrillator lead removal in an attempt to improve symptomatic tricuspid regurgitation. Europace 2013;15(3):409–13.

38. Iskandar SB, Ann Jackson S, Fahrig S, et al. Tricuspid valve malfunction and ventricular pacemaker lead: case report and review of the literature. Echocardiography 2006;23(8):692–7.

39. Al-Mohaissen MA, Chan KL. Prevalence and mechanism of tricuspid regurgitation following implantation of endocardial leads for pacemaker or cardioverter-defibrillator. J Am Soc Echocardiogr 2012;25(3):245–52.

40. Cullen MW, Cabalka AK, Alli OO, et al. Transvenous, antegrade Melody valve-in-valve implantation for bioprosthetic mitral and tricuspid valve dysfunction: a case series in children and adults. JACC Cardiovasc Interv 2013;6(6):598–605.

41. Heo YH, Kim SJ, Lee SY, et al. A case demonstrating a percutaneous closure using the Amplatzer duct occluder for paravalvular leakage after tricuspid valve replacement. Korean Circ J 2013; 43(4):273–6.

42. Chikwe J, Anyanwu AC. Surgical strategies for functional tricuspid regurgitation. Semin Thorac Cardiovasc Surg 2010;22(1):90–6.

43. Thapa R, Dawn B, Nath J. Tricuspid regurgitation: pathophysiology and management. Curr Cardiol Rep 2012;14(2):190–9.

44. Singh SK, Tang GH, Maganti MD, et al. Midterm outcomes of tricuspid valve repair versus replacement for organic tricuspid disease. Ann Thorac Surg 2006;82(5):1735–41 [discussion: 1741].

45. van Slooten YJ, Freling HG, van Melle JP, et al. Long-term tricuspid valve prosthesis-related complications in patients with congenital heart disease. Eur J Cardiothorac Surg 2013. [Epub ahead of print].

46. Garatti A, Nano G, Bruschi G, et al. Twenty-five year outcomes of tricuspid valve replacement comparing mechanical and biologic prostheses. Ann Thorac Surg 2012;93(4):1146–53.

47. da Silva JP, Baumgratz JF, da Fonseca L, et al. The cone reconstruction of the tricuspid valve in Ebstein's anomaly. The operation: early and midterm results. J Thorac Cardiovasc Surg 2007; 133(1):215–23.

48. Carpentier A, Chauvaud S, Macé L, et al. A new reconstructive operation for Ebstein's anomaly of the tricuspid valve. J Thorac Cardiovasc Surg 1988;96(1):92–101.

49. Danielson GK, Fuster V. Surgical repair of Ebstein's anomaly. Ann Surg 1982;196(4):499–504.

50. Stulak JM, Dearani JA, Puga FJ, et al. Right-sided maze procedure for atrial tachyarrhythmias in congenital heart disease. Ann Thorac Surg 2006; 81(5):1780–4 [discussion: 1784–5].

Heart Failure Caused by Congenital Left-Sided Lesions

Eric V. Krieger, MD[a],*, Susan M. Fernandes, LPD, PA-C[b]

KEYWORDS

- Coarctation • Shone syndrome • Bicuspid aortic valve • Heart failure
- Left ventricular noncompaction • Cor triatriatum

KEY POINTS

- Depending on the location, left-sided lesions can obstruct left ventricular inflow, obstruct left ventricular outflow, cause left-sided valvular regurgitation, or affect ventricular myocardial performance directly.
- Left-sided lesions are often found in combination, whereas bicuspid aortic valve and coarctation often coexist and can be associated with more complex multilevel obstruction, which can markedly increase left ventricular workload.
- Left ventricular noncompaction is a difficult diagnosis because of marked phenotypic variability in left ventricular trabeculation. The prognosis of isolated left ventricular noncompaction is not well understood but seems to be poor in patients with systolic dysfunction and good in those with preserved ejection fraction.

INTRODUCTION

There are diverse mechanisms by which congenital left-sided cardiac lesions can precipitate heart failure. Left heart outflow obstruction can occur at, below, or above the aortic valve, imposing abnormal pressure load on the left ventricle, inducing adverse remodeling, hypertrophy, and diastolic and systolic dysfunction. Abnormalities in left ventricular inflow can occur in the pulmonary veins and within the left atrium, as well as in the region of the mitral valve, increasing pulmonary venous pressure and predisposing to pulmonary edema. In addition, inborn abnormalities in left ventricular myocardial structure and function can impair both systolic and diastolic function and manifest as heart failure later in life. In this article, the different mechanisms, outcomes, and treatments of heart failure in patients with congenital left-sided lesions are discussed.

Even with remarkable advancements in treatment of pediatric heart disease in the last 50 years, patients with repaired congenital heart disease (CHD) have reduced survival.[1,2] Most patients who die early with CHD die from cardiovascular causes. Heart failure continues to be the dominant mode of death in patients with repaired CHD, accounting for more than 40% of CHD-related death. Of the congenital left-sided lesions, coarctation of the aorta (CoA), and congenital aortic stenosis account for the highest proportion of premature mortality.[3,4]

AORTIC VALVE DYSFUNCTION
Bicuspid Aortic Valve

Bicuspid aortic valve (BAV) is present in 0.5% to 2% of the general population and represents the

Disclosures: None.
[a] Division of Cardiology, Seattle Adult Congenital Heart Service, Seattle Children's Hospital, University of Washington Medical Center, University of Washington School of Medicine, 1959 Northeast Pacific Street, Seattle, WA 98109, USA; [b] Adult Congenital Heart Program at Stanford, Lucile Packard Children's Hospital, Stanford Hospital and Clinics, Stanford University School of Medicine, 750 Welch Road, Suite 321, Palo Alto, CA 94304, USA
* Corresponding author.
E-mail address: ekrieger@u.washington.edu

Heart Failure Clin 10 (2014) 155–165
http://dx.doi.org/10.1016/j.hfc.2013.09.015
1551-7136/14/$ – see front matter © 2014 Elsevier Inc. All rights reserved.

most common congenital heart lesion.[5–7] It is more common in males than females (3:1) and can be found in isolation or in association with a wide range of other congenital heart lesions.[8] BAV can be found in association with almost all types of CHD and is common in patients with other left heart obstructive lesions, with more than 50% of patients with aortic coarctation having a BAV.[9]

Most BAVs have 3 leaflets but only 2 well-developed commissures, resulting in 2 functional leaflets.[10–12] Fusion of the right coronary and left coronary leaflets (absence of the intercoronary commissure) is the most common morphology (70%) followed by fusion of the right coronary and noncoronary leaflets. Fusion of the left coronary and noncoronary leaflets is rare (1.4%).[9] A recent study by Fernández and colleagues[13] suggested that right coronary and left coronary leaflet fusion may have different developmental underpinnings from BAVs with fusion of the right coronary and noncoronary leaflets. This suggestion is supported by clinical findings that suggest that children with fusion of the right coronary and non-coronary leaflets are significantly more likely to have progression of aortic stenosis and regurgitation compelling intervention than children with fusion of the right coronary and left coronary leaflets.[14] However, studies in adults with BAV suggest that BAV morphology does not seem to be a strong predictor of valve dysfunction.[15] This distinction is likely related to the impact of calcific changes noted in adulthood, which are more likely to drive valve dysfunction, and the fact that right coronary and noncoronary leaflet fusion are less likely than right coronary and left coronary leaflet fusion to be without significant valve dysfunction until adulthood.[14]

Although patients with BAV can present in infancy with severe aortic stenosis, in most cases, the BAV functions well until later in life, when calcific changes cause progression of stenosis or regurgitation.[15] There is a well-documented association between BAV and progressive dilation of the ascending aorta, the cause of which is not completely understood and seems to be independent of the degree of aortic stenosis.[16,17] Several studies have suggested that not only do patients with BAV without significant valvular dysfunction have associated aortic dilation, but these patients also have abnormal left ventricular mechanics and performance.[18,19] This finding suggests that BAV is unlikely to represent isolated valvular disease, which may have significant implications on long-term ventricular function even in the absence of significant aortic stenosis or regurgitation.

Other Causes of Congenital Aortic Stenosis

BAV is the most common cause of aortic stenosis, but the valve morphology in rare cases can be quadricuspid ($\sim$0.005% of the general population)[20] or unicuspid ($\sim$0.02%) with only 1 functioning leaflet.[21] The latter often presents with severe obstruction in infancy.[22] In addition to obstruction at the level of the aortic valve, there can be obstruction below the aortic valve because of a discrete membrane or fibromuscular tunnel or ridge or there can be significant narrowing above the valve (supravalvar). Supravalvar aortic stenosis is commonly associated with William syndrome, and the level of the obstruction is typically above the aortic root.[23]

Regardless of the level of obstruction, compensatory left ventricular hypertrophy is required to meet the physiologic demands of pressure afterload caused by aortic stenosis. The increase in left ventricular mass can be inadequate for the degree of wall stress, resulting in left ventricular systolic dysfunction and decreased cardiac output.[24] Even when left ventricular hypertrophy seems adequate, chronically increased pressure load can lead to myocardial damage, negatively affecting both left ventricular systolic and diastolic function. Such deleterious effects often result in symptoms of angina, exercise intolerance, near syncope or syncope, and heart failure, which have been associated with significant morbidity and mortality in patients with aortic stenosis.[25,26] Once symptoms are present, the mean survival is only 2 to 3 years.[27] Continuous assessment of cardiac symptoms, aortic stenosis severity, and left ventricular performance as well as ensuring appropriate timing of intervention seems important to ensure long-term well-being.

Indications for intervention in symptomatic patients with severe valvar aortic stenosis and for asymptomatic patients with left ventricular dysfunction or exercise-induced symptoms or hypotension are well defined.[27–29] The timing of intervention in the remainder of asymptomatic patients with significant valvar aortic stenosis can be more difficult.[30] Although its role is not fully defined, stress echocardiography may be helpful in determining timing of intervention in this subset of patients. Studies suggest that a significant increase in the aortic valve gradient, the presence of exercise-induced pulmonary hypertension, and changes in ventricular function (increased left ventricular volume and stiffness) can identify those patients at increased risk of cardiac events.[29,31,32]

Aortic Regurgitation

Isolated congenital aortic regurgitation is rare. Typically, it is associated with abnormal morphology of the aortic valve, but it can also be seen in a host of congenital lesions, including truncus arteriosus and ventricular septal defect.[33] Aortic regurgitation can also be caused by aortic dilation itself in the setting of a normal-appearing aortic valve, such as in patients with connective tissue disorders.[34] Most patients with aortic regurgitation experience a slow progression that results in progressive left ventricular dilation, eccentric hypertrophy, and increased compliance. As the degree of aortic regurgitation increases, the balance between preload, afterload, and hypertrophy can become mismatched, resulting in a decline in left ventricular systolic function.[22,27] Although many patients are asymptomatic for years despite severe aortic regurgitation, dyspnea and exercise intolerance may be early indicators of disease progression. Serial echocardiograms can help identify patients with changes in left ventricular size and function. Patients with progressive increase in end-systolic left ventricular volume and a decrease in ejection fraction are more likely to develop symptoms prompting intervention.[35] When aortic regurgitation progresses without intervention, the left ventricle can decompensate, resulting in an increase in left ventricular end-diastolic volume and pressure and even an increase in left atrial and right-sided heart pressures, resulting in symptoms of both right-sided and left-sided heart failure.[22] Timing of aortic valve replacement in patients with significant aortic regurgitation has been well established,[27,28] the goal of which is to intervene when left ventricular recovery is still possible, because left ventricular dilation and function at timing of intervention are of prognostic importance.[35] The ideal candidates for surgical aortic valve replacement/repair are those patients with severe aortic regurgitation who have preserved and stable left ventricular function and size (left ventricular end-diastolic volume $\leq$75 mm, left ventricular end-systolic volume $\leq$55 mm) and who are asymptomatic, with good exercise tolerance.[28] Patients with poor exercise tolerance and ejection fraction less than 50% at time of aortic valve replacement/repair are at significant risk for postoperative mortality or progressive left ventricular dysfunction and clinical symptoms of progressive heart failure.[22,36]

The observation of changes in left ventricular parameters over time offers important information that guides not only timing of the need for intervention in patients with aortic valve disease but offers meaningful information about operative risk and long-term prognosis.[37] Therefore, serial assessment of these parameters in patients with significant aortic valve disease seems warranted and may help avoid the deleterious consequences of progressive ventricular dysfunction and symptomatic heart failure.

COARCTATION OF THE AORTA
Anatomy and Associated Lesions

CoA is an anatomically simple lesion with complex physiologic consequences. Typically, CoA is a discrete fibrotic narrowing at the aortic isthmus in the region of the ligamentum arteriosus. However, CoA can also involve long-segment hypoplasia and involve the transverse aortic arch. CoA is often accompanied by other left-sided lesions, including BAV, mitral stenosis, ventricular septal defect, and complex CHD.

Arterial Dysfunction and Ventricular Interaction

The pathophysiology of unrepaired CoA involves upper extremity hypertension and, to a lesser extent, hypoperfusion distal to the arch obstruction. Infants with CoA commonly present with heart failure from left ventricular pressure overload, and physical examination may show diminished femoral pulses or a posterior murmur. When diagnosed in infancy, CoA should be repaired promptly. However, CoA can often remain undiagnosed until adulthood, when patients may present with refractory hypertension.

Even after early successful repair, adults with CoA have persistent abnormalities in vascular function, which predispose to hypertension and ventricular dysfunction.[38–40] Patients with CoA have increased vascular stiffness, decreased arterial elasticity, and impaired endothelial function.[41–46] Impairments to arterial compliance and accelerated pulse-wave velocity lead to augmented systolic blood pressure. Stiff proximal conduit arteries do not provide adequate cushioning to pulsatile flow, further raising vascular impedance and ventricular afterload.[47,48] For these reasons, hypertension is common in patients with repaired coarctation,[49–52] and many patients with repaired CoA with normal resting blood pressure can have ambulatory or exercise-induced hypertension.[53–56]

Because the left ventricle is coupled to this abnormal arterial tree, myocardial remodeling occurs. The presence of hypertension leads to left ventricular hypertrophy, a response that normalizes ventricular wall stress.[57–59] For this reason, left ventricular mass is increased in many patients with repaired CoA.[38] Even in normotensive patients, increased arterial stiffness can increase concentric remodeling, leading to increases in relative wall thickness.[53,60]

Ventricular Dysfunction and Heart Failure in CoA

Left ventricular diastolic dysfunction is common after repair of CoA. Invasive hemodynamic studies[61] have shown an upward shift in the pressure-volume relation curve, which is believed to be caused by persistent left ventricular hypertrophy. Early diastolic filling is reduced, with an increased dependence on late diastolic filling, and this pattern is accentuated in patients with residual arch obstruction or worse hypertrophy.[62] Relief of even mild residual obstruction can improve diastolic filling and decrease left ventricular end-diastolic pressure.[63]

Left ventricular systolic function is usually normal or hyperdynamic after successful coarctation repair.[61,62] This finding is likely explained by compensatory hypertrophy, which decreases left ventricular wall stress (afterload). Increased left ventricular contractility has been shown to be increased in normotensive patients with repaired CoA as well, which has been speculated to be caused by persistent hypertrophy in the absence of ongoing pressure overload.[64,65] Patients with systolic dysfunction after repair are more likely to have been repaired at an older age.[66] Despite overall normal (or increased) contractility, tissue Doppler measurements of left ventricular longitudinal shortening have been shown to be abnormal in many patients with repaired CoA.[66]

Survival after CoA repair is good, with more than 90% surviving at least 15 years.[4] Approximately 10% to 25% of the cardiovascular deaths in patients with repaired CoA are caused by heart failure. The prognosis is worse in those with concomitant aortic valve disease or ventricular septal defect.[1,2] These contemporary numbers compare favorably with early studies,[67] which reported high rates of premature mortality from heart failure, vascular disease, cerebral hemorrhage, and endocarditis.

Patients with unrepaired CoA are at increased risk for heart failure as a result of a chronic ventricular pressure load. Patients with repaired CoA have persistent disturbances of vascular function, which alters ventricular-vascular coupling, predisposing to ventricular remodeling, hypertrophy, and diastolic dysfunction. These findings are most common in those with residual arch obstruction and older age of repair.

SHONE COMPLEX (SYNDROME)

Anatomy

Shone complex is a rare constellation of 4 congenital heart lesions first described by Shone and colleagues[68] in 1963. The complete form includes CoA, supramitral ring, parachute mitral valve, and subaortic narrowing. The more common incomplete form is variably defined and usually includes 2 or 3 of these components.[69]

Mitral valve obstruction is typically the most critical lesion, and the severity of mitral valve obstruction has been correlated with surgical and long-term outcomes.[70,71] The mitral valve obstruction is usually related to morphologic abnormalities of the mitral valve, which include shortened and thickened chordae and insertion of the mitral valve leaflets into a single papillary muscle (posterior medial).[68,70] This mitral anomaly, referred to as a parachute mitral valve, restricts leaflet motion, resulting in varying degrees of mitral stenosis. Most patients do not have significant obstruction, and the degree of obstruction tends to remain stable and does not require valvotomy.[71] The supravalvar mitral ring is a circumferential ridge of connective tissue that is at or just above the mitral annulus, which results in varying degrees of obstruction to left ventricular inflow.[68,72] The supravalvar mitral ring is believed to be the result of incomplete division of the endocardial cushion during embryologic development, which differentiates it from cor triatriatum (see later discussion).[73] Anatomically, the supravalvar mitral ring is close to the mitral valve annulus, and the left atrial appendage is above the supravalvar mitral ring.[74] Patients with significant obstruction often undergo surgical resection in early childhood, but caution should be noted in the adult patient, because recurrence of the supravalvar mitral ring has been reported.[75]

Subaortic stenosis in Shone complex can be related to either a thin, discrete membrane or a fibromuscular ridge, which results in obstruction to flow out of the left ventricular outflow tract.[68] The degree of obstruction is highly variable, and although rapid progression of the obstruction can be common in children, the progression of obstruction in adulthood is generally gradual.[76] Flow acceleration across the left ventricular outflow tract, even when minimal, causes turbulent flow across the aortic valve leaflets,[77] which can damage the aortic valve over time, resulting in progressive aortic regurgitation. Risk factors for the development of aortic regurgitation include maximal left ventricular outflow tract gradient greater than 30 mm Hg, closeness of the membrane to aortic valve, and extension of the membrane to the anterior leaflet of the mitral valve.[78] In childhood, resection of the membrane at onset of aortic regurgitation has been advocated to prevent progressive aortic regurgitation,[76] but indications and timing of resection in adulthood are less clear. A study of adults with subaortic obstruction suggests that aortic regurgitation is common (81%) but it is usually of mild severity, and was more common in patients who had previous subvalvar aortic obstruction resection.[76] The membrane can recur after resection in some patients, and the need for reoperation, especially in patients with Shone complex, is not uncommon.[79]

Impact on Left Ventricular Function

Most reports in the literature regarding Shone complex address intervention in small samples of infants and children. However, most patients with either partial or complete Shone complex require several surgical interventions over their lifetime. The outcomes of these interventions are dependent on the specific lesions and burden of associated lesions.[71] Nearly all patients have some residual hemodynamic burden, which can decrease left ventricular preload and increase volume and pressure afterload, resulting in a decrease in left ventricular performance. Even mild residual obstruction, if at various levels, likely contributes to greater damage to left ventricular function than in isolation. Consideration of treatment strategies in Shone complex must incorporate the impact of all residual lesions on left ventricular performance.

LEFT VENTRICULAR NONCOMPACTION
Anatomy and Physiology

Left ventricular noncompaction (LVNC) is a rare primary genetic cardiomyopathy characterized by abnormal persistence of spongy myocardium with deep intertrabecular recesses that communicate with the ventricular cavity.[80,81] The mechanism is believed to be caused by interruption of endomyocardial morphogenesis and failure of the spongy avascular myocardium to compress into compact myocardium between weeks 5 and 8 of embryogenesis, a process normally associated with development of myocardial capillary beds.[82,83] Because this compression progresses from the epicardium to the endocardium and from the base to the apex, LVNC is typically most prominent in the apical portions of the left ventricle and is also frequently seen in the lateral wall.[84] LNVC is often associated with other congenital cardiac anomalies, such as Ebstein anomaly of the tricuspid valve, Barth syndrome, and septal defects.[85–89] Forms of acquired LVNC have been described; the cause is unknown.[90]

Many cases of LVNC are believed to be caused by genetic predisposition, because 18% to 33% of patients have documented familial involvement. Numerous genes have been implicated, including G4.5, ZASP, CSX, and several genes encoding mitochondrial and sarcomere proteins. Both autosomal-dominant and X-linked (eg, Barth syndrome) inheritance have been described.[83,84,88,91,92]

Diagnosis

Definitive diagnosis of LVNC is challenging, because there exist numerous diagnostic criteria and there is considerable phenotypic variability in normal and noncompacted myocardium. Derivation studies are small, and some[93] but not all definitions have been validated. In addition, there is no agreed gold standard diagnostic confirmatory test, making it difficult to evaluate diagnostic criteria.

Diagnosis of LVNC requires evidence of excessive noncompacted myocardium by noninvasive imaging and evidence of hypertrabeculation that communicates with the left ventricular cavity. Different diagnostic criteria using echocardiography and cardiac magnetic resonance have been proposed and are summarized in **Box 1**. However, there is poor reproducibility of echocardiographic diagnostic criteria, with only 67% reproducibility among blinded readers in a controlled study.[89] There is concern that diagnostic criteria for LVNC are insufficiently specific. Because it easier to identify noncompacted myocardium with modern imaging technology, there is concern that LVNC is overdiagnosed in normal patients with prominent apical trabeculations; approximately 8% of apparently normal controls fulfill diagnostic criteria for LVNC.[94] For this reason, some have suggested that strict diagnostic criteria be abandoned and a qualitative assessment be used instead, in which the diagnosis is reserved for those with a thick, bilayered myocardium with prominent ventricular trabeculations with deep intratrabecular recesses.[95,96]

Clinical Manifestations

The natural history of LVNC is characterized by heart failure, ventricular arrhythmias, and thromboembolic complications. Not all patients have a rapidly progressive clinical course. The rate of adverse outcomes depends on the population studied and varies widely across the literature. Patients with baseline reduced ejection fraction at diagnosis have considerably worse prognosis than those with preserved systolic function. One study of 34 patients[84] found only 53% free of death or transplant at 44 months of follow-up. Ventricular arrhythmias occurred in 41% and thromboembolic events in 24%. All patients in this study had significant diastolic dysfunction as

Box 1
Different published diagnostic criteria for LVNC

Chin and colleagues[80]

- Echocardiographic appearance of numerous, excessively prominent trabeculations
- Ratio of noncompacted/compacted myocardium progressively increases from the papillary muscles to the apex and is less than 0.5 at the apex

Jenni and colleagues[106]

- Echocardiographic 2-layered appearance of myocardium with a compacted epicardial layer and thicker noncompacted endocardial layer
- Deep endomyocardial spaces
- End-systolic ratio of noncompacted/compacted layers greater than 2
- Doppler evidence of deep perfused intratrabecular recesses

Stöllberger and Finsterer[107]

- Echocardiographic or magnetic resonance imaging appearance of more than 3 prominent trabeculations apical to the papillary muscle and simultaneously visible in a single imaging plane
- Doppler evidence that the trabecular recesses are profused from the left ventricular cavity
- Trabeculations have synchronous movement with compacted layer

Petersen and colleagues[108]

- Magnetic resonance imaging ratio of noncompacted/compacted myocardium greater than 2.3 in end-diastole

Jacquier and colleagues[109]

- Trabeculated myocardial mass greater than 20% of total myocardial mass

Adapted from Paterick TE, Umland MM, Jan MF, et al. Left ventricular noncompaction: a 25-year odyssey. J Am Soc Echocardiogr 2012;25:368; with permission.

measured by echocardiography. However, these patients were unwell at the time of diagnosis: mean left ventricular ejection fraction was 33%, and more than one-third of the patients experienced New York Heart Association class III/IV heart failure symptoms. A subsequent prospective study of 45 patients with a milder LVNC phenotype showed a more favorable prognosis. Mean survival from death or transplant was 97% at 46 months, and the rate of thromboembolic complications was only 4% over the study duration. None of the patients with normal ejection fraction at baseline progressed to clinical heart failure.[97] A third study of 65 patients with echocardiographic criteria of LVNC[98] again showed that asymptomatic patients had a benign clinical course, whereas those with symptoms at baseline were more likely to die, have arrhythmia, thromboembolic complication, or require transplantation. Whether these findings are caused by lead-time bias or whether there are distinct phenotypes with variable progression is unknown.

Treatment

There are limited data on optimal medical treatment of LVNC. Patients with systolic dysfunction are typically treated according to established guidelines for those with reduced systolic function or ejection fraction.[99] Similarly, supportive measures are recommended for patients with LVNC and diastolic dysfunction. However, whether these treatments are effective in patients with LVNC is unknown. Mechanical circulatory support and transplantation have been used in patients with LVNC who are refractory to conventional therapy.

There is no consensus on whether anticoagulation is indicated for all patients with LVNC. As discussed earlier, there is a theoretic risk of thrombus formation within the deep intratrabecular recesses, which could lead to systemic thromboembolic complications. However, thromboembolic risk is low in patients without a previous event, normal ejection fraction, and no atrial arrhythmias.[97,98] Therefore, it may be reasonable to provide systemic anticoagulation only for those with risk factors for thromboembolic disease.

COR TRIATRIATUM
Anatomy and Definition

Cor triatriatum sinister (cor triatriatum) is a rare congenital anomaly resulting from incomplete incorporation of the pulmonary veins into the body of the left atrium. As a consequence, the pulmonary veins enter an accessory chamber, which communicates with the left atrium via an orifice, which typically restricts flow (**Fig. 1**).

The anatomy of cor triatriatum is variable. In the classic form, all of the pulmonary veins enter into the pulmonary venous confluence, which communicates exclusively with the left atrium via a restrictive membrane (see **Fig. 1**). Partial cor triatriatum, in which 1 lung drains normally to the left atrium and the other lung drains into the accessory chamber, is also possible. Although the accessory chamber usually communicates exclusively with the left atrium, in both the complete and partial

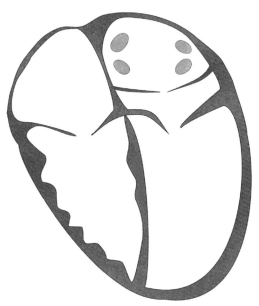

Fig. 1. Complete cor triatriarum where all 4 pulmonary veins drain to an accessory chamber, which communicates via a stenotic orifice to the left atrium.

forms, the accessory chamber can communicate with the right atrium via an atrial septal defect or decompress via a vertical vein to the superior or inferior vena cava.[100]

The physiology and clinical significance of cor triatriatum depends on the anatomy. If the connection between the pulmonary venous confluence and the left atrium is obstructed and there is no other egress (atrial septal defect or decompressing vein), pulmonary venous hypertension develops and the patient contracts pulmonary edema. In partial cor triatriatum, pulmonary edema is asymmetric, present only in the lung, which drains abnormally. If there is communication with the right heart via decompressing vein or atrial septal defect, then the physiology is of a left-to-right pretricuspid shunt, with volume overload of the right heart.

Although most patients with cor triatriatum present in childhood with signs of left-sided heart failure, late diagnosis is possible in those with mild obstruction between the pulmonary venous confluence and left atrium.[101,102] Some patients with mild obstruction may have modest increases in pulmonary venous pressure in early childhood. However, chronic pulmonary venous hypertension results in pulmonary vascular remodeling, and pulmonary arterial hypertension can develop later in life (World Health Organization group II pulmonary hypertension).

Cor triatriatum can be diagnosed by echocardiography[103] or cardiac magnetic resonance imaging.[104] The goals of imaging examination should

be to determine which veins are committed to the accessory chamber, to determine the anatomy of the membrane, and to calculate a mean diastolic gradient across the membrane. Cor triatriatum should be distinguished from a supravalvular mitral ring, because cor triatriatum is usually curvilinear, remote form the mitral valve, and may have a wind-sock appearance.[105] At the time of catheterization, pulmonary capillary wedge pressure is increased in the presence of low left ventricular end-diastolic pressure. Pulmonary arterial hypertension is often present as a result of vascular remodeling. If partial cor triatriatum is present, bilateral pulmonary artery and pulmonary capillary wedge pressures should be measured.

The treatment of cor triatriatum is surgical and should be performed by an experienced congenital heart surgeon. Supportive therapy with diuretics should be used until definitive surgical management is possible.

REFERENCES

1. Lamour JM, Kanter KR, Naftel DC, et al. The effect of age, diagnosis, and previous surgery in children and adults undergoing heart transplantation for congenital heart disease. J Am Coll Cardiol 2009; 54:160–5.
2. Verheugt CL, Uiterwaal CS, van der Velde ET, et al. Mortality in adult congenital heart disease. Eur Heart J 2010;31:1220–9.
3. Lamour JM, Hsu DT, Quaegebeur JM, et al. Heart transplantation to a physiologic single lung in patients with congenital heart disease. J Heart Lung Transplant 2004;23:948–53.
4. Speziali G, Driscoll DJ, Danielson GK, et al. Cardiac transplantation for end-stage congenital heart defects: the Mayo Clinic experience. Mayo Cardiothoracic Transplant Team. Mayo Clin Proc 1998;73: 923–8.
5. Hoffman JI, Kaplan S. The incidence of congenital heart disease. J Am Coll Cardiol 2002;39:1890–900.
6. Yener N, Oktar L, Erer D, et al. Bicuspid aortic valve. Ann Thorac Cardiovasc Surg 2002;8:264–7.
7. Basso C, Boschello M, Perrone C, et al. An echocardiographic survey of primary school children for bicuspid aortic valve. Am J Cardiol 2004;93: 661–3.
8. Siu S, Silversides CK. Bicuspid aortic valve disease. J Am Coll Cardiol 2010;55:2789–800.
9. Fernandes SM, Sanders SP, Khairy P, et al. Morphology of bicuspid aortic valve in children and adolescents. J Am Coll Cardiol 2004;44: 1648–51.
10. Sanders SP, Morris Simonds H, Jameson SM. Noninvasive evaluation of aortic valve anatomy. Echocardiography 1996;13:315–23.

11. Roberts WC. The congenitally bicuspid aortic valve: a study of 85 autopsy cases. Am J Cardiol 1970;26:72–83.

12. Kang JW, Song HG, Yang DH, et al. Association between bicuspid aortic valve phenotype and patterns of valvular dysfunction and bicuspid aortopathy: comprehensive evaluation using MDCT and echocardiography. JACC Cardiovasc Imaging 2013;6:150–61.

13. Fernández B, Durán AC, Fernández-Gallego T, et al. Bicuspid aortic valves with different spatial orientations of the leaflets are distinct etiological entities. J Am Coll Cardiol 2009;54:2312–8.

14. Fernandes SM, Khairy P, Sanders SP, et al. Bicuspid aortic valve morphology and interventions in the young. J Am Coll Cardiol 2007;49:2211–4.

15. Michelena HI, Desjardins VA, Avierinos JF, et al. Natural history of asymptomatic patients with normally functioning or minimally dysfunctional bicuspid aortic valve in the community. Circulation 2008; 117:2776–84.

16. Thanassoulis G, Yip JW, Filion K, et al. Retrospective study to identify predictors of the presence and rapid progression of aortic dilatation in patients with bicuspid aortic valves. Nat Clin Pract Cardiovasc Med 2008;5:821–8.

17. Bonow RO. Bicuspid aortic valves and dilated aortas: a critical review of the critical review of the ACC/AHA practice guidelines recommendations. Am J Cardiol 2008;102:111–4.

18. Kurt M, Tanboga I, Bilen E, et al. Abnormal left ventricular mechanics in isolated bicuspid aortic valve disease may be independent of aortic distensibility: 2D strain imaging study. J Heart Valve Dis 2012;21(5):608–14.

19. Bilen E, Akçay M, Bayram NA, et al. Aortic elastic properties and left ventricular diastolic function in patients with isolated bicuspid aortic valve. J Heart Valve Dis 2012;21:189.

20. di Pino A, Gitto P, Silvia A, et al. Congenital quadricuspid aortic valve in children. Cardiol Young 2008;18:324–7.

21. Brantley HP, Nekkanti R, Anderson CA, et al. Three-dimensional echocardiographic features of unicuspid aortic valve stenosis correlate with surgical findings. Echocardiography 2012;29:E204–7.

22. Otto CM, Bonow RO. Valvular heart disease. In: Bonow RO, Mann DL, Zipes DP, et al, editors. Braunwald's heart disease–a textbook of cardiovascular medicine. Philadelphia: Elsevier; 2012. p. 1468–88.

23. Keane JF, Lock JE, Fyler DC. Nadas' pediatric cardiology. Philadelphia: Elsevier; 2006.

24. Carabello BA. Introduction to aortic stenosis. Circ Res 2013;113:179–85.

25. Bonow RO. Exercise hemodynamics and risk assessment in asymptomatic aortic stenosis. Circulation 2012;126:803–5.

26. Park SJ, Enriquez-Sarano M, Chang SA, et al. Hemodynamic patterns for symptomatic presentations of severe aortic stenosis. JACC Cardiovasc Imaging 2013;6:137–46.

27. Bonow RO, Carabello BA, Chatterjee K, et al. ACC/AHA 2006 guidelines for the management of patients with valvular heart disease: a report of the American College of Cardiology/American Heart Association Task Force on Practice Guidelines (writing committee to revise the 1998 Guidelines for the Management of Patients with Valvular Heart Disease): developed in collaboration with the Society of Cardiovascular Anesthesiologists: endorsed by the Society for Cardiovascular Angiography and Interventions and the Society of Thoracic Surgeons. Circulation 2006;114:e84–231.

28. Members AT, Vahanian A, Alfieri O, et al, Joint Task Force on the Management of Valvular Heart Disease of the European Society of Cardiology (ESC) and the European Association for Cardio-Thoracic Surgery (EACTS). Guidelines on the management of valvular heart disease (version 2012). Eur Heart J 2012;33:2451–96.

29. Lancellotti P, Magne J, Pierard LA. The role of stress testing in evaluation of asymptomatic patients with aortic stenosis. Curr Opin Cardiol 2013;28:531–9.

30. Henkel DM, Malouf JF, Connolly HM, et al. Asymptomatic left ventricular systolic dysfunction in patients with severe aortic stenosis: characteristics and outcomes. J Am Coll Cardiol 2012;60:2325–9.

31. Miller LE, Miller VM, Acers LD. Asymptomatic severe aortic stenosis with left ventricular dysfunction: watchful waiting or valve replacement? Clin Med Res 2013;11:51–3.

32. Lancellotti P, Magne J, Donal E, et al. Determinants and prognostic significance of exercise pulmonary hypertension in asymptomatic severe aortic stenosis. Circulation 2012;126:851–9.

33. Hoffman JI. The natural and unnatural history of congenital heart disease. Hoboken (NJ): Wiley-Blackwell; 2009.

34. Tierney ES, Levine JC, Chen S, et al. Echocardiographic methods, quality review, and measurement accuracy in a randomized multicenter clinical trial of Marfan syndrome. J Am Soc Echocardiogr 2013;26:657–66.

35. Bonow RO, Lakatos E, Maron BJ, et al. Serial long-term assessment of the natural history of asymptomatic patients with chronic aortic regurgitation and normal left ventricular systolic function. Circulation 1991;84:1625–35.

36. Tornos P, Sambola A, Permanyer-Miralda G, et al. Long-term outcome of surgically treated aortic regurgitation: influence of guideline adherence toward early surgery. J Am Coll Cardiol 2006;47:1012–7.

37. Smucker ML, Manning SB, Stuckey TD, et al. Preoperative left ventricular wall stress, ejection fraction, and aortic valve gradient as prognostic indicators in aortic valve stenosis. Cathet Cardiovasc Diagn 1989;17:133–43.

38. Ou P, Celermajer DS, Jolivet O, et al. Increased central aortic stiffness and left ventricular mass in normotensive young subjects after successful coarctation repair. Am Heart J 2008;155:187–93.

39. Vogt M, Kuhn A, Baumgartner D, et al. Impaired elastic properties of the ascending aorta in newborns before and early after successful coarctation repair: proof of a systemic vascular disease of the prestenotic arteries? Circulation 2005;111:3269–73.

40. Krieger EV, Stout K. The adult with repaired coarctation of the aorta. Heart 2010;96:1676–81.

41. Brili S, Tousoulis D, Antoniades C, et al. Effects of ramipril on endothelial function and the expression of proinflammatory cytokines and adhesion molecules in young normotensive subjects with successfully repaired coarctation of aorta: a randomized cross-over study. J Am Coll Cardiol 2008;51:742–9.

42. Brili S, Tousoulis D, Antoniades C, et al. Evidence of vascular dysfunction in young patients with successfully repaired coarctation of aorta. Atherosclerosis 2005;182:97–103.

43. Senzaki H, Iwamoto Y, Ishido H, et al. Ventricular-vascular stiffening in patients with repaired coarctation of aorta: integrated pathophysiology of hypertension. Circulation 2008;118:S191–8.

44. de Divitiis M, Pilla C, Kattenhorn M, et al. Vascular dysfunction after repair of coarctation of the aorta: impact of early surgery. Circulation 2001;104:I165–70.

45. Gardiner HM, Celermajer DS, Sorensen KE, et al. Arterial reactivity is significantly impaired in normotensive young adults after successful repair of aortic coarctation in childhood. Circulation 1994;89:1745–50.

46. Gidding SS, Rocchini AP, Moorehead C, et al. Increased forearm vascular reactivity in patients with hypertension after repair of coarctation. Circulation 1985;71:495–9.

47. O'Rourke M. Mechanical principles in arterial disease. Hypertension 1995;26:2–9.

48. Chirinos JA, Segers P. Noninvasive evaluation of left ventricular afterload: part 1: pressure and flow measurements and basic principles of wave conduction and reflection. Hypertension 2010;56:555–62.

49. Krieger EV, Landzberg MJ, Economy KE, et al. Comparison of risk of hypertensive complications of pregnancy among women with versus without coarctation of the aorta. Am J Cardiol 2011;107:1529–34.

50. O'Sullivan JJ, Derrick G, Darnell R. Prevalence of hypertension in children after early repair of coarctation of the aorta: a cohort study using casual and 24 hour blood pressure measurement. Heart 2002;88:163–6.

51. Hager A, Kanz S, Kaemmerer H, et al. Coarctation long-term assessment (COALA): significance of arterial hypertension in a cohort of 404 patients up to 27 years after surgical repair of isolated coarctation of the aorta, even in the absence of restenosis and prosthetic material. J Thorac Cardiovasc Surg 2007;134:738–45.

52. Toro-Salazar OH, Steinberger J, Thomas W, et al. Long-term follow-up of patients after coarctation of the aorta repair. Am J Cardiol 2002;89:541–7.

53. Krieger EV, Clair M, Opotowsky AR, et al. Correlation of exercise response in repaired coarctation of the aorta to left ventricular mass and geometry. Am J Cardiol 2013;111(3):406–11.

54. Morgan GJ, Lee KJ, Chaturvedi R, et al. Systemic blood pressure after stent management for arch coarctation implications for clinical care. JACC Cardiovasc Interv 2013;6:192–201.

55. Luijendijk P, Bouma BJ, Vriend JW, et al. Usefulness of exercise-induced hypertension as predictor of chronic hypertension in adults after operative therapy for aortic isthmic coarctation in childhood. Am J Cardiol 2011;108:435–9.

56. Vriend JW, van Montfrans GA, Romkes HH, et al. Relation between exercise-induced hypertension and sustained hypertension in adult patients after successful repair of aortic coarctation. J Hypertens 2004;22:501–9.

57. Grossman W, Jones D, McLaurin LP. Wall stress and patterns of hypertrophy in the human left ventricle. J Clin Invest 1975;56:56–64.

58. Ou P, Celermajer DS, Raisky O, et al. Angular (gothic) aortic arch leads to enhanced systolic wave reflection, central aortic stiffness, and increased left ventricular mass late after aortic coarctation repair: evaluation with magnetic resonance flow mapping. J Thorac Cardiovasc Surg 2008;135:62–8.

59. Pacileo G, Pisacane C, Russo MG, et al. Left ventricular remodeling and mechanics after successful repair of aortic coarctation. Am J Cardiol 2001;87:748–52.

60. Roman MJ, Ganau A, Saba PS, et al. Impact of arterial stiffening on left ventricular structure. Hypertension 2000;36:489–94.

61. Krogmann ON, Rammos S, Jakob M, et al. Left ventricular diastolic dysfunction late after coarctation repair in childhood: influence of left ventricular hypertrophy. J Am Coll Cardiol 1993;21:1454–60.

62. Moskowitz WB, Schieken RM, Mosteller M, et al. Altered systolic and diastolic function in children after "successful" repair of coarctation of the aorta. Am Heart J 1990;120:103–9.

63. Marshall AC, Perry SB, Keane JF, et al. Early results and medium-term follow-up of stent implantation

for mild residual or recurrent aortic coarctation. Am Heart J 2000;139:1054–60.

64. Krogmann ON, Kramer HH, Rammos S, et al. Noninvasive evaluation of left ventricular systolic function late after coarctation repair: influence of early vs late surgery. Eur Heart J 1993;14:764–9.

65. Kimball TR, Reynolds JM, Mays WA, et al. Persistent hyperdynamic cardiovascular state at rest and during exercise in children after successful repair of coarctation of the aorta. J Am Coll Cardiol 1994;24:194–200.

66. Lam YY, Mullen MJ, Kaya MG, et al. Left ventricular long axis dysfunction in adults with "corrected" aortic coarctation is related to an older age at intervention and increased aortic stiffness. Heart 2009; 95:733–9.

67. Maron BJ, Humphries JO, Rowe RD, et al. Prognosis of surgically corrected coarctation of the aorta. A 20-year postoperative appraisal. Circulation 1973;47:119–26.

68. Shone JD, Sellers RD, Anderson RC, et al. The developmental complex of "parachute mitral valve," supravalvular ring of left atrium, subaortic stenosis, and coarctation of aorta. Am J Cardiol 1963;11:714–25.

69. Popescu BA, Jurcut R, Serban M, et al. Shone's syndrome diagnosed with echocardiography and confirmed at pathology. Eur J Echocardiogr 2008; 9:865–7.

70. Brown JW, Ruzmetov M, Vijay P, et al. Operative results and outcomes in children with Shone's anomaly. Ann Thorac Surg 2005;79:1358–65.

71. Schaverien MV, Freedom RM, McCrindle BW. Independent factors associated with outcomes of parachute mitral valve in 84 patients. Circulation 2004; 109:2309–13.

72. Vaideeswar P, Baldi MM, Warghade S. An analysis of 24 autopsied cases with supramitral rings. Cardiol Young 2009;19:70–5.

73. Brown JW, Ruzmetov M, Rodefeld MD, et al. Surgical strategies and outcomes in patients with supraannular mitral ring: a single-institution experience. Eur J Cardiothorac Surg 2010;38:556–60.

74. Collison SP, Kaushal SK, Dagar KS, et al. Supramitral ring: good prognosis in a subset of patients with congenital mitral stenosis. Ann Thorac Surg 2006;81:997–1001.

75. Tulloh RM, Bull C, Elliot MJ, et al. Supravalvar mitral stenosis: risk factors for recurrence or death after resection. Br Heart J 1995;73:164–8.

76. Oliver JM, González A, Gallego P, et al. Discrete subaortic stenosis in adults: increased prevalence and slow rate of progression of the obstruction and aortic regurgitation. J Am Coll Cardiol 2001;38: 835–42.

77. DiSessa TG, Hagan AD, Isabel-Jones JB, et al. Two-dimensional echocardiographic evaluation of discrete subaortic stenosis from the apical long axis view. Am Heart J 1981;101:774–82.

78. McMahon CJ, Gauvreau K, Edwards JC, et al. Risk factors for aortic valve dysfunction in children with discrete subvalvar aortic stenosis. Am J Cardiol 2004;94:459–64.

79. Geva A, McMahon CJ, Gauvreau K, et al. Risk factors for reoperation after repair of discrete subaortic stenosis in children. J Am Coll Cardiol 2007; 50:1498–504.

80. Chin TK, Perloff JK, Williams RG, et al. Isolated noncompaction of left ventricular myocardium. A study of eight cases. Circulation 1990;82: 507–13.

81. Maron BJ, Towbin JA, Thiene G, et al, American Heart Association, Council on Clinical Cardiology Heart Failure and Transplantation Committee, Quality of Care and Outcomes and Functional Genomics and Translational Biology Interdisciplinary Working Groups, Council on Epidemiology and Prevention. Contemporary definitions and classification of the cardiomyopathies: an American Heart Association Scientific Statement from the Council on Clinical Cardiology, Heart Failure and Transplantation Committee; Quality of Care and Outcomes Research and Functional Genomics and Translational Biology Interdisciplinary Working Groups; and Council on Epidemiology and Prevention. Circulation 2006;113:1807–16.

82. Sedmera D, Pexieder T, Vuillemin M, et al. Developmental patterning of the myocardium. Anat Rec 2000;258:319–37.

83. Weiford BC, Subbarao VD, Mulhern KM. Noncompaction of the ventricular myocardium. Circulation 2004;109:2965–71.

84. Oechslin EN, Attenhofer Jost CH, Rojas JR, et al. Long-term follow-up of 34 adults with isolated left ventricular noncompaction: a distinct cardiomyopathy with poor prognosis. J Am Coll Cardiol 2000; 36:493–500.

85. Burke A, Mont E, Kutys R, et al. Left ventricular noncompaction: a pathological study of 14 cases. Hum Pathol 2005;36:403–11.

86. Krieger EV, Valente AM. Diagnosis and management of Ebstein anomaly of the tricuspid valve. Curr Treat Options Cardiovasc Med 2012;14: 594–607.

87. Attenhofer Jost CH, Connolly HM, Warnes CA, et al. Noncompacted myocardium in Ebstein's anomaly: initial description in three patients. J Am Soc Echocardiogr 2004;17:677–80.

88. Lilje C, Razek V, Joyce JJ, et al. Complications of non-compaction of the left ventricular myocardium in a paediatric population: a prospective study. Eur Heart J 2006;27:1855–60.

89. Saleeb SF, Margossian R, Spencer CT, et al. Reproducibility of echocardiographic diagnosis of left

ventricular noncompaction. J Am Soc Echocardiogr 2012;25:194–202.

90. Stollberger C, Finsterer J. Pitfalls in the diagnosis of left ventricular hypertrabeculation/non-compaction. Postgrad Med J 2006;82:679–83.

91. Aras D, Tufekcioglu O, Ergun K, et al. Clinical features of isolated ventricular noncompaction in adults long-term clinical course, echocardiographic properties, and predictors of left ventricular failure. J Card Fail 2006;12:726–33.

92. Sarma RJ, Chana A, Elkayam U. Left ventricular noncompaction. Prog Cardiovasc Dis 2010;52:264–73.

93. Frischknecht BS, Attenhofer Jost CH, Oechslin EN, et al. Validation of noncompaction criteria in dilated cardiomyopathy, and valvular and hypertensive heart disease. J Am Soc Echocardiogr 2005;18:865–72.

94. Kohli SK, Pantazis AA, Shah JS, et al. Diagnosis of left-ventricular non-compaction in patients with left-ventricular systolic dysfunction: time for a reappraisal of diagnostic criteria? Eur Heart J 2008;29:89–95.

95. Finsterer J, Stollberger C. No rationale for a diagnostic ratio in left ventricular hypertrabeculation/noncompaction. Int J Cardiol 2011;146:91–2.

96. Paterick TE, Umland MM, Jan MF, et al. Left ventricular noncompaction: a 25-year odyssey. J Am Soc Echocardiogr 2012;25:363–75.

97. Murphy RT, Thaman R, Blanes JG, et al. Natural history and familial characteristics of isolated left ventricular non-compaction. Eur Heart J 2005;26:187–92.

98. Lofiego C, Biagini E, Pasquale F, et al. Wide spectrum of presentation and variable outcomes of isolated left ventricular non-compaction. Heart 2007;93:65–71.

99. Yancy CW, Jessup M, Bozkurt B, et al. 2013 ACCF/AHA guideline for the management of heart failure: a report of the American College of Cardiology Foundation/American Heart Association Task Force on Practice Guidelines. Circulation 2013. [Epub ahead of print].

100. Lai WW. Echocardiography in pediatric and congenital heart disease: from fetus to adult. Oxford (United Kingdom): Wiley-Blackwell; 2009.

101. Vallakati A, Nerella N, Chandra P, et al. Incidental diagnosis of cor triatriatum in 2 elderly patients. J Am Coll Cardiol 2012;59:e43.

102. Slight RD, Nzewi OC, Mankad PS. Echocardiographic diagnosis of cor triatriatum sinister in the adult. Heart 2004;90:63.

103. Lai WW, Mertens LL, Cohen MS, et al. Echocardiography in pediatric and congenital heart disease: from fetus to adult. 2009.

104. Elagha AA, Fuisz AR, Weissman G. Cardiac magnetic resonance imaging can clearly depict the morphology and determine the significance of cor triatriatum. Circulation 2012;126:1511–3.

105. Allen HD. Moss and Adams heart disease in infants, children, and adolescents: including the fetus and young adult. Philadelphia: Wolters Kluwer Health/Lippincott Williams & Wilkins; 2013.

106. Jenni R, Oechslin E, Schneider J, et al. Echocardiographic and pathoanatomical characteristics of isolated left ventricular non-compaction: a step towards classification as a distinct cardiomyopathy. Heart 2001;86:666–71.

107. Stöllberger C, Finsterer J. Left ventricular hypertrabeculation/noncompaction. J Am Soc Echocardiogr 2004;17:91–100.

108. Petersen SE, Selvanayagam JB, Wiesmann F, et al. Left ventricular non-compaction: insights from cardiovascular magnetic resonance imaging. J Am Coll Cardiol 2005;46:101–5.

109. Jacquier A, Thuny F, Jop B, et al. Measurement of trabeculated left ventricular mass using cardiac magnetic resonance imaging in the diagnosis of left ventricular non-compaction. Eur Heart J 2010;31:1098–104.

Medical Therapy in Adults with Congenital Heart Disease

Wendy M. Book, MD[a],*, Robert E. Shaddy, MD[b]

KEYWORDS

- Heart failure • Congenital heart disease • Medical therapy • β-blockers
- Angiotensin-converting enzyme inhibitor

KEY POINTS

- Clinical heart failure is associated with increased morbidity and mortality in adults with congenital heart disease.
- The onset of clinical heart failure should prompt the treating physician to look for residual hemodynamically important anatomic defects that may be amenable to intervention.
- Because of heterogeneity and insufficient patients number for randomized controlled trials, extrapolation and expert opinion guide medical therapy.

INTRODUCTION

The development of heart failure (HF) is a clinically important event in patients with adult congenital heart disease (ACHD). Hospitalization for HF identifies a population of ACHD patients at risk for subsequent hospitalizations and mortality over the next 3 years. In a recent study, incidence for first HF admission in young patients with congenital heart disease (CHD) was 1.2 per 1000 patient-years, more than 10-fold higher than that in the general population of the same age. Following a first admission for HF, mortality was high, 24% at 1 year and 35% at 3 years, and primarily of cardiovascular causes,[1] emphasizing the importance of the onset of HF in an ACHD patient. Despite the significant contribution of HF to premature morbidity and mortality in the ACHD population, no adequately powered clinical trials have been done to understand the role of medical therapies in ACHD patients with clinical HF.

Although many patients with ACHD meet the clinical definition of HF,[2] patients with ACHD have been excluded from clinical trials of medical therapy in HF and, because of consequently limited specific data, from the HF guidelines.

Patients with ACHD are at risk for complications related to the original defect and/or subsequent repairs. In addition, some patients with univentricular circulations or Eisenmenger syndrome develop dysfunction involving multiple organ systems. Therefore ACHD patients with evidence of clinical signs and symptoms of HF need evaluation for residual hemodynamically significant defects, including valvular dysfunction, shunts, pulmonary vascular disease, obstruction of conduits and baffles, and other potentially correctable anatomic lesions.

In conjunction with correction of residual anatomic lesions, medical therapy may be of benefit for the management of ventricular dysfunction in the ACHD patient. This article reviews the

Disclosures: Dr W.M. Book receives research funding from Actelion, and funding from the Centers for Disease Control and Prevention; Dr R.E. Shaddy is a consultant for Bayer and Novartis.
[a] Department of Internal Medicine, Division of Cardiology, Emory Adult Congenital Heart Center, School of Medicine, Emory University, 1365 Clifton Road Northeast, Suite A2447, Atlanta, GA 30322, USA; [b] The Children's Hospital of Philadelphia, Perelman School of Medicine, University of Pennsylvania, 34th Street & Civic Center Boulevard, Room 8 NW 90, 8th Floor, Northwest Tower, Main Philadelphia, PA 19104, USA
* Corresponding author.
E-mail address: wbook@emory.edu

heartfailure.theclinics.com

applicability of the current HF guidelines to an ACHD population, and reviews medical therapies for HF in specific patient populations, including biventricular repair with normal connections, subaortic right ventricle in a two-ventricle circulation, and single-ventricle (SV) circulations.

THE HF GUIDELINES: RATIONALE FOR MEDICAL THERAPY

Similarities in clinical presentation make it tempting to broadly extrapolate the HF guidelines to patients with ACHD. Challenges in extrapolating heart guidelines to a heterogeneous ACHD population range from difficulties in recognizing exercise intolerance, quantifying ventricular dysfunction, lack of diagnostic criteria, and lack of consensus recommendations on management.

Neurohormonal activation may also be seen in ACHD patients with a variety of surgically repaired and unrepaired heart defects,[3] similar to that described in a population with acquired HF.[3–8] Therefore the use of therapies that are known to improve outcomes in acquired left ventricular (LV) systolic dysfunction (HF with reduced ejection fraction, or HFrEF) may be of benefit in carefully selected patients with ACHD.

Cardiac remodeling is the final common pathway by which an initial injury or stressor to the ventricle leads to progressive structural changes of the ventricle, which is driven by a variety of neurohormonal stimuli,[9,10] cytokines,[11] changes in calcium handling,[12,13] signaling pathways,[14] extracellular matrix,[15] autoimmunity,[16] oxidative stress, and substrate utilization.[17]

The clinical importance of neurohormonal pathways, particularly the sympathetic nervous system (SNS) and renin-angiotensin-aldosterone system (RAAS), has been demonstrated in numerous clinical trials in HFrEF, demonstrating survival benefit with blockade of these pathways. Therapies that reverse or slow the remodeling process improve survival in patients with HFrEF.[18–26] Similarly, the Studies of Left Ventricular Dysfunction (SOLVD) investigators demonstrated a significant delay in the time to development of clinical HF and hospitalization in patients with asymptomatic LV systolic dysfunction treated with the angiotensin-converting enzyme inhibitor (ACEI) enalapril.[27]

However, as has been learned from the HF experience, these benefits may not be realized in populations of patients with HF of differing etiology, such as HF with preserved ejection fraction (HFpEF), despite a similar clinical event rate.[28–32] The recent observation that 24 weeks of sildenafil did not improve quality of life (QOL) or exercise capacity in patents with HFpEF, despite prior studies

suggesting a hemodynamic benefit,[33] serves as a cautionary tale for clinical application of medications in a population based on small single-center studies focused on acute hemodynamic benefit, without study of long-term effectiveness. **Table 1** outlines current knowledge about the use of HF medications in different populations.

PREVENTING HF: RISK-FACTOR MODIFICATION

Identification of patients with modifiable risk factors may delay or prevent HF in certain at-risk populations. Application of basic cardiology practices to the ACHD population makes sense given the prevalence of modifiable risk factors (eg, hypertension, diabetes mellitus, obesity, atherosclerosis, sedentary lifestyle) in our contemporary population. The recently updated HF guidelines also recommend exercise training or regular physical activity, education focusing on self-care, and identification and discontinuation of cardiotoxins.[2] Early intervention in those at risk should also include patients with ACHD.

EXTRAPOLATION FROM THE HF GUIDELINES: INITIAL ASSESSMENT OF THE SYMPTOMATIC PATIENT

In addition to evaluation for important residual anatomic lesions, assessment of patients with ACHD and signs of clinical HF should include the same thorough history and physical examination described in the HF guidelines.[2] Recommendations for assessment of functional class, volume status, changes in orthostatic blood pressure, weight, body mass index, laboratory studies, 12-lead electrocardiogram, chest radiograph, and 2-dimensional echocardiography with Doppler[2] are generally applicable to an ACHD population.

DIURETICS

Diuretics should be considered for all patients with signs of fluid retention. Patients unresponsive to oral loop diuretics should be given intravenous diuretics to relieve congestion. Aldosterone antagonists can be considered in patients with systolic LV dysfunction and a prior hospitalization for congestive HF, or symptoms of New York Heart Association functional class III to IV, who are appropriate candidates (estimated glomerular filtration rate >30 mL/min/1.73 m^2 and serum potassium <5 mEq/L).[2] Baseline laboratory studies and routine monitoring of renal function and electrolytes should be performed for all patients on diuretics.

Table 1
Comparison of medical therapies for acquired heart failure in patients with structurally normal hearts and those with congenital heart defects

Medication	HFrEF	HFpEF	Valvular Heart Disease	ACHD: Normal Connections, Two Ventricles, Systemic LV	ACHD: Subaortic RV, Two Ventricles	ACHD: Single Ventricle
ACEI and ARB	Benefit	Benefit for the management of hypertension and in patients with diabetes	No known benefit	Possible beneficial effect on remodeling	Possible beneficial effect on remodeling	Unknown
β-Blockers	Benefit	Benefit for management of hypertension	Possible beneficial effect on remodeling	Possible beneficial effect on remodeling	Limited data, possible benefit	Unknown
Aldosterone antagonists	Benefit	Benefit for management of hypertension	Unknown	Unknown	Not studied	Unknown
PDE5 inhibitors	No benefit	No benefit	Not studied	Not studied	Not studied	Possible benefit on exercise tolerance

Abbreviations: ACEI, angiotensin-converting enzyme inhibitors; ACHD, adult congenital heart disease; ARB, angiotensin receptor blockers; HFpEF, heart failure with preserved ejection fraction; HFrEF, heart failure with reduced ejection fraction; LV, left ventricle; PDE5, phosphodiesterase 5; RV, right ventricle.

Fluid Retention: Additional Considerations

Patients who present with evidence of congestion are candidates for diuretics, with rare exceptions. The finding of elevated central venous pressure and ascites, without hepatomegaly, in patients with long-standing right HF should prompt consideration of hepatic fibrosis or cirrhosis as the cause of their ascites. This situation is most commonly seen in patients with Fontan circulations, or in those with dextro-transposition of the great arteries (dTGA) status post (s/p) atrial switch procedure with obstructed baffles of the inferior vena cava, and should prompt evaluation for possible anatomic obstruction of right-sided blood flow and evaluation for concomitant hepatic disease.

Medical therapy for ACHD patients: Biventricular circulations with normal connections (following repair)

Included in This Category

Left-sided

- Left ventricular outflow tract obstruction
- Other left-sided valvular disease
- Coronary reimplantations
- Coarctation of the aorta

Right-sided

- Tetralogy of Fallot, with or without pulmonary atresia
- Truncus arteriosus
- Ebstein anomaly
- Right ventricular outflow tract obstruction

Shunts

- Atrial septal defect
- Ventricular septal defect
- Patent ductus arteriosus

EVALUATION OF THE ACHD PATIENT WITH HF

The ACHD patient who presents with signs and symptoms consistent with HF requires evaluation in a center with expertise in managing patients with ACHD to exclude and/or correct residual anatomic lesions, as described in the section on left-sided lesions. Management of left-sided valvular heart disease is also well discussed in the American Heart Association/American College of Cardiology guidelines on valvular heart disease,[34] and are not reiterated here. Management of the ACHD patient with LV failure includes a complete assessment for residual anatomic issues that may be affecting LV function, including assessment for coronary obstructions and ischemia in patients with previous reimplantation of the coronary arteries. Initial treatment of the symptomatic patient should focus on identification and relief of residual obstruction and/or regurgitation lesions by an appropriate imaging technique.[35] However, not all ACHD patients with HFrEF will be candidates for surgical repair.

MEDICAL THERAPY FOR HF: LEFT-SIDED LESIONS AND/OR REPAIRED SEPTAL DEFECTS

Once residual hemodynamically important anatomic lesions have been assessed in the ACHD patient with HFrEF, extrapolation of the HF guidelines to this ACHD population with systolic LV dysfunction includes appropriate use of diuretics to manage volume, ACEI and aldosterone antagonists when indicated, and initiation and appropriate titration of β-blockers (bisoprolol, metoprolol, or carvedilol). Management of comorbidities as per the HF guidelines is also recommended, including the use of ACEI and β-blockers in appropriate patients with HF Stage A and Stage B.[2] Based on the current understanding of neurohormonal activation in HFrEF, extrapolation of the HF guidelines to patients with ACHD and normal connections, LV systolic dysfunction, and no residual correctable anatomic defects makes sense.

USE OF β-BLOCKERS IN REGURGITANT LEFT-SIDED VALVULAR LESIONS

Although there are no specific data regarding the use of HF therapies in patients with left-sided CHD, there are several studies demonstrating the benefit of β-blockers in patients with aortic valve regurgitation and mitral valve regurgitation in preserving ventricular function and slowing remodeling in the volume-loaded left ventricle. Preliminary data suggest a benefit of β-blockers, such as carvedilol, in aortic regurgitation[36,37] and, possibly, mitral regurgitation (MR),[38] by slowing LV dilatation, decreasing hypertrophy, decreasing fibrosis, decreasing filling pressures and improving the ejection fraction, although a rat model of MR did not suggest benefit.[39] These data suggest a potential role for β-blockers in patients with volume-loaded left ventricles from residual left-to-right shunts across a ventricular septal defect or patent ductus arteriosus, who are not candidates for closure.

RIGHT-SIDED LESIONS WITH NORMAL CONNECTIONS

Patients with ACHD with initial right-sided lesions and normal connections are also at risk for the development of biventricular HF. The etiology is often multifactorial, and includes remodeling related to prior volume load from previous or residual shunts, ischemic injury at the time of initial repair, coronary anomalies, ventricular myotomy, and volume load of the right ventricle.

Right ventricular (RV) failure, resulting from pressure or volume loading, may affect LV function,[40] and may be seen following repair of tetralogy of Fallot (rTOF),[40] pulmonary atresia, Ebstein anomaly, and pulmonary valvotomy for congenital pulmonary stenosis. Therefore, a thorough evaluation at a center specializing in CHD is recommended to identify and correct any hemodynamically significant lesions contributing to HF.

HF IN REPAIRED TETRALOGY OF FALLOT

Although no study has specifically assessed HF incidence in rTOF, the reported HF rates in pediatric studies are low, ranging from 1% to 3% over the long-term follow-up.[41–43] The low event rate in the pediatric group will limit any studies of medical therapy unless the trial design includes follow-up over decades. Despite a low prevalence of HF in pediatric patients, adults with rTOF followed in a tertiary setting have a higher prevalence of LV dysfunction (by ejection fraction), estimated at around 20%.[44] Several studies suggest that pulmonary valve replacement (PVR) improves LV function, suggesting that LV dysfunction is related to RV dysfunction, whereas randomized trials with β-blockers[45–47] and ACEI in rTOF patients pre-PVR have not shown any beneficial effects on LV function.[47] Therefore, the preferred therapy for appropriate surgical candidates presenting with LV dysfunction and severe pulmonary valve regurgitation with RV dilatation is PVR.

MEDICAL THERAPY FOR RTOF WITH COMPETENT PULMONARY VALVE AND HFREF

Heart failure in patients with rTOF and a competent pulmonary valve is rare; in a recent post-PVR patient series, there was only 1 case reported from 90 patients after 8.5 years,[43] with low rates of HF noted in another long-term series as well.[48] Therefore, data on outcomes with ACEI and β-blockers in rTOF patients following PVR who have persistent LV systolic dysfunction are limited.

However, anecdotal experience suggests that patients who have persistent LV systolic dysfunction following correction of residual valvular lesions in rTOF may benefit from traditional HF therapies, including diuretics for volume management, ACEI, aldosterone antagonists, and β-blockers.

SUBAORTIC (SYSTEMIC) RV DYSFUNCTION IN PATIENTS WITH TWO-VENTRICLE CIRCULATION

This population primarily consists of patients with:

- dTGA s/p atrial switch procedures (Senning or Mustard)
- Congenitally corrected transposition of the great arteries (CCTGA)

Data on the management of ventricular dysfunction in patients with systemic right ventricle are lacking, despite the high incidence of late clinical HF and sudden death in this population.[49–51] Clinical definitions of "normal" versus "abnormal" systemic RV function are poorly defined, as is the best method of assessing ventricular function,[52,53] which makes challenging the comparison of single-center studies, interpretation of literature, and clinical trial design. Prognostic markers for late development of HF and/or sudden death are also limited.[5]

Despite the clinical importance of HF limiting late outcomes in this population, few studies have addressed the use of HF therapies. The right ventricle differs from the left ventricle not only architecturally but also regarding adaptability in neonatal life.[54] It is unclear whether there are differences at the cellular level that might affect the response to medical therapies.

MEDICAL THERAPY: CAUTION ADVISED

Use of β-blockers is associated with a higher risk in this population because of sinus node dysfunction (dTGA s/p atrial switch) and heart block (CCTGA). Baffle stenosis (dTGA s/p atrial switch), and reduced venous capacitance due to atrial baffles (dTGA s/p atrial switch) may lead to unintended consequences with the use of ACEI and vasodilators in certain patients.

β-BLOCKERS

Several small single-center studies have suggested a potential benefit of β-blockade in patients with systemic right ventricle, associated with improvement in symptoms, less (systemic) tricuspid regurgitation, improved functional status, and positive effects on RV remodeling.[55–57] In the dTGA s/p atrial switch population, treatment with β-blockers may protect against arrhythmic events.[50] Anecdotal case reports comprise the remaining published literature.[58] However, other investigators have failed to demonstrate a benefit in a randomized controlled trial in a heterogeneous pediatric HF population.[59]

ACEI AND ANGIOTENSIN RECEPTOR BLOCKERS

In patients with acquired HFrEF, the use of chronic ACEI has been shown to improve long-term outcomes (time to clinical HF, improved functional status, reduction in hospitalizations and mortality). However, acute treatment with ACEI did not improve exercise capacity in the population with acquired LV dysfunction,[60] whereas chronic therapy does improve exercise tolerance, supporting multiple studies demonstrating that benefits of ACEI are related to reversal of remodeling, not acute hemodynamic effects.

Studies evaluating ACEI in ACHD patients with systemic RV dysfunction are lacking. Small single-center studies to date have used exercise parameters as a surrogate end point. A retrospective study of lisinopril in 14 patients with TGA did not show improvement in RV ejection fraction (RVEF) or peak oxygen consumption.[61] Small, uncontrolled, underpowered case series are not sufficient to determine whether ACEI benefit patients with systemic RV dysfunction.

Several prospective, randomized, double-blind, controlled clinical trials of angiotensin receptor blockers (ARB)[62,63] and ACEI[64] have produced varying results. A small prospective cross-over study of the ARB losartan in patients with TGA demonstrated improved ejection fraction and exercise duration in an adolescent/young-adult population.[63] A randomized placebo-controlled trial of the ACEI ramipril in 17 adults s/p atrial switch for dTGA did not demonstrate a change in RVEF or RV end-diastolic volume after 1 year of treatment.[64] However, the largest of these studies evaluated 44 patients, and no study has evaluated clinically important end points such as mortality or HF hospitalization.

Although there are theoretical rationales to support the use of β-blockers and ACEI/ARB in asymptomatic patients with systemic right ventricle, routine use of these medications cannot be recommended until further understanding of the pathophysiology of systemic right ventricle has been better elucidated and adequately powered randomized studies have been completed. For patients with systemic right ventricle and clinical symptomatic HF, use of HF therapies can be considered once anatomic, surgical, and arrhythmic (including chronotropic incompetence) issues have been addressed.

CCTGA: Special Considerations

Many patients with CCTGA have an abnormal tricuspid valve (systemic atrioventricular valve) with resultant regurgitation, and may require tricuspid valve replacement to reduce volume load on the susceptible right ventricle. Surgical replacement of the tricuspid valve in CCTGA should be considered on an individual basis, based on severity of tricuspid regurgitation (TR) and RV dysfunction.[65] However, some anecdotal experience suggests that medical therapy with β-blockers and ACEI may also improve HF symptoms and TR in patients with CCTGA who seem to have primarily functional TR.

FUTURE NEEDS

In addition to difficulties in identifying exercise intolerance in patients with systemic right ventricle data on normal RVEF, size, and optimal imaging assessment of the right ventricle are lacking. Once the clinical syndrome of HF has been identified in the patient with a systemic right ventricle and residual anatomic lesions have been addressed, there are few data to guide medical therapy. Studies in this population will be limited by small patient numbers and heterogeneity, making it difficult to properly power these studies.

SINGLE-VENTRICLE CIRCULATION

The appropriate medical management of HF in ACHD patients with SV circulation is complicated by the lack of large, prospective, randomized trials from which to derive evidence-based guidelines. Although numerous drug trials in adults with HFrEF have demonstrated the beneficial effects of ACEI/ARB, β-blockers, aldosterone antagonists, and other medications for the treatment of HF, none of these studies included patients with SV physiology. Therefore, the best one can do is to either extrapolate from these trials and/or base one's treatment decisions on small nonrandomized reports or expert opinion. The overwhelming majority of adult patients with SV circulations have undergone some form of the Fontan operation, so subsequent discussions in this section are limited to these patients. Patients after the Fontan operation can have symptoms of HF arising from one of two very distinct problems: there is either systemic ventricular dysfunction, or there are hemodynamic abnormalities of the Fontan circuit, or there are both.

HF Caused by Reduced Systemic Ventricular Ejection Fraction

In patients with SV circulation, the morphology of the systemic SV can be that of LV, RV, or indeterminate morphology. It is tempting to think that those patients after the Fontan operation with systemic left ventricle (eg, tricuspid atresia or double-inlet left ventricle) may be comparable with adults with structurally normal hearts and HFrEF. It may be reasonable to follow the HF guidelines for the management of chronic HF in adults for patients after the Fontan operation with a systemic left ventricle (ACEI/ARB, β-blockers, aldosterone antagonists, and so forth).[2] Unfortunately, efficacy of medications in this setting remains unproven, and there are ventricular-ventricular interactions in a biventricular heart that are lacking in a univentricular heart. These differences may significantly alter the response of a single left ventricle to medications proven to work in HFrEF with biventricular anatomy.

In those patients after the Fontan operation with an SV that is not of LV morphology, management strategies of chronic HFrEF has been extrapolated from guidelines for adults with ischemic or nonischemic causes of HF.[2] Diuretics are indicated in patients with fluid overload. The choice of diuretics should be similar to those used in biventricular hearts: loop diuretics with consideration of addition of thiazide diuretics if refractory. There are no studies to support or refute the use of ACEI in this situation. Kouatli and colleagues[66] performed a randomized trial of enalapril in a small group of stable children after the Fontan operation, and measured their exercise tolerance after 6 weeks of therapy. Not only was there no improvement in exercise performance in the enalapril group compared with the placebo group, but the average increase in cardiac index from rest to maximal exercise was actually decreased in the enalapril group, suggesting possible deleterious effects of enalapril in this population. In a larger prospective randomized trial of enalapril in infants with SV anatomy (before the Fontan operation), the investigators were unable to discern any benefit of enalapril over placebo in the primary end point of weight-for-age z-score, nor was there any benefit in any of the secondary end points including echocardiographic parameters, symptoms, or brain natriuretic peptide.[67] The role of ARBs, β-blockers, aldosterone antagonists, and digoxin in patients after the Fontan operation is similarly unclear. There are no reports on the use of these agents in this population. Thus it may be reasonable to consider these medications for those patients who meet the standard criteria for the use of these medications in adults with ischemic or nonischemic chronic HFrEF. However, in this setting one may wish to consider counseling the patients as to the off-label use of these drugs and their unknown efficacy and/or adverse effects.

HF Caused by the Failing Fontan Circuit and Relatively Preserved Systemic Ventricular Ejection Fraction

Management strategies in this clinical situation are directed toward optimizing pulmonary blood flow, optimizing systemic blood flow, and reducing systemic venous congestion. Manifestations of a failing Fontan circuit are variable. Some patients present with evidence of systemic venous congestion, whereas others may present with protein-losing enteropathy (PLE) or plastic bronchitis. Although it is unclear as to why some patients develop these signs and symptoms and others do not, it is presumed that these are all manifestations of the failing Fontan circuit. It is important to make every effort to diagnose the cause of the failing Fontan circuit, and direct therapy accordingly. For instance, heart catheterization is necessary to assess hemodynamics and exclude any mechanical obstructions within the Fontan circuit that would benefit from transcatheter or surgical intervention. If there is no mechanical obstruction, or if there are persistent symptoms after relief of obstruction, one must consider other treatment options, which includes creating (if absent) or enlarging (if oxygen saturations allow) a fenestration in the Fontan circuit to reduce right-sided pressures and increase cardiac output, at the expense of a right-to-left shunt with decrease in systemic oxygen saturation. Pulmonary vasodilators such as oxygen, nitric oxide, and/or phosphodiesterase type 5 (PDE5) inhibitors, such as sildenafil, can be considered to help improve pulmonary blood flow and relieve right-sided congestion. PDE5 inhibitors may benefit both pulmonary mechanics and ventricular function in these patients,[68] although larger trials are needed (and are planned) to determine their utility and safety.

In patients with plastic bronchitis or PLE these measures may be effective, but additional diagnostic and treatment measures may also be necessary.[69] For plastic bronchitis the use of thrombolytic agents, such as inhaled tissue plasminogen activator, may be beneficial.[70,71] In patients with PLE, some institutions are recommending endoscopy to look for evidence of inflammation that may be responsive to anti-inflammatory medications such as budesonide.[69,72] Intermittent albumin infusions may help alleviate symptoms, but this does not represent a long-term solution. Although these types of measures may palliate some patients with plastic bronchitis or PLE, many of these patients continue to have symptoms that would classify them as Class D HF: that is, HF requiring special interventions such as inotropes, mechanical support, or heart transplantation. In the setting of preserved ventricular function, inotropes have little role in HF management in these patients. Mechanical circulatory support may be considered, but presents significant anatomic challenges. Heart transplantation is a reasonable option, but these patients are at higher risk than the patient with failing Fontan and reduced ejection fraction. In general, patients with SV circulations, and signs or symptoms of HF, benefit from evaluation and management at an ACHD center that has a multidisciplinary team experienced in caring for the multitude of complex medical issues faced by these patients.

Management of acute decompensated HF

Management strategies of acute decompensated HF in ACHD patients with HFrEF are also derived from adult HF recommendations. Diuretics are the mainstay of therapy. Addition of inotropes can be considered, but data supporting their use is lacking. Mechanical circulatory support in CHD patients can be challenging, and may require creative surgical revision to ensure adequate blood flow in the circuit of a ventricular assist device, as outlined in the articles by Mulukutla and colleagues as well as Stewart and Meyer elsewhere in this issue.[73–75] Although there are only anecdotal reports to date, a total artificial heart may be an option for some CHD patients who fail medical management.[76] Heart transplantation is an option for appropriate candidates, particularly in those whose symptoms are due to systemic ventricular dysfunction.[77,78] There are reports of the use of heart-liver transplantation in SV patients who suffer damage to the liver caused by the failing Fontan circulation.[79,80]

OVERCOMING CHALLENGES: DEVELOPING AN EVIDENCE BASE FOR MANAGEMENT OF HF IN ACHD

The hallmark method for developing an evidence base for the medical management of any disease is the multicenter, prospective, randomized, placebo-controlled, parallel-group trial. These trials are very expensive and are often difficult to carry out. Identifying the appropriate patient population is critically important, as is the choice of the primary end point.

In large adult HF trials, the patient population has generally been composed of patients with acquired HF, with either reduced or preserved ejection fraction. These patients are dissimilar from ACHD patients; patients in the larger HF trials have structurally normal hearts and are generally 55 to 75 years old, with a higher incidence of diabetes mellitus, hypertension, and atrial fibrillation.[81–83] By contrast, ACHD patients with HF are generally much younger and have less comorbidity, with heterogeneity of anatomic defects and surgical repairs. Recruiting adequate numbers of ACHD patients for large multicenter HF trials will be challenging because of the small recruitment base. In addition, the choice of primary end point is critically important in performing an adequate randomized trial. In the large adult HF trials, end points such as mortality (all-cause or HF mortality), hospitalizations (all-cause or HF hospitalizations), or symptom and/or QOL assessment have been successfully used. However, when using these types of end points, large numbers of patients are required. For example, most major β-blocker adult HF trials enrolled between 1000 and 4000 patients.[20,21,26] Such enrollment would be extremely difficult for ACHD patients because of the smaller number of such patients and the heterogeneity of the ACHD population. Thus, consideration should be given to surrogate or intermediate end points to assess the efficacy and safety of HF therapies in patients with ACHD and HF. Investigators have argued that the use of remodeling end points such as LV end-diastolic dimension or volume would be a reliable end point in HF trials because this measurement correlates so well with mortality, hospitalizations, and symptoms.[84] Of interest, in the randomized trial of valsartan in ACHD patients with systemic right ventricle, the primary end point failed to show any benefit of valsartan over placebo, whereas the secondary remodeling end points of RV volume and RV mass both demonstrated improvement in the valsartan group.[62] Thus, validation and creative use of true surrogate end points is warranted in developing a useful evidence base for the management of HF in ACHD patients.

In addition to randomized trials, the use of comparative effectiveness research for developing evidence bases has recently gained in popularity.[85] In general, this requires the existence of an accurate, audited database that can be examined to assess the safety and efficacy of different treatments. These analyses offer advantages over randomized trials in that they are not limited to the narrow entry criteria often needed for randomized trials, thus making the analysis more representative of the "real-world" patient population.[86] More work is needed to better define the optimal use of these types of analyses, but the treatment of HF in ACHD patients may be well suited for such methodology. Of course, development and maintenance of a strong database is essential to success. Given the importance of clinical HF in an ACHD population, identification of medical therapies that may benefit these patients is imperative.

REFERENCES

1. Zomer AC, Vaartjes I, van der Velde ET, et al. Heart failure admissions in adults with congenital heart disease; risk factors and prognosis. Int J Cardiol 2013;168(3):2487–93.
2. Yancy CW, Jessup M, Bozkurt B, et al. 2013 ACCF/AHA Guideline for the Management of Heart Failure: A Report of the American College of Cardiology Foundation/American Heart Association Task Force on Practice Guidelines. J Am Coll Cardiol 2013;62(16):e147–239.
3. Bolger AP, Sharma R, Li W, et al. Neurohormonal activation and the chronic heart failure syndrome in adults with congenital heart disease. Circulation 2002;106:92–9.
4. Tulevski II, Groenink M, van Der Wall EE, et al. Increased brain and atrial natriuretic peptides in patients with chronic right ventricular pressure overload: correlation between plasma neurohormones and right ventricular dysfunction. Heart 2001;86:27–30.
5. Book WM, Hott BJ, McConnell M. B-type natriuretic peptide levels in adults with congenital heart disease and right ventricular failure. Am J Cardiol 2005;95:545–6.
6. Daliento L, Folino AF, Menti L, et al. Adrenergic nervous activity in patients after surgical correction of tetralogy of Fallot. J Am Coll Cardiol 2001;38:2043–7.
7. Ohuchi H, Negishi J, Miyake A, et al. Long-term prognostic value of cardiac autonomic nervous activity in postoperative patients with congenital heart disease. Int J Cardiol 2011;151:296–302.
8. Leuchte HH, Holzapfel M, Baumgartner RA, et al. Clinical significance of brain natriuretic peptide in primary pulmonary hypertension. J Am Coll Cardiol 2004;43:764–70.
9. Schrier RW. Effects of adrenergic nervous-system and catecholamines on systemic and renal hemodynamics, sodium and water excretion and renin secretion. Kidney Int 1974;6:291–306.
10. Schrier RW, Abraham WT. Hormones and hemodynamics in heart failure. N Engl J Med 1999;341:577–85.
11. El-Menyar AA. Cytokines and myocardial dysfunction: state of the art. J Card Fail 2008;14:61–74.
12. Respress JL, van Oort RJ, Li N, et al. Role of RyR2 phosphorylation at S2814 during heart failure progression. Circ Res 2012;110:1474–83.
13. Yano M, Kobayashi S, Kohno M, et al. FKBP12.6-mediated stabilization of calcium-release channel (ryanodine receptor) as a novel therapeutic strategy against heart failure. Circulation 2003;107:477–84.
14. Kehat I, Molkentin JD. Molecular pathways underlying cardiac remodeling during pathophysiological stimulation. Circulation 2010;122:2727–35.
15. Chapman RE, Spinale FG. Extracellular protease activation and unraveling of the myocardial interstitium: critical steps toward clinical applications. Am J Physiol Heart Circ Physiol 2004;286(1):H1–10.
16. Lappe JM, Pelfrey CM, Tang WH. Recent insights into the role of autoimmunity in idiopathic dilated cardiomyopathy. J Card Fail 2008;14:521–30.
17. Ashrafian H, Frenneaux MP, Opie LH. Metabolic mechanisms in heart failure. Circulation 2007;116:434–48.
18. Effect of enalapril on survival in patients with reduced left ventricular ejection fractions and congestive heart failure. The SOLVD Investigators. N Engl J Med 1991;325:293–302.
19. Pitt B, Zannad F, Remme WJ, et al. The effect of spironolactone on morbidity and mortality in patients with severe heart failure. Randomized Aldactone Evaluation Study Investigators. N Engl J Med 1999;341:709–17.
20. Bristow MR, Gilbert EM, Abraham WT, et al. Carvedilol produces dose-related improvements in left ventricular function and survival in subjects with chronic heart failure. MOCHA Investigators. Circulation 1996;94:2807–16.
21. Packer M, Bristow MR, Cohn JN, et al. The effect of carvedilol on morbidity and mortality in patients with chronic heart failure. U.S. Carvedilol Heart Failure Study Group. N Engl J Med 1996;334:1349–55.
22. Fowler MB. Carvedilol prospective randomized cumulative survival (COPERNICUS) trial: carvedilol in severe heart failure. Am J Cardiol 2004;93:35b–9b.
23. Hjalmarson A, Goldstein S, Fagerberg B, et al. Effects of controlled-release metoprolol on total mortality, hospitalizations, and well-being in patients with heart failure: the Metoprolol CR/XL Randomized Intervention Trial in congestive heart failure (MERIT-HF). MERIT-HF Study Group. JAMA 2000;283:1295–302.
24. The Cardiac Insufficiency Bisoprolol Study II (CIBIS-II): a randomised trial. Lancet 1999;353:9–13.
25. Packer M, Poole-Wilson PA, Armstrong PW, et al. Comparative effects of low and high doses of the angiotensin-converting enzyme inhibitor, lisinopril, on morbidity and mortality in chronic heart failure. ATLAS Study Group. Circulation 1999;100:2312–8.
26. Effect of metoprolol CR/XL in chronic heart failure: Metoprolol CR/XL Randomised Intervention Trial in Congestive Heart Failure (MERIT-HF). Lancet 1999;353:2001–7.

27. Effect of enalapril on mortality and the development of heart failure in asymptomatic patients with reduced left ventricular ejection fractions. The SOLVD Investigators. N Engl J Med 1992; 327:685–91.

28. Yancy CW, Lopatin M, Stevenson LW, et al. Clinical presentation, management, and in-hospital outcomes of patients admitted with acute decompensated heart failure with preserved systolic function: a report from the Acute Decompensated Heart Failure National Registry (ADHERE) Database. J Am Coll Cardiol 2006;47:76–84.

29. Lam CS, Donal E, Kraigher-Krainer E, et al. Epidemiology and clinical course of heart failure with preserved ejection fraction. Eur J Heart Fail 2011;13: 18–28.

30. Massie BM, Carson PE, McMurray JJ, et al. Irbesartan in patients with heart failure and preserved ejection fraction. N Engl J Med 2008;359:2456–67.

31. Cleland JG, Tendera M, Adamus J, et al. The perindopril in elderly people with chronic heart failure (PEP-CHF) study. Eur Heart J 2006;27:2338–45.

32. Yusuf S, Pfeffer MA, Swedberg K, et al. Effects of candesartan in patients with chronic heart failure and preserved left-ventricular ejection fraction: the CHARM-Preserved Trial. Lancet 2003;362: 777–81.

33. Redfield MM, Chen HH, Borlaug BA, et al. Effect of phosphodiesterase-5 inhibition on exercise capacity and clinical status in heart failure with preserved ejection fraction: a randomized clinical trial. JAMA 2013;309:1268–77.

34. Nishimura RA, Carabello BA, Faxon DP, et al. ACC/AHA 2008 guideline update on valvular heart disease: focused update on infective endocarditis: a report of the American College of Cardiology/American Heart Association Task Force on Practice Guidelines: endorsed by the Society of Cardiovascular Anesthesiologists, Society for Cardiovascular Angiography and Interventions, and Society of Thoracic Surgeons. Circulation 2008; 118:887–96.

35. El-Segaier M, Lundin A, Hochbergs P, et al. Late coronary complications after arterial switch operation and their treatment. Catheter Cardiovasc Interv 2010;76:1027–32.

36. Zendaoui A, Lachance D, Roussel E, et al. Usefulness of carvedilol in the treatment of chronic aortic valve regurgitation. Circ Heart Fail 2011;4:207–13.

37. Plante E, Lachance D, Champetier S, et al. Benefits of long-term beta-blockade in experimental chronic aortic regurgitation. Am J Physiol Heart Circ Physiol 2008;294:H1888–95.

38. Ennis DB, Rudd-Barnard GR, Li B, et al. Changes in mitral annular geometry and dynamics with ss-blockade in patients with degenerative mitral valve disease. Circ Cardiovasc Imaging 2010;3:687–93.

39. Pu M, Gao Z, Pu DK, et al. Effects of early, late, and long-term nonselective beta-blockade on left ventricular remodeling, function, and survival in chronic organic mitral regurgitation. Circ Heart Fail 2013;6:756–62.

40. Davlouros PA, Kilner PJ, Hornung TS, et al. Right ventricular function in adults with repaired tetralogy of Fallot assessed with cardiovascular magnetic resonance imaging: detrimental role of right ventricular outflow aneurysms or akinesia and adverse right-to-left ventricular interaction. J Am Coll Cardiol 2002;40:2044–52.

41. Katz NM, Blackstone EH, Kirklin JW, et al. Late survival and symptoms after repair of tetralogy of Fallot. Circulation 1982;65:403–10.

42. Harrison DA, Siu SC, Hussain F, et al. Sustained atrial arrhythmias in adults late after repair of tetralogy of Fallot. Am J Cardiol 2001;87:584–8.

43. Scherptong RW, Hazekamp MG, Mulder BJ, et al. Follow-up after pulmonary valve replacement in adults with tetralogy of Fallot: association between QRS duration and outcome. J Am Coll Cardiol 2010;56:1486–92.

44. Broberg CS, Aboulhosn J, Mongeon FP, et al. Prevalence of left ventricular systolic dysfunction in adults with repaired tetralogy of Fallot. Am J Cardiol 2011;107:1215–20.

45. Norozi K, Bahlmann J, Raab B, et al. A prospective, randomized, double-blind, placebo controlled trial of beta-blockade in patients who have undergone surgical correction of tetralogy of Fallot. Cardiol Young 2007;17:372–9.

46. Norozi K, Buchhorn R, Wessel A, et al. Beta-blockade does not alter plasma cytokine concentrations and ventricular function in young adults with right ventricular dysfunction secondary to operated congenital heart disease. Circ J 2008;72:747–52.

47. Babu-Narayan SV, Uebing A, Davlouros PA, et al. Randomised trial of ramipril in repaired tetralogy of Fallot and pulmonary regurgitation: the APPROPRIATE study (Ace inhibitors for Potential PRevention Of the deleterious effects of Pulmonary Regurgitation In Adults with repaired TEtralogy of Fallot. Int J Cardiol 2012;154:299–305.

48. Nollert G, Fischlein T, Bouterwek S, et al. Long-term survival in patients with repair of tetralogy of Fallot: 36-year follow-up of 490 survivors of the first year after surgical repair. J Am Coll Cardiol 1997;30: 1374–83.

49. Kammeraad JA, van Deurzen CH, Sreeram N, et al. Predictors of sudden cardiac death after Mustard or Senning repair for transposition of the great arteries. J Am Coll Cardiol 2004;44:1095–102.

50. Khairy P, Harris L, Landzberg MJ, et al. Sudden death and defibrillators in transposition of the great arteries with intra-atrial baffles: a multicenter study. Circ Arrhythm Electrophysiol 2008;1:250–7.

51. Wilson NJ, Clarkson PM, Barratt-Boyes BG, et al. Long-term outcome after the mustard repair for simple transposition of the great arteries. 28-year follow-up. J Am Coll Cardiol 1998;32:758–65.

52. Moroseos T, Mitsumori L, Kerwin WS, et al. Comparison of Simpson's method and three-dimensional reconstruction for measurement of right ventricular volume in patients with complete or corrected transposition of the great arteries. Am J Cardiol 2010;105:1603–9.

53. Salehian O, Schwerzmann M, Merchant N, et al. Assessment of systemic right ventricular function in patients with transposition of the great arteries using the myocardial performance index: comparison with cardiac magnetic resonance imaging. Circulation 2004;110:3229–33.

54. Zhang L, Allen J, Hu L, et al. Cardiomyocyte architectural plasticity in fetal, neonatal, and adult pig hearts delineated with diffusion tensor MRI. Am J Physiol Heart Circ Physiol 2013;304:H246–52.

55. Josephson CB, Howlett JG, Jackson SD, et al. A case series of systemic right ventricular dysfunction post atrial switch for simple D-transposition of the great arteries: the impact of beta-blockade. Can J Cardiol 2006;22:769–72.

56. Giardini A, Piva T, Picchio FM, et al. Impact of transverse aortic arch hypoplasia after surgical repair of aortic coarctation: an exercise echo and magnetic resonance imaging study. Int J Cardiol 2007;119:21–7.

57. Doughan AR, McConnell ME, Book WM. Effect of beta blockers (carvedilol or metoprolol XL) in patients with transposition of great arteries and dysfunction of the systemic right ventricle. Am J Cardiol 2007;99:704–6.

58. Lindenfeld J, Keller K, Campbell DN, et al. Improved systemic ventricular function after carvedilol administration in a patient with congenitally corrected transposition of the great arteries. J Heart Lung Transplant 2003;22:198–201.

59. Shaddy RE, Boucek MM, Hsu DT, et al. Carvedilol for children and adolescents with heart failure: a randomized controlled trial. JAMA 2007;298:1171–9.

60. Osaki S, Kinugawa T, Ogino K, et al. Effects of acute and chronic alacepril treatment on exercise capacity and hemodynamics in patients with heart failure: a preliminary study. Int J Clin Pharmacol Ther 2002;40:69–74.

61. Hechter SJ, Fredriksen PM, Liu P, et al. Angiotensin-converting enzyme inhibitors in adults after the Mustard procedure. Am J Cardiol 2001;87:660–3 A11.

62. van der Bom T, Winter MM, Bouma BJ, et al. Effect of valsartan on systemic right ventricular function: a double-blind, randomized, placebo-controlled pilot trial. Circulation 2013;127:322–30.

63. Lester SJ, McElhinney DB, Viloria E, et al. Effects of losartan in patients with a systemically functioning morphologic right ventricle after atrial repair of transposition of the great arteries. Am J Cardiol 2001;88:1314–6.

64. Therrien J, Provost Y, Harrison J, et al. Effect of angiotensin receptor blockade on systemic right ventricular function and size: a small, randomized, placebo-controlled study. Int J Cardiol 2008;129:187–92.

65. Mongeon FP, Connolly HM, Dearani JA, et al. Congenitally corrected transposition of the great arteries ventricular function at the time of systemic atrioventricular valve replacement predicts long-term ventricular function. J Am Coll Cardiol 2011;57:2008–17.

66. Kouatli AA, Garcia JA, Zellers TM, et al. Enalapril does not enhance exercise capacity in patients after Fontan procedure. Circulation 1997;96:1507–12.

67. Hsu DT, Zak V, Mahony L, et al. Enalapril in infants with single ventricle: results of a multicenter randomized trial. Circulation 2010;122:333–40.

68. Goldberg DJ, French B, McBride MG, et al. Impact of oral sildenafil on exercise performance in children and young adults after the Fontan operation: a randomized, double-blind, placebo-controlled, crossover trial. Circulation 2011;123:1185–93.

69. Ostrow AM, Freeze H, Rychik J. Protein-losing enteropathy after Fontan operation: investigations into possible pathophysiologic mechanisms. Ann Thorac Surg 2006;82:695–700.

70. Heath L, Ling S, Racz J, et al. Prospective, longitudinal study of plastic bronchitis cast pathology and responsiveness to tissue plasminogen activator. Pediatr Cardiol 2011;32:1182–9.

71. Gibb E, Blount R, Lewis N, et al. Management of plastic bronchitis with topical tissue-type plasminogen activator. Pediatrics 2012;130:e446–50.

72. Thacker D, Patel A, Dodds K, et al. Use of oral budesonide in the management of protein-losing enteropathy after the Fontan operation. Ann Thorac Surg 2010;89:837–42.

73. Nathan M, Baird C, Fynn-Thompson F, et al. Successful implantation of a Berlin heart biventricular assist device in a failing single ventricle. J Thorac Cardiovasc Surg 2006;131:1407–8.

74. Ricci M, Gaughan CB, Rossi M, et al. Initial experience with the TandemHeart circulatory support system in children. ASAIO J 2008;54:542–5.

75. VanderPluym CJ, Rebeyka IM, Ross DB, et al. The use of ventricular assist devices in pediatric patients with univentricular hearts. J Thorac Cardiovasc Surg 2011;141:588–90.

76. Kirsch ME, Nguyen A, Mastroianni C, et al. SynCardia temporary total artificial heart as bridge to transplantation: current results at La Pitie Hospital. Ann Thorac Surg 2013;95:1640–6.

77. Karamlou T, Gelow J, Diggs BS, et al. Mechanical circulatory support pathways that maximize post-heart transplant survival. Ann Thorac Surg 2013; 95:480–5 [discussion: 5].

78. Griffiths ER, Kaza AK, Wyler von Ballmoos MC, et al. Evaluating failing Fontans for heart transplantation: predictors of death. Ann Thorac Surg 2009; 88:558–63 [discussion: 63–4].

79. Hollander SA, Reinhartz O, Maeda K, et al. Intermediate-term outcomes after combined heart-liver transplantation in children with a univentricular heart. J Heart Lung Transplant 2013;32:368–70.

80. Vallabhajosyula P, Komlo C, Wallen TJ, et al. Combined heart-liver transplant in a situs-ambiguous patient with failed Fontan physiology. J Thorac Cardiovasc Surg 2013;145:e39–41.

81. Krum H, Gilbert RE. Demographics and concomitant disorders in heart failure. Lancet 2003;362:147–58.

82. Publication Committee for the VMAC Investigators (Vasodilatation in the Management of Acute CHF). Intravenous nesiritide vs nitroglycerin for treatment of decompensated congestive heart failure: a randomized controlled trial. JAMA 2002;287: 1531–40.

83. Adams KF Jr, Fonarow GC, Emerman CL, et al. Characteristics and outcomes of patients hospitalized for heart failure in the United States: rationale, design, and preliminary observations from the first 100,000 cases in the Acute Decompensated Heart Failure National Registry (ADHERE). Am Heart J 2005;149:209–16.

84. Konstam MA, Udelson JE, Anand IS, et al. Ventricular remodeling in heart failure: a credible surrogate endpoint. J Card Fail 2003;9:350–3.

85. Eapen ZJ, McBroom AJ, Gray R, et al. Priorities for comparative effectiveness reviews in cardiovascular disease. Circ Cardiovasc Qual Outcomes 2013; 6:139–47.

86. Concato J. Is it time for medicine-based evidence? JAMA 2012;307:1641–3.

Percutaneous Options for Heart Failure in Adults with Congenital Heart Disease

Darren Mylotte, MB MRCPI, MD[a],
Giuseppe Martucci, MD, FRCPC[a],*,
Nicolo Piazza, MD, PhD, FRCPC, FESC[a], Doff McElhinney, MD[b]

KEYWORDS

- Adult congenital heart disease • Percutaneous intervention • Transcatheter intervention
- Heart failure

KEY POINTS

- Transcatheter interventions have evolved considerably in recent years and now play a key role in the treatment of heart failure (HF) in adult patients with congenital heart disease (CHD).
- These innovative procedures, when performed successfully and in a timely fashion, can lead to reversal of ventricular dilatation and dysfunction.
- Percutaneous interventions complement medical and surgical therapies and together form a comprehensive therapeutic approach for the treatment of HF in adults with CHD.

INTRODUCTION

Heart failure (HF) is a complex biochemical and physiologic response to the inability of the heart to meet the metabolic demands of the body. Hemodynamically, HF results from a decrease in cardiac output, a function of both heart rate and stroke volume (SV). The SV is determined by preload, afterload, and ventricular contractility, and derangement of 1 or a combination of these elements can reduce the SV. In patients with congenital heart disease (CHD), a variety of cardiac and extracardiac anatomic defects can initiate pathophysiologic change, culminating in reduced SV and HF. These defects can be categorized as either ventricular pressure- or volume-loaded states.

Transcatheter interventions play a critical role in the treatment of HF in adult patients with CHD (ACHD). These procedures complement the more traditional medical and surgical therapies to form a comprehensive therapeutic approach for the treatment of HF in ACHD. An in-depth review of all transcatheter interventions performed by the adult interventional congenital cardiologist is beyond the scope of this article. Hence, the most commonly encountered CHD lesions associated with HF and their transcatheter treatments are described: atrial septal defect (ASD), ventricular septal defect (VSD), and patent ductus arteriosus (PDA); right-sided obstructive and regurgitant lesions, including pulmonary regurgitation (PR) and stenosis; and left-sided obstructive lesions, such as aortic coarctation. These lesions are organized anatomically into those that predominantly affect the right ventricle (RV) and those affecting the left ventricle (LV). Of course, this practical and simplified approach does not account for the principles of ventricular interdependence, nor does it take into consideration that many patients with CHD have complex anatomies, with more than 1 lesion competing for physiologic dominance.

[a] Department of Interventional Cardiology, McGill University Health Centre, Royal Victoria Hospital, 687, Pine Avenue West, Montréal H3A-1A1, Québec, Canada; [b] Department of Pediatrics, Langone Medical Center, New York University, 550 First Avenue, New York, NY 10016, USA
* Corresponding author. McGill Adult Unit for Congenital Heart Disease (MAUDE Unit), 687 Pine Avenue West, Montréal, Québec H3A 1A1, Canada.
E-mail address: joe-martucci@hotmail.com

Heart Failure Clin 10 (2014) 179–196
http://dx.doi.org/10.1016/j.hfc.2013.09.018
1551-7136/14/$ – see front matter © 2014 Elsevier Inc. All rights reserved.

LESIONS PREDOMINANTLY AFFECTING THE RV

ASDs

ASDs are the most common form of CHD in adults, accounting for up to one-third of all cases. They may be classified anatomically (**Table 1**): ostium primum in the lower part of the atrial septum; ostium secundum in the region of the fossa ovalis; sinus venosus with overriding of the atrial septum by the superior or inferior vena cava; and coronary sinus defects. Ostium secundum are the most common defects (75%), followed by ostium primum (15%), and sinus venosus defects (10%). ASDs may present as isolated lesions or may be associated with other cardiac abnormalities.[1]

ASDs allow shunting of blood from 1 atrium to the other. The direction and magnitude of the shunt are determined by the size of the ASD and the relative compliance of the ventricles.[2] Small shunts (<5 mm) may be inconsequential, whereas large shunts may produce considerable hemodynamic consequences. In most cases of an isolated ASD, the RV is more compliant than the LV, and hence, blood is shunted from the left to right atrium. Over time, significant shunts increase pulmonary blood flow, thereby inducing RV and pulmonary arterial dilatation. Unchecked, the volume-loaded RV dilates and RV function decreases, resulting in right-sided HF.

Adult patients typically present with RV dilatation, right-sided HF, pulmonary hypertension, atrial arrhythmias, or systemic embolism.[3,4] The anatomic position, hemodynamic consequences, and associated lesions of the ASD are confirmed by echocardiography, and the magnitude of shunting can be quantification by cardiac catheterization by calculating the pulmonary/systemic blood flow ratio (Qp/Qs).

Transcatheter ASD Closure

Indications for transcatheter ASD closure

Patients with small shunts (<5 mm) and normal RV dimensions are usually asymptomatic and require no further therapy. ASD closure may be performed for defects greater than 5 mm in diameter with evidence of RV dilatation with or without symptoms, if there is a history of paradoxic embolism (regardless of defect size), or if there is evidence of platypnea-orthodeoxia. ASD closure may also be performed in the presence of left-to-right shunt associated with increased pulmonary arterial pressures, where the pulmonary arterial pressure is less

---

Table 1
ASDs: classification, indications for closure, and reported transcatheter complications

Classification	Frequency (%)	Location
Ostium primum	15	Lower atrial septum
Ostium secundum	75	Fossa ovalis
Sinus venosus	10	At junction of SVC or IVC and atrial septum

Indications for closure
Defect >5 mm diameter and
1. RV or right atrial dilatation with or without symptoms
2. A history of paradoxic embolism (regardless of defect size)
3. Left to right shunt with increased PAP, if PAP < two-thirds systemic pressure, PVR < two-thirds SVR, or if responsive to pulmonary vasodilator therapy or test occlusion of the defect
4. Platypnea-orthodeoxia
Complications of transcatheter closure
Acute
  Embolization: (0.5%) associated with device undersizing, inadequate rims (<5 mm), and technical issues; percutaneous retrieval can be successfully achieved in up to three-quarters of cases
  Cardiac perforation: rare and usually related to wire perforation
  Arrhythmia: atrial arrhythmias are usually transient; heart block in 0.3% of cases
  Implant failure: implant fails in 1–3% of cases, most commonly because of large defects, unstable or inadequate positioning
Chronic
  Thrombosis: uncommon (1.2%); most cases (85%) resolve with systemic anticoagulation
  Arrhythmia: 5.2% within 4 mo: 4.8% with atrial tachyarrhythmias and 0.3% with heart block
  Erosion: (0.1–0.3%) associated with deficient aortic or superior rims; most present with symptoms within 72 h; surgical repair required

Abbreviations: IVC, inferior vena cava; PAP, pulmonary artery pressure; PVR, pulmonary vascular resistance; SVC, superior vena cava; SVR, systemic vascular resistance.

than two-thirds systemic pressure, pulmonary vascular resistance (PVR) is less than two-thirds systemic vascular resistance (SVR), or if the patient is responsive to pulmonary vasodilator therapy or test occlusion of the defect.[5] Contraindications to transcatheter ASD closure include nonsecundum ASD, coexisting congenital cardiac defects requiring surgical repair, irreversible pulmonary hypertension, defects greater than 40 mm in diameter, and inadequate rims.

Transcatheter ASD closure devices

Transcatheter ASD closure was first described by King and colleagues in 1974.[6,7] Today, the 2 most common devices used for ASD closure are the Amplatzer septal occluder (ASO) (St Jude Medical, St Paul, MN), and more recently, the Helex septal occluder (HSO) (W.L. Gore, Flagstaff, AZ). The ASO is a self-expanding nitinol wire mesh prosthesis that was developed in 1997 and approved by the US Food and Drug Administration (FDA) in 2001.[8] The ASO consists of 2 self-expandable round disks made of nitinol and linked together by a short connecting waist (**Fig. 1**). The disks and connecting waist are filled with Dacron fabric to facilitate thrombosis. The HSO received FDA approval in 2006. It is a nitinol wire covered with a polytetrafluoroethylene membrane that forms 2 disks on either side of the atrial septum on deployment.[9,10]

Safety, efficacy, and complications of transcatheter ASD closure

The pivotal ASO study was a multicenter nonrandomized trial that assigned 142 patients with secundum ASD to closure with the ASO device, and 154 patients to surgical closure.[11] Patients were deemed suitable for inclusion if they had a secundum ASD (diameter <38 mm for the device

group), a left to right shunt with a Qp/Qs of more than 1.5:1 or presence of RV volume overload, or symptoms in patients with minimal shunt. The reported incidence of major adverse event was 1.6% in the device group and 5.2% in the surgical group. A persistent clinically significant ASD was determined in 0% of surgical candidates and in 1.2% of device recipients at 12-month follow-up.

Similarly, the HSO pivotal study was a multicenter nonrandomized trial that enrolled 119 and 128 patients to device or surgical closure, respectively.[10] Inclusion criteria were similar to the ASO pivotal trial, but included balloon occlusion defect diameter less than 22 mm and the presence of adequate septal rims. The major adverse event rate was 5.9% for the device group and 10.9% for the surgical group. Closure success, defined as complete closure or a clinically insignificant residual shunt, was similar in both groups. A persistent clinically significant ASD was determined in 0% of surgical candidates and in 1.9% of device recipients at 12-month follow-up.

Complications related to transcatheter ASD closure may be classified as acute or chronic. Acute complications include device embolization, cardiac perforation, arrhythmia, and deployment failure. Chronic complications may include device infection, thrombosis, and erosion. Device embolization of the ASO has been reported in 0.55% of cases.[12,13] Factors associated with embolization include device undersizing, inadequate rims (<5 mm), and technical operator-related issues. Heart block and atrial arrhythmias may complicate transcatheter ASD closure. Clinically significant arrhythmias have been reported in 5.2% of cases in the 4 months after device placement, including 4.8% with atrial tachyarrhythmias and 0.3% with heart block.[14] The incidence of device-related

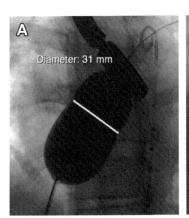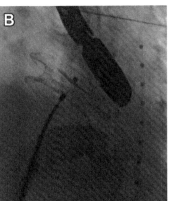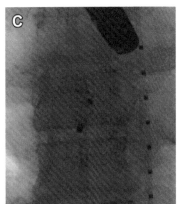

Fig. 1. Transcatheter ASD closure. (*A*) The ASD was sized at 31 mm with a sizing balloon. (*B*) Subsequently, a 34-mm ASO was positioned and (*C*) deployed. There was no residual shunt after release of the ASO device.

thrombosis is low (1.2%).[15] Most cases (85%) resolve with systemic anticoagulation. Erosion leading to cardiac perforation is a rare event, occurring in 0.1% to 0.28% of patients treated with the ASO.[8] The most commonly observed associated factor is deficient aortic or superior rims. Most patients present with symptoms within 72 hours of ASO implantation; however, late erosion up to 3 years has been reported.[13,16] Treatment involves surgical repair of the perforation or fistulous connection. Recent data suggest that patient mortality from erosion may be as high as 11.9%.[17] Erosion of the HSO device has not been reported.

After successful percutaneous ASD closure, the volume-loaded dilated RV usually remodels and returns to normal or near normal size.[18] Given the high success of transcatheter ASD closure and the low rates of periprocedural complications, most patients are offered a percutaneous rather than surgical approach to secundum ASD closure.[19–21]

RV Outflow Tract Dysfunction: Pulmonary Outflow Obstruction and PR

One of the most common conditions that may contribute to HF in ACHD is chronic postoperative RV outflow tract (RVOT) dysfunction, consisting of obstruction, PR, or mixed disease. In congenital heart defects such as tetralogy of Fallot (TOF), truncus arteriosus, double-outlet RV, some forms of transposition of the great arteries, and pulmonary atresia or stenosis associated with other complex anomalies, surgical repair includes augmentation or reconstruction of the connection of the pulmonary ventricle to the pulmonary artery. This situation is also true for patients with congenital aortic valve disease who undergo a Ross procedure (ie, pulmonary autograft replacement of the aortic valve). Reconstruction of the pulmonary outflow tract in these patients takes various forms, depending on the underlying defect and several other factors, and can include patching or augmenting the outflow tract without implanting a valve, or inserting some form of prosthetic conduit or valve to connect the ventricle with the pulmonary arteries.

Although RVOT reconstruction accomplishes the primary goal of providing a secure form of blood flow to the lungs, it is generally not a definitive long-term solution for these patients. All prosthetic conduits and valves used for RVOT reconstruction, whether in children or adults, are composed of either synthetic material or nonviable homograft or xenograft tissue. Thus, they cannot grow with the patient, which becomes a major limitation when they are implanted in small children, and they are subject to progressive degeneration and dysfunction. Depending on the method of reconstructing the RVOT, the pathway may become obstructed, which introduces a pressure load on the RV, or there may be progressively severe PR, which results in chronic volume overload of the RV. These lesions and the extra work they impose on the RV can be variably well tolerated over time, and often become fairly advanced before the onset of symptoms, but regardless of the clinical manifestations and pathophysiologic timeline, they are detrimental to the RV, and to the patient, contributing to right-sided and sometimes left-sided (ie, through ventricular interaction) HF. Transcatheter interventions are available to treat both RVOT obstruction and PR in many circumstances.

RVOT Obstruction

Pulmonary outflow obstruction in ACHD is most often caused by obstruction of a surgically implanted RVOT conduit or valve. It may also be caused by congenital stenosis of the pulmonary valve or subvalvar outflow tract, which was not repaired/treated earlier in life or which recurred after a previous surgical or balloon valvotomy.

Congenital pulmonary valve stenosis

Congenital pulmonary valve stenosis (PS), a common form of CHD, can vary substantially in its severity and clinical presentation.[22] Although PS severe enough to merit treatment tends to present in early childhood, it may come to attention later in life, and the obstruction can progress over time, so development of symptoms and treatment in adulthood are not rare. The first-line treatment of valvar PS at any age is balloon pulmonary valvotomy (**Fig. 2**). First reported 30 years ago,[23] balloon dilation of the pulmonary valve is usually effective at reducing the RVOT gradient and RV pressure, and in most cases should be sufficient anatomic treatment of HF symptoms related to this condition. There are some circumstances in which balloon dilation does not relieve PS, most notably when the valve leaflets are thick and dysplastic. This condition is not commonly encountered in adults with valvar PS, but even when it is, an attempt at balloon dilation is indicated before proceeding to surgical therapy.

There are several published reports on outcomes after balloon pulmonary valvotomy specifically in adults,[24–26] and adults are included in other larger series as well. Aside from the need for larger balloons (and sometimes a double-balloon technique, with simultaneous inflation of 2 balloons in parallel), there is nothing unique about the technical aspects

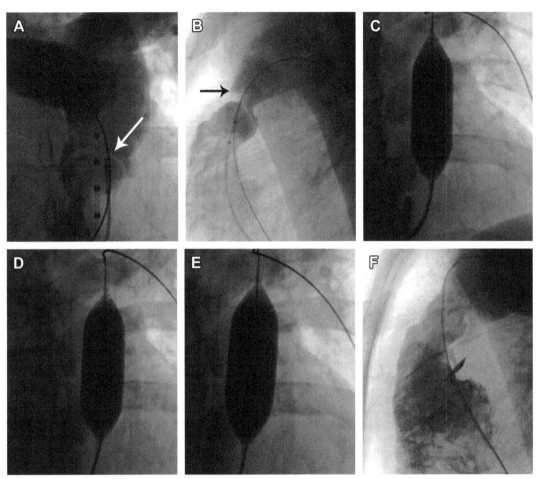

Fig. 2. Balloon pulmonary valvotomy. Sequential balloon pulmonary valvotomy in a patient with severe PS (transvalvular gradient 160 mm Hg). (*A*) Anteroposterior and (*B*) lateral views of the stenotic valve. Note doming of the valve leaflets (*arrow*). Balloon valvuloplasty with (*C*) 15 × 60 mm Z-Med (NuMed Hopkington, New York), (*D*) 18 × 40 mm Mullins (NuMed Hopkington, New York), and (*E*) 22 × 40 Mullins balloons. (*F*) Acceptable final result, with final peak transvalvular gradient of 20 mm Hg.

of the procedure in adults compared with younger patients. Hemodynamic outcomes after valvuloplasty are generally excellent in older patients, similar to those that are achieved in children. One potential concern in adult patients who have chronic RVOT obstruction and RV hypertrophy is that relief of the valvar stenosis may result in exacerbation of dynamic subvalvular muscular obstruction. This situation does occur in a subset of patients but generally resolves and does not cause important residual obstruction.[25,26] Stent implantation has been reported for dynamic subvalvular muscular RVOT obstruction and persistent symptoms after pulmonary valvotomy in several adults with congenital PS, but this is not a common scenario.[27]

With proper technique and balloon sizing, procedural complications related to balloon pulmonary

valvotomy are rare. However, balloon dilation of the pulmonary valve often results in some degree of PR, which can become significant and contribute to RV enlargement and exercise cardiopulmonary dysfunction over time.[28]

Postoperative RVOT obstruction

A more common form of RVOT obstruction in adults occurs when a surgically implanted pulmonary conduit or valve becomes obstructed. This situation may be caused by remodeling of the conduit in vivo, characterized by contraction, calcification, and thickening or fusion of the valve leaflets. Alternatively, RVOT conduit obstruction may simply be the result of size discordance, because the nonviable conduit cannot enlarge to match somatic growth, which is a common occurrence when children with conduits grow into adulthood. There are other factors that may contribute to the functional obstruction of a pulmonary valve or conduit, including the geometry of its implant, its location within the mediastinum, and the material of the prosthesis. Obstruction related to compression within the confined space of the mediastinum is important in some cases, a phenomenon that can be exacerbated by features that can be found with conontruncal heart defects, such as the presence of a large ascending aorta, malposition or rotation of the cardiac axis or position, and the relation and orientation of the great arteries.

In many cases, RVOT conduit or valve obstruction can be treated using one of several percutaneous methods. Angioplasty of obstructed conduits may yield some benefit, but often there is significant residual obstruction.[29] Angioplasty followed by implantation of a bare metal stent is more likely to reduce the RVOT gradient and RV pressure to acceptable levels than angioplasty alone, and for many years, stent implantation was the best transcatheter option for relieving postoperative RVOT obstruction.[30,31] One of the primary limitations of stent therapy for RVOT obstruction is that it typically results in severe PR. Obstruction of RVOT conduits is frequently at the level of the valve, and even if the valve leaflets are mobile and functional, which is not the norm, placement of the stent across the obstruction covers and immobilizes the leaflets, and there is free PR. Thus, treatment of RVOT obstruction with a bare metal stent generally entails trading obstruction for PR. Although the RV in patients with primary RVOT obstruction is often hypertrophied and able to handle the PR without acute dilation or dysfunction, this outcome is suboptimal.

A recently introduced alternative to bare metal stenting for RVOT obstruction is transcatheter pulmonary valve (TPV) replacement (or percutaneous pulmonary valve implantation), first reported by Bonhoeffer and colleagues[32] in 2000. TPV replacement, which allows treatment of obstructed or regurgitant RVOT conduits without the consequent PR that is associated with bare metal stent placement, has become an important option in the management of adults with postoperative RVOT dysfunction. A focused discussion of TPV replacement follows the section on postoperative PR; a more comprehensive review of this therapy can be found elsewhere.[33]

PR

PR with resulting RV dilation and dysfunction may be the most common contributor to the pathophysiology of HF in adults with TOF and related anomalies.[34,35] For several years after TOF repair became routine, the general belief was that chronic postoperative PR was well tolerated and of limited consequence. Patients could survive and function well for several decades with even severe PR. However, as more patients with severe chronic PR reached adulthood, it became increasingly apparent that PR and consequent RV enlargement could be associated with manifold adverse outcomes.[34–36]

Implantation of a prosthetic pulmonary valve can effectively reduce PR and RV volume overload, but with the growing application of cardiac magnetic resonance imaging, which facilitated more reliable and accurate quantification of RV volume and function, it became apparent that dilation and dysfunction of the RV were not necessarily reversible with pulmonary valve replacement if the process was too advanced.[34] It was also recognized that pulmonary valve replacement at these late stages did not always improve survival or other significant outcomes. Thus, in an effort to prevent irreversible changes in the RV and to reduce the risk of adverse long-term outcomes, there has been a recent trend toward earlier pulmonary valve replacement in this patient population. However, because replacement valves and conduits are subject to time-related degeneration and dysfunction, earlier surgical pulmonary valve replacement is not an ideal solution, given that open-heart surgery is inevitably associated with morbidity and risk.

Until recently, the only means of eliminating PR was surgical pulmonary valve replacement. Thus, the development of percutaneous TPV replacement offers an exciting alternative that has the potential to revolutionize the therapeutic landscape for patients with postoperative PR.

TPV replacement

As noted earlier, TPV replacement was first reported in 2000 using a valved segment of bovine jugular vein sutured to a balloon expandable stent.[32] Within several years, the Melody TPV (Medtronic, Minneapolis, MN) was being implanted at several centers in Europe and Canada (**Fig. 3**). In 2007, a prospective nonrandomized multicenter investigational device exemption (IDE) trial of the device began in the United States, and enrollment was completed 3 years later, around the same time the device was officially approved in the United States under a Humanitarian Device Exemption. The Sapien transcatheter heart valve (Edwards Lifesciences, Irvine, CA), primarily developed and used for acquired aortic stenosis, is available on an investigational basis for TPV replacement in the United States and is being implanted in the pulmonary position commercially in Canada and Europe.[37–39] The following section

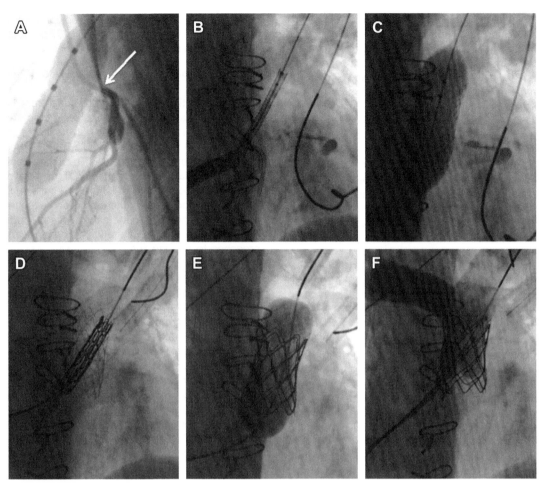

Fig. 3. TPV replacement. TPV replacement with the Melody (Medtronic, Minn, USA) valve. (*A*) Left main coronary angiography shows that the left main (*arrow*) is not compromised while an 18 × 30 mm Z-Med balloon (NuMed, Hopkington, New York, USA) was inflated in the RV to pulmonary artery (RV-PA) conduit (Contegra, Medtronic, Minn, USA). The conduit was severely stenosed with a gradient of 63 mm Hg. (*B*) A 21 × 30 mm Andrastent (Andramed, Reutlingen, Germany) was hand crimped onto an 18 × 35 mm Numed BIB (NuMed, Hopkington, New York, USA), positioned and (*C*) expanded in the RV-PA conduit. (*D*) The Melody valve is positioned within the stented conduit, (*E*) implanted, and postdilated with a 20 × 40 mm Mullins balloon (NuMed, Hopkington, New York, USA). (*F*) Acceptable final angiographic and hemodynamic results with no significant valvular regurgitation and a transvalvular gradient of 11 mm Hg.

focuses on the hemodynamic, cardiac, and functional outcomes of TPV replacement. A comprehensive review of TPV therapy in ACHD would include discussion of other factors, including technical considerations, early and late adverse events, durability of the TPV, but those issues, which are presented elsewhere,[33] are beyond the scope of this overview.

Hemodynamic and cardiac functional outcomes
Reports from the Melody valve IDE trial population, along with updates published by Bonhoeffer's group and isolated single and multicenter reports from other countries, comprise the primary literature documenting the experience with TPV

technology.[40–47] Although TPV replacement is performed in patients across a wide age range, adults comprise a large proportion of most published studies, which have consistently found that the Melody valve can be implanted in the intended location in the RVOT with few serious procedural complications and promising hemodynamic and functional results.[40–47] Specifically, TPV replacement acutely relieves RVOT obstruction, although the gradient is not eliminated completely in many patients with important conduit stenosis before TPV implant. In most patients, RVOT gradients remain fairly stable for at least 2 to 3 years, beyond which adequate data are not yet available.[43] In addition, TPV replacement eliminates PR in essentially all patients, and the longest published follow-up studies report sustained pulmonary valve competence for 3 or more years. Elimination of PR by TPV replacement also leads to reduction of RV end-diastolic and end-systolic volumes, and improvement in absolute and effective RV SVs. Similar to studies of surgical pulmonary valve replacement, data on changes in RV ejection fraction after TPV are mixed. There is convincing evidence that RV and LV mechanical efficiency improves, with augmentation of absolute and effective SVs after a TPV is implanted.[48–51] RV systolic function improves in some patients after TPV replacement, particularly in those with primary RVOT obstruction but generally not in those with primary PR,[48,51] and there is some suggestion of RV diastolic functional improvement.[52] Although limited, there is evidence that TPV replacement may result in improved LV systolic and diastolic function as well.[48,49,51,53]

Functional outcomes

Symptomatic status has been one of the fundamental outcome measures included in studies of TPV replacement. Without exception, studies in which change in symptomatic status has been reported have documented a significant improvement in New York Heart Association (NHYA) class among the cohort, which has largely been maintained for the duration of follow-up.[40,42,45,47,50,53] Most patients are in NYHA class II or III before treatment, and virtually all experience improvement, although some remain in class II. There is no published information on the need for HF medications before or changes in such therapy after TPV replacement.

Exercise cardiopulmonary function is frequently abnormal in patients with complex CHD, because of a variety of factors, and is often figured into decision making about intervention in patients with RVOT dysfunction. Peak oxygen consumption and other metabolic parameters have been evaluated in several studies of patients undergoing TPV replacement.[48–51,54] In general, preintervention measures of exercise cardiopulmonary function vary considerably in these studies, and there is usually not a significant change overall in the short-term after TPV replacement. However, because of the variable preintervention physiology (ie, some patients with primary RVOT obstruction, some with primary PR), general assessment of TPV replacement cohorts may not reveal important differences related to preintervention physiologic parameters. For example, several studies found that various measures of cardiopulmonary function (including peak oxygen consumption, ventilatory efficiency, and anaerobic oxygen consumption) improve after TPV replacement in patients with primary or significant RVOT obstruction, but not in patients with primary PR.[48–51,54]

Expanded applications and the future of TPV replacement

Most adults with repaired CHD who suffer from HF symptoms related to postoperative PR do not have a conduit or bioprosthetic valve suitable for treatment with a currently available TPV. Rather, the most common scenario is PR after incision and patch enlargement of the RVOT as part of the initial surgical repair, which often results in an RVOT that is too large for current balloon expandable TPV devices. There are several case reports and small series in the literature of creative approaches to treating RVOT failure using existing TPV technology in a variety of different nonconduit anatomies,[55–57] but these techniques have not been widely used. Newer experimental technologies, such as the Medtronic Native Outflow Tract device,[58] hold promise and may represent future treatment alternatives for patients with a large RVOT. However, the surgically augmented RVOT can vary considerably in geometry and dimensions and frequently undergoes complex deformation during the cardiac cycle, which can present unique challenges for the development of devices that are applicable to a broad population of patients.[58,59] Early preclinical experience with other TPV devices designed for large outflow tracts has been reported as well.[60–63]

LESIONS THAT PREDOMINANTLY AFFECT THE LV
VSDs

VSD is the most common congenital heart lesion in infants and children (**Table 2**).[64] VSDs are classified anatomically according to site of the defect in the interventricular septum: membranous septum, muscular septum, subaortic, and between the junction of the mitral and tricuspid valves (atrioventricular canal defects). Many defects involve more than 1 component of the ventricular septum. Membranous VSDs are the most common (70%), followed by muscular (20%), subaortic (5%), and atrioventricular canal defects (5%).[64]

The hemodynamic consequences of VSDs are determined by the size of the VSD and the relative impedance of the systemic and pulmonary arterial beds. Small defects have minimal impact on pulmonary blood flow and are therefore of little consequence. However, in large defects, because the LV systolic pressure exceeds RV systolic pressure and SVR exceeds PVR, there is left to right

Table 2
VSDs: classification, indications for closure, and reported transcatheter complications

Classification	Frequency (%)	Location
Membranous	70	Adjacent to the commissure between the anterior and septal leaflets of the tricuspid valve
Muscular	20	Anywhere in the muscular interventricular septum
Subaortic	3	Lies between the conal and muscular interventricular septum
Sub pulmonary	2	Immediately below the pulmonary valve
Atrioventricular canal	5	Below the septal leaflet of the tricuspid valve

Indications for closure
Most adults with VSD are asymptomatic. Closure is indicated if
1. Qp/Qs >2.0 with evidence of LV volume overload
2. Qp/Qs >1.5 with LV systolic or diastolic dysfunction
3. Qp/Qs >1.5 if PAP < two-thirds systemic pressure and PVR < two-thirds SVR
4. History of infective endocarditis
5. VSDs inducing progressive aortic valve disease should be considered for closure
Complications of transcatheter closure
   Vascular complications: significant complications occur in 0.3%
   Embolization: uncommon: (1.2%) most can be recaptured percutaneously
   Arrhythmia: persistent complete heart block in 1.1%–3.9% and permanent pacemaker required in 2.4%
   Valvular regurgitation: 3.4% and 6.5% of patients develop aortic or tricuspid regurgitation, respectively; usually mild and without sequelae
   Thrombosis: uncommon (1.1%); most cases resolve with systemic anticoagulation

Abbreviation: PAP, pulmonary artery pressure.

shunting with corresponding pulmonary artery, left atrial, and LV volume overload with resultant LV dilatation and failure. In patients with increased PVR, RVOT obstruction, or PS, the magnitude of the shunt is limited and may even be right to left. In many patients with large VSD, PVR increases and may exceed SVR with reversal of blood flow across the VSD and right to left shunting. This physiology is the Eisenmenger syndrome and is associated with systemic desaturation, cyanosis, and secondary erythrocytosis (see article elsewhere in this issue).

The clinical impact of VSD depends on the size of the defect. Most patients with isolated small VSDs have normal pulmonary arterial pressure and are unlikely to develop symptoms, LV dysfunction, or pulmonary vascular disease.[65] In contrast, patients with uncorrected large VSDs develop LV dilatation and failure, pulmonary hypertension, and associated RV failure.[66] The presence and location of the VSD is confirmed by echocardiography and the magnitude of shunting, and the PVR can be quantified by cardiac catheterization.[67]

Indications for VSD closure
Most adult patients with VSDs have small defects and do not require intervention. Indications for

VSD closure include: (1) Qp/Qs greater than 2.0:1 with evidence of LV volume overload; (2) Qp/Qs greater than >1.5:1 with LV systolic or diastolic dysfunction; (3) Qp/Qs greater than 1.5:1 if pulmonary artery pressure is less than two-thirds systemic pressure and PVR is less than two-thirds SVR; and (3) history of infective endocarditis.[5] VSDs inducing progressive aortic valve disease are also considered for closure. Furthermore, adults with previous surgical VSD closure require close surveillance, because residual defects occur in up to 30% of cases.[68] In such patients, LV volume overload and progressive aortic regurgitation are indications for reintervention. VSD closure is contraindicated in patients with severe irreversible pulmonary arteriolar hypertension.[5]

Transcatheter VSD closure
Although surgical VSD closure is considered to be the gold standard treatment of VSD, it can be associated with significant morbidity and mortality.[69,70]

Transcatheter VSD closure devices
In 1987, Lock and colleagues[71] reported experience using the Rashkind double-umbrella device in patients who were declined surgical VSD closure. More recently, the Amplatzer muscular

and perimembranous VSD occluders (St Jude Medical, St Paul, MN) have been introduced.[72–74] These more operator-friendly devices are specifically designed for VSD closure, are available in a range of sizes, and can be recaptured and repositioned.[75]

Safety, efficacy, and complications of transcatheter VSD closure

Several case series have reported acceptable safety and efficacy data for the Amplatzer muscular and perimembranous VSD occluders.[75–81] Procedural mortality is rare. Successful delivery of the device can be achieved in more than 95% of cases.[75,77,78,80] Both devices show impressive efficacy, with immediate complete VSD closure rates of 60% or more, increasing to 90% to 100% at 6 months follow-up.[72,73,77–82] Residual shunts are usually trivial/mild with curative surgery required in 0.7%.[75]

Significant complications associated with transcatheter VSD closure occur in up to 6.5% of cases.[75] Vascular complications were reported in 0.3% in a large European registry.[75] The reported incidence of persistent complete heart block with transcatheter perimembranous VSD closure is between 1.07% and 3.9%, and up to 2.4% require implantation of a permanent pacemaker.[75,77,78,80] Late heart block, not infrequently occurring up to 3 years after transcatheter VSD closure, has recently prompted a redesign of the Amplatzer perimembranous VSD occluder.[83] Device embolization has been reported in up to 1.2% of cases.[75] Up to 3.4% and 6.5% of patients develop aortic or tricuspid regurgitation, respectively.[75] In most cases, valvular regurgitation is trivial/mild, with infrequent surgery required for aortic insufficiency.[75,81]

Outcomes after successful percutaneous VSD closure show significant improvement in NYHA functional class. In addition, there is significant remodeling of the volume-loaded LV, such that, in most patients, the LV dimension and LV function return to normal.[80,81]

PDA

In fetal life, the ductus arteriosus is a vital conduit, connecting the left pulmonary artery with the descending aorta (distal to the left subclavian artery). The ductus permits pulmonary arterial blood to bypass the unexpanded lungs, enter the descending aorta, and perfuse the lower body. Normally, the ductus arteriosus closes within 48 hours of birth, but in some cases, spontaneous closure does not occur, and there is continuous left to right shunting from the aorta to the pulmonary artery. PDA accounts for approximately 10% of all CHD

lesions and occurs more commonly in pregnancies complicated by perinatal hypoxemia or maternal rubella. The most common associated lesions are VSDs or ASDs.

A PDA rarely closes spontaneously after infancy.[84] Again, the hemodynamic impact of a PDA depends on the magnitude of shunting. Small PDAs result in minimal left to right shunting, are unlikely to causes symptoms, and hence have a negligible impact on life expectancy. Moderate-size PDAs may remain undetected during childhood and present with congestive HF or arrhythmia in adulthood.[85] Large shunts tend to present early with LV dilatation and failure; and if uncorrected, pulmonary arterial hypertension ensues, with reversal of shunt direction when the PVR exceeds the SVR.[86]

The diagnosis of PDA may be suggested by clinical features and confirmed by transthoracic echocardiography. The anatomic features of the PDA, the magnitude of the shunt, and the PVR can be evaluated at cardiac catheterization.

Indications for PDA closure

PDA closure is indicated in the presence of LV enlargement and in the presence of pulmonary arterial hypertension if there is net left to right shunting (**Box 1**).[5] Although some clinicians believe that transcatheter PDA closure is deemed to be a reasonable strategy in asymptomatic patients with small PDA because of the increased risk of infective endarteritis, this approach is controversial and most do not advocate prophylactic closure of small silent PDA. Previous endarteritis is however, an indication for PDA closure. PDA closure is not

---

Box 1
PDA: indications for closure and reported transcatheter complications

Indications for closure

Closure is indicated if

1. There is evidence of left atrial or LV enlargement

2. The presence significant pulmonary arterial hypertension

3. Net left to right shunting

4. History of infective endocarditis

5. Considered reasonable in asymptomatic patients with small PDA because of the risk of infective endocarditis

Complications of transcatheter closure

Embolization: infrequent (<0.5%)

recommended in patients with pulmonary arterial hypertension and net right to left shunt.

Transcatheter PDA closure

The first reported transcatheter PDA closure was performed in 1967.[87] However, the procedure did not become routine until the development of the Rashkind umbrella device in the 1980s.[88] The Gianturco and Flipper coils (Cook, Bloomington, IN) are the most commonly used transcatheter coil devices for PDA closure.[89–92] Successful coil PDA closure is determined by size of the defect, with higher failure rates and coil embolization occurring in PDAs larger than 3.0 mm to 3.5 mm.[93]

The Amplatzer ductal occluder (ADO) I (St Jude Medical, St Paul, MN) is the most commonly used device. The ADO I is a self-expanding nitinol frame device, which was adapted from the Amplatzer ASO device. The device is delivered from the pulmonary artery and has a retention disk at the aortic end. More recently, the ADO II device was introduced. This nitinol device has a central waist and 2 symmetric disks. This device may be delivered from either the systemic venous (pulmonary artery) or the systemic arterial (aorta) side and is more flexible than its predecessor.

Current guidelines recommend transcatheter closure of isolated PDAs over surgical closure in adult patients because of the frequency of friable or calcified ductal tissue, atherosclerosis, aneurysm formation, and the presence of comorbid conditions that may increase operative risk.[5,94]

Safety, efficacy, and complications of transcatheter PDA closure

Transcatheter PDA occlusion is a safe and effective therapy. Initial procedural success with the ADO devices is reported in almost 100% of cases.[95] Complications such as coil or device embolization occur infrequently, and long-term complete closure rates usually exceed 95%.[95,96]

Aortic Coarctation

Aortic coarctation usually consists of a discrete ridge of tissue that extends into the lumen of the aorta just distal to the left subclavian artery at the site of the aortic ductal attachment (ligamentum arteriosum). Infrequently, the coarctation may be found proximal to the left subclavian artery, involving narrowing of the aortic arch or isthmus. Collateral vessels may arise proximal to the stenosis and provide compensatory distal blood flow. Coarctation occurs more frequently in men and is associated with bicuspid aortic valve, subaortic stenosis, mitral valve abnormalities, VSD, PDA, gonadal dysgenesis, and aneurysms of the circle of Willis.[2]

Aortic coarctation results in systemic arterial hypertension proximal to the coarctation and resultant LV pressure overload. LV hypertrophy, increasing vascular and ventricular stiffness, and diastolic dysfunction are intermediate steps that progress to cause HF if inadequately treated.[97]

Most adults with aortic coarctation are asymptomatic, and the diagnosis is often reached after investigation for systemic arterial hypertension. Physical examination may reveal a myriad of clinical signs suggestive of coarctation. The electrocardiogram typically shows LV hypertrophy, and rib notching or the reversed E sign may be apparent on chest radiograph. The diagnosis is usually confirmed on echocardiography, and further precise anatomic information (location and length of the coarctation; diameter of aorta proximal and distal to the coarctation) may be determined using contrast angiography, computed tomography, or magnetic resonance imaging.

Indication for coarctation repair

In patients with uncorrected coarctation, survival is considerably reduced: historically, there is a reported mean life expectancy of 35 years, with 75% mortality by 46 years.[98] Death is usually a consequence of systemic hypertension, accelerated atherosclerotic coronary heart disease, stroke, aortic dissection, or congestive HF.[5]

Current guidelines recommend coarctation repair in the presence of a peak-to-peak coarctation gradient of 20 mm Hg or greater (**Box 2**).[5] Importantly, the presence of significant collateral blood flow may reduce the gradient across the obstruction and mask the severity of the coarctation. In cases in which there is clear evidence of abundant collateral flow and a gradient of 20 mm Hg or less, the presence of LV dysfunction, or progressive hypertrophy, coarctation repair should be considered.

Transcatheter coarctation stenting

The decision to proceed to either transcatheter or surgical coarctation repair should be made in consultation with a team of expert ACHD specialists, interventional cardiologists, and ACHD surgeons. Specific anatomic or patient characteristics may favor either the transcatheter or surgical approach in individual patients. In adults, balloon angioplasty, with stent placement, is recognized as an acceptable alternative to surgical repair as a primary intervention for localized discrete coarctation of the native aorta.

In cases of recurrent coarctation after surgical repair, transcatheter intervention is recognized to be the preferred strategy in the absence of confounding anatomic features such as aneurysm or

Box 2
Aortic coarctation: indications for intervention and reported transcatheter complications

Indications for intervention

Intervention is indicated if

1. Peak-to-peak coarctation gradient 20 mm Hg or greater

2. In cases in which there is clear evidence of abundant collateral flow and a gradient of 20 mm Hg or less, the presence of LV dysfunction, or progressive hypertrophy, coarctation repair should be considered

Complications of transcatheter coarctation stenting

Aortic rupture or extensive dissection: rarely (<0.5%) and usually associated with intervention in elderly patients

Nonocclusive intimal tears ($\approx$1.5%)

Nonextensive dissection ($\approx$1.5%)

Stent migration ($\approx$5%)

Aneurysm formation ($\approx$1%)

Vascular access injury ($\approx$2.5%)

Stroke (<1.0%)

pseudoaneurysm formation or the involvement of adjacent aortic arch vessels.[5] The transcatheter approach is also deemed preferable in patients at increased surgical risk because of the presence of significant LV dysfunction or other comorbid conditions. In contrast, the transcatheter approach is deemed less suitable in the context of long segment or tortuous aortic coarctation.

Transcatheter balloon angioplasty of congenital aortic coarctation was first introduced in the early 1980s.[99,100] The aim of this procedure is to increase the diameter of the lesion by disrupting the aortic intima and media. In most cases, elastic recoil occurred after balloon dilatation, and inadequate relief of the obstruction resulted in the requirement for reintervention in many patients. Rarely, balloon overexpansion causes devastating aortic rupture.

Although infrequent, acute aortic wall injury (dissection or aneurysm formation) and restenosis hastened the development of aortic coarctation stenting in the 1990s.[101] Stents reduce the acute elastic recoil associated with balloon dilatation, minimize trauma to the aortic wall, control dissection flaps, and reduce late restenosis. Coarctation stenting is now the dominant transcatheter technique and may be performed with

a variety of stainless steel, cobalt chromium, nitinol self-expanding, and covered stents.[102] The introduction of the Palmaz XL 10-series bare metal stents (Cordis Endovascular, Miami, FL) in 1999 allowed more complex, longer lesions to be addressed percutaneously and for the management of complications arising from balloon angioplasty.

Nitinol self-expanding stents are a potentially less traumatic option than traditional balloon expandable stents. Furthermore, these prostheses are more likely to preserve the functional elasticity of the native aortic wall. Small case series have suggested that these stents are both safe and efficacious.[102,103]

Covered stents were initially developed as a bailout therapy for aortic wall injury encountered during balloon dilatation or bare metal stenting (**Fig. 4**). However, the indications for using these devices have increased in recent years and they are now considered to be the stent of choice in patients with an aneurysmal aortic wall, a severe primary coarctation at high risk of rupture, in the presence of an associated arterial duct, and in older patients with noncompliant aortas.[104,105]

Safety, efficacy, and complications of transcatheter coarctation intervention

Early acute procedural results with balloon aortic angioplasty were encouraging; however, up to 10% of patients had persistent poststenting gradients of more than 20 mm Hg.[106,107] Procedural and long-term mortality is low (<1%).[108,109] Late aneurysm formation has been observed in up to 20% of cases, although restenosis is infrequent in adults with a successful procedure (final gradient <10 mm Hg).

In the absence of randomized trials, it is difficult to compare the results of balloon angioplasty and stenting. However, stenting has become the dominant strategy in most institutions, with acceptable acute procedural results. Aneurysm formation after stenting seems to occur less frequently than in the balloon angioplasty era (<5%). In the largest series published to date (n = 565),[110] acute procedural success was achieved in 98% of cases. Successful coarctation stenting improves blood pressure in most patients, reduces LV mass, and improves LV function.[111-113] However, up to one-third of patients have persistent hypertension after transcatheter coarctation intervention.[114,115]

Careful patient selection and preprocedural anatomic screening are essential for optimal patient outcomes. Aortic rupture and extensive dissection are the most feared complications of transcatheter coarctation intervention, but these dramatic events occur rarely (<0.5%) and are usually associated

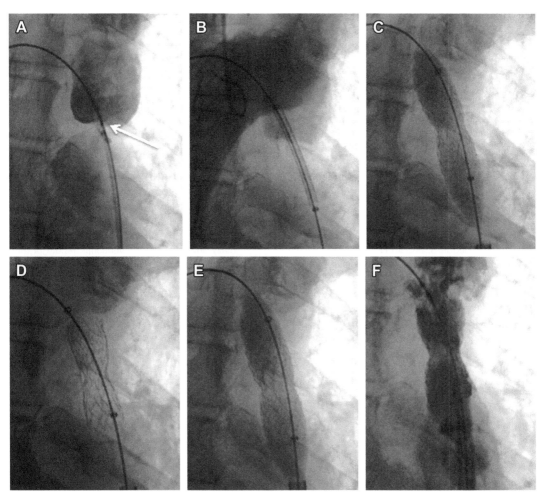

Fig. 4. Aortic coarctation stenting. (*A*) Severe aortic coarctation (*arrow*; 0.6 mm diameter and simultaneous gradient = 50 mm Hg). (*B*) A Medtronic Atrium (Medtronic, Minn, USA) V12 (16 × 41 mm) covered stent is positioned across the coarctation and inflated (*C*). Residual stenosis (*D*) is postdilated with a (*E*) Numed BIB (NuMed, Hopkington, New York, USA) (20 × 40 mm). (*F*) Acceptable final angiographic result with residual gradient less than 5 mm Hg.

with intervention in elderly patients.[110] Stent and balloon oversizing, repeated after dilatation, and attempts to flare the stent ends to ensure apposition to the aortic wall should be avoided. Covered stents or stent grafts should be readily accessible to treat aortic rupture or dissection, and on-site surgical backup is mandatory.

Less dramatic complications have been reported in up to 14% of cases: stent migration (≈5%), vascular access injury (≈2.5%), intimal tears (≈1.5%), dissection (≈1.5%), and aneurysm formation (≈1%).[110] Stroke has also been reported after transcatheter coarctation intervention (<1%). The reported incidence of complications from coarctation stenting has decreased in recent years, because of increasing physician experience and enhanced balloon and stent design.[110]

SUMMARY

Transcatheter interventions have evolved considerably over recent years and now play a key role in the treatment of HF in ACHD. These innovative procedures, when performed successfully and in a timely fashion, can lead to reversal of ventricular dilatation and dysfunction. Percutaneous interventions complement medical and surgical therapies and together form a comprehensive therapeutic approach for the treatment of HF in ACHD.

REFERENCES

1. Van Praagh S, Carrera ME, Sanders SP, et al. Sinus venosus defects: unroofing of the right pulmonary veins–anatomic and echocardiographic findings and surgical treatment. Am Heart J 1994;128(2): 365–79.

2. Brickner ME, Hillis LD, Lange RA. Congenital heart disease in adults. First of two parts. N Engl J Med 2000;342(4):256–63.

3. Craig RJ, Selzer A. Natural history and prognosis of atrial septal defect. Circulation 1968;37(5):805–15.

4. Campbell M. Natural history of atrial septal defect. Br Heart J 1970;32(6):820–6.

5. Warnes CA, Williams RG, Bashore TM, et al. ACC/AHA 2008 guidelines for the management of adults with congenital heart disease. J Am Coll Cardiol 2008;52(23):e143–263.

6. King TD, Thompson SL, Steiner C, et al. Secundum atrial septal defect. Nonoperative closure during cardiac catheterization. JAMA 1976;235(23):2506–9.

7. King T, Mills N. Historical perspectives on ASD device closure. Minneapolis (MN): Cardiotext; 2010.

8. Moore J, Hegde S, El-Said H, et al. Transcatheter device closure of atrial septal defects: a safety review. JACC Cardiovasc Interv 2013;6(5):433–42.

9. Zahn EM, Wilson N, Cutright W, et al. Development and testing of the Helex septal occluder, a new expanded polytetrafluoroethylene atrial septal defect occlusion system. Circulation 2001;104(6):711–6.

10. Jones TK, Latson LA, Zahn E, et al. Results of the U.S. multicenter pivotal study of the HELEX septal occluder for percutaneous closure of secundum atrial septal defects. J Am Coll Cardiol 2007;49(22):2215–21.

11. Du ZD, Hijazi ZM, Kleinman CS, et al. Comparison between transcatheter and surgical closure of secundum atrial septal defect in children and adults: results of a multicenter nonrandomized trial. J Am Coll Cardiol 2002;39(11):1836–44.

12. Levi DS, Moore JW. Embolization and retrieval of the Amplatzer septal occluder. Catheter Cardiovasc Interv 2004;61(4):543–7.

13. DiBardino DJ, McElhinney DB, Kaza AK, et al. Analysis of the US Food and Drug Administration Manufacturer and User Facility Device Experience database for adverse events involving Amplatzer septal occluder devices and comparison with the Society of Thoracic Surgery congenital cardiac surgery database. J Thorac Cardiovasc Surg 2009;137(6):1334–41.

14. Johnson JN, Marquardt ML, Ackerman MJ, et al. Electrocardiographic changes and arrhythmias following percutaneous atrial septal defect and patent foramen ovale device closure. Catheter Cardiovasc Interv 2011;78(2):254–61.

15. Krumsdorf U, Ostermayer S, Billinger K, et al. Incidence and clinical course of thrombus formation on atrial septal defect and patient foramen ovale closure devices in 1,000 consecutive patients. J Am Coll Cardiol 2004;43(2):302–9.

16. Amin Z, Hijazi ZM, Bass JL, et al. Erosion of Amplatzer septal occluder device after closure of secundum atrial septal defects: review of registry of complications and recommendations to minimize future risk. Catheter Cardiovasc Interv 2004;63(4):496–502.

17. US FDA. FDA Executive Summary Memorandum–May 24 C, Occluders: SAPMTA, Clinical Update and Review of Events [pdf]. May 24 Aa, et al.

18. Walters DL, Boga T, Burgtow D, et al. Percutaneous ASD closure in a large Australian series: short and long-term outcomes. Heart Lung Circ 2012;21(9):572–5.

19. Kotowycz MA, Therrien J, Ionescu-Ittu R, et al. Long-term outcomes after surgical versus transcatheter closure of atrial septal defects in adults. JACC Cardiovasc Interv 2013;6(5):497–503.

20. Formigari R, Di Donato RM, Mazzera E, et al. Minimally invasive or interventional repair of atrial septal defects in children: experience in 171 cases and comparison with conventional strategies. J Am Coll Cardiol 2001;37(6):1707–12.

21. Thomson JD, Aburawi EH, Watterson KG, et al. Surgical and transcatheter (Amplatzer) closure of atrial septal defects: a prospective comparison of results and cost. Heart 2002;87(5):466–9.

22. Cuypers JA, Witsenburg M, van der Linde D, et al. Pulmonary stenosis: update on diagnosis and therapeutic options. Heart 2013;99:339–47.

23. Kan JS, White RI Jr, Mitchell SE, et al. Percutaneous balloon valvuloplasty: a new method for treating congenital pulmonary-valve stenosis. N Engl J Med 1982;307:540–2.

24. Chen CR, Cheng TO, Huang T, et al. Percutaneous balloon valvuloplasty for pulmonic stenosis in adolescents and adults. N Engl J Med 1996;335:21–5.

25. Fawzy ME, Hassan W, Fadel BM, et al. Long-term results (up to 17 years) of pulmonary balloon valvuloplasty in adults and its effects on concomitant severe infundibular stenosis and tricuspid regurgitation. Am Heart J 2007;153:433–8.

26. Taggart NW, Cetta F, Cabalka AK, et al. Outcomes for balloon pulmonary valvuloplasty in adults: comparison with a concurrent pediatric cohort. Catheter Cardiovasc Interv 2013. http://dx.doi.org/10.1002/ccd.24973. [Epub ahead of print].

27. Steadman CD, Clift PF, Thorne SA, et al. Treatment of dynamic subvalvar muscular obstruction in the native right ventricular outflow tract by percutaneous stenting in adults. Congenit Heart Dis 2009;4:494–8.

28. Harrild DM, Powell AJ, Trang TX, et al. Long-term pulmonary regurgitation following balloon valvuloplasty for pulmonary stenosis: risk factors and relationship to exercise capacity and ventricular volume and function. J Am Coll Cardiol 2010;55:1041–7.

29. Lloyd TR, Marvin WJ Jr, Mahoney LT, et al. Balloon dilation valvuloplasty of bioprosthetic valves in extracardiac conduits. Am Heart J 1987;114:268–74.

30. Peng LF, McElhinney DB, Nugent AW, et al. Endovascular stenting of obstructed right ventricle-to-pulmonary artery conduits: a fifteen-year experience. Circulation 2006;113:2598–605.

31. Sugiyama H, Williams W, Benson LN. Implantation of endovascular stents for the obstructive right ventricular outflow tract. Heart 2005;91:1058–63.

32. Bonhoeffer P, Boudjemline Y, Saliba Z, et al. Percutaneous replacement of pulmonary valve in a right-ventricle to pulmonary-artery prosthetic conduit with valve dysfunction. Lancet 2000;356:1403–5.

33. Gillespie MJ, McElhinney DB. Transcatheter pulmonary valve replacement: a current review. Curr Pediatr Rep 2013;1:83–91.

34. Geva T. Indications and timing of pulmonary valve replacement after tetralogy of Fallot repair. Semin Thorac Cardiovasc Surg Pediatr Card Surg Annu 2006;11–22.

35. Gregg D, Foster E. Pulmonary insufficiency is the nexus of late complications in tetralogy of Fallot. Curr Cardiol Rep 2007;9:315–22.

36. Tweddell JS, Simpson P, Li SH, et al. Timing and technique of pulmonary valve replacement in the patient with tetralogy of Fallot. Semin Thorac Cardiovasc Surg Pediatr Card Surg Annu 2012; 15:27–33.

37. Kenny D, Hijazi ZM, Kar S, et al. Percutaneous implantation of the Edwards SAPIEN transcatheter heart valve for conduit failure in the pulmonary position: early phase 1 results from an international multicenter clinical trial. J Am Coll Cardiol 2011; 58:2248–56.

38. Boone RH, Webb JG, Horlick E, et al. Transcatheter pulmonary valve implantation using the Edwards SAPIEN transcatheter heart valve. Catheter Cardiovasc Interv 2010;75:286–94.

39. Haas NA, Moysich A, Neudorf U, et al. Percutaneous implantation of the Edwards SAPIEN(™) pulmonic valve: initial results in the first 22 patients. Clin Res Cardiol 2013;102:119–28.

40. Khambadkone S, Coats L, Taylor AM, et al. Transcatheter pulmonary valve implantation in humans: initial results in 59 consecutive patients. Circulation 2005;112:1189–97.

41. Lurz P, Coats L, Khambadkone S, et al. Percutaneous pulmonary valve implantation: impact of evolving technology and learning curve on clinical outcome. Circulation 2008;117:1964–72.

42. McElhinney DB, Hellenbrand WE, Zahn EM, et al. Short- and medium-term outcomes after transcatheter pulmonary valve placement in the expanded multicenter U.S. Melody valve trial. Circulation 2010;122:507–16.

43. McElhinney DB, Cheatham JP, Jones TK, et al. Stent fracture, valve dysfunction, and right ventricular outflow tract reintervention after transcatheter pulmonary valve implantation: patient-related and procedural risk factors in the US Melody valve trial. Circ Cardiovasc Interv 2011;4:602–14.

44. Eicken A, Ewert P, Hager A, et al. Percutaneous pulmonary valve implantation: two-centre experience with more than 100 patients. Eur Heart J 2011;32:1260–5.

45. Demkow M, Biernacka EK, Spiewak M, et al. Percutaneous pulmonary valve implantation preceded by routine presenting with a bare metal stent. Catheter Cardiovasc Interv 2011;77:381–9.

46. Gillespie MJ, Rome JJ, Levi DS, et al. Melody® valve implant within failed bioprosthetic valves in the pulmonary position: a multicenter experience. Circ Cardiovasc Interv 2012;5:862–70.

47. Butera G, Milanesi O, Spadoni I, et al. Melody transcatheter pulmonary valve implantation. Results from the registry of the Italian Society of Pediatric Cardiology. Catheter Cardiovasc Interv 2013; 81:310–6.

48. Coats L, Khambadkone S, Derrick G, et al. Physiological and clinical consequences of relief of right ventricular outflow tract obstruction late after repair of congenital heart defects. Circulation 2006;113: 2037–44.

49. Coats L, Khambadkone S, Derrick G, et al. Physiological consequences of percutaneous pulmonary valve implantation: the different behaviour of volume- and pressure-overloaded ventricles. Eur Heart J 2007;28:1886–93.

50. Lurz P, Nordmeyer J, Giardini A, et al. Early versus late functional outcome after successful percutaneous pulmonary valve implantation: are the acute effects of altered right ventricular loading all we can expect? J Am Coll Cardiol 2011;57:724–31.

51. Lurz P, Giardini A, Taylor AM, et al. Effect of altering pathologic right ventricular loading conditions by percutaneous pulmonary valve implantation on exercise capacity. Am J Cardiol 2010;105:721–6.

52. Romeih S, Kroft LJ, Bokenkamp R, et al. Delayed improvement of right ventricular diastolic function and regression of right ventricular mass after percutaneous pulmonary valve implantation in patients with congenital heart disease. Am Heart J 2009;158:40–6.

53. Lurz P, Puranik R, Nordmeyer J, et al. Improvement in left ventricular filling properties after relief of right ventricle to pulmonary artery conduit obstruction: contribution of septal motion and interventricular mechanical delay. Eur Heart J 2009;30:2266–74.

54. Batra AS, McElhinney DB, Wang W, et al. Cardiopulmonary exercise function among patients undergoing transcatheter pulmonary valve implantation in the US Melody valve investigational trial. Am Heart J 2012;163:280–7.

55. Gillespie MJ, Dori Y, Harris MA, et al. Bilateral branch pulmonary artery melody valve implantation for treatment of complex right ventricular

outflow tract dysfunction in a high-risk patient. Circ Cardiovasc Interv 2011;4:e21–3.

56. Boudjemline Y, Brugada G, Van-Aerschot I, et al. Outcomes and safety of transcatheter pulmonary valve replacement in patients with large patched right ventricular outflow tracts. Arch Cardiovasc Dis 2012;105:404–13.

57. Boudjemline Y, Legendre A, Ladouceur M, et al. Branch pulmonary artery jailing with a bare metal stent to anchor a transcatheter pulmonary valve in patients with patched large right ventricular outflow tract. Circ Cardiovasc Interv 2012;5:e22–5.

58. Schievano S, Taylor AM, Capelli C, et al. First-in-man implantation of a novel percutaneous valve: a new approach to medical device development. EuroIntervention 2010;5:745–50.

59. Capelli C, Taylor AM, Migliavacca F, et al. Patient-specific reconstructed anatomies and computer simulations are fundamental for selecting medical device treatment: application to a new percutaneous pulmonary valve. Philos Trans A Math Phys Eng Sci 2010;368:3027–38.

60. Mollet A, Basquin A, Stos B, et al. Off-pump replacement of the pulmonary valve in large right ventricular outflow tracts: a transcatheter approach using an intravascular infundibulum reducer. Pediatr Res 2007;62:428–33.

61. Attmann T, Quaden R, Jahnke T, et al. Percutaneous pulmonary valve replacement: 3-month evaluation of self-expanding valved stents. Ann Thorac Surg 2006;82:708–13.

62. Zong GJ, Bai Y, Jiang HB, et al. Use of a novel valve stent for transcatheter pulmonary valve replacement: an animal study. J Thorac Cardiovasc Surg 2009;137:1363–9.

63. Amahzoune B, Szymansky C, Fabiani JN, et al. A new endovascular size reducer for large pulmonary outflow tract. Eur J Cardiothorac Surg 2010; 37:730–2.

64. Graham TJ, Gutgesell H. Ventricular septal defects. Baltimore (MD): Williams & Wilkins; 1995.

65. Kidd L, Driscoll DJ, Gersony WM, et al. Second natural history study of congenital heart defects. Results of treatment of patients with ventricular septal defects. Circulation 1993;87(Suppl 2): I38–51.

66. Perloff J. Survival patterns without cardiac surgery or interventional catheterization: a narrowing base. 2nd edition. Philadelphia: WB Saunders; 1998.

67. Boehrer JD, Lange RA, Willard JE, et al. Advantages and limitations of methods to detect, localize, and quantitate intracardiac left-to-right shunting. Am Heart J 1992;124(2):448–55.

68. Nygren A, Sunnegardh J, Berggern H. Preoperative evaluation and surgery in isolated ventricular septal defects: a 21 year perspective. Heart 2000;83(2):198–204.

69. Yeager SB, Freed MD, Keane JF, et al. Primary surgical closure of ventricular septal defect in the first year of life: results in 128 infants. J Am Coll Cardiol 1984;3(5):1269–76.

70. Gaynor JW, O'Brien JE Jr, Rychik J, et al. Outcome following tricuspid valve detachment for ventricular septal defects closure. Eur J Cardiothorac Surg 2001;19(3):279–82.

71. Lock JE, Block PC, McKay RG, et al. Transcatheter closure of ventricular septal defects. Circulation 1988;78(2):361–8.

72. Hijazi ZM, Hakim F, Haweleh AA, et al. Catheter closure of perimembranous ventricular septal defects using the new Amplatzer membranous VSD occluder: initial clinical experience. Catheter Cardiovasc Interv 2002;56(4):508–15.

73. Thanopoulos BD, Tsaousis GS, Konstadopoulou GN, et al. Transcatheter closure of muscular ventricular septal defects with the Amplatzer ventricular septal defect occluder: initial clinical applications in children. J Am Coll Cardiol 1999;33(5):1395–9.

74. Velasco-Sanchez D, Tzikas A, Ibrahim R, et al. Transcatheter closure of perimembranous ventricular septal defects: initial human experience with the Amplatzer® membranous VSD occluder 2. Catheter Cardiovasc Interv 2013;82(3):474–9.

75. Carminati M, Butera G, Chessa M, et al. Transcatheter closure of congenital ventricular septal defects: results of the European Registry. Eur Heart J 2007;28(19):2361–8.

76. Knauth AL, Lock JE, Perry SB, et al. Transcatheter device closure of congenital and postoperative residual ventricular septal defects. Circulation 2004; 110(5):501–7.

77. Masura J, Gao W, Gavora P, et al. Percutaneous closure of perimembranous ventricular septal defects with the eccentric Amplatzer device: multicenter follow-up study. Pediatr Cardiol 2005; 26(3):216–9.

78. Carminati M, Butera G, Chessa M, et al. Transcatheter closure of congenital ventricular septal defect with Amplatzer septal occluders. Am J Cardiol 2005;96(12A):52L–8L.

79. Fu YC, Bass J, Amin Z, et al. Transcatheter closure of perimembranous ventricular septal defects using the new Amplatzer membranous VSD occluder: results of the US phase I trial. J Am Coll Cardiol 2006;47(2):319–25.

80. Al-Kashkari W, Balan P, Kavinsky CJ, et al. Percutaneous device closure of congenital and iatrogenic ventricular septal defects in adult patients. Catheter Cardiovasc Interv 2011;77(2):260–7.

81. Holzer R, de Giovanni J, Walsh KP, et al. Transcatheter closure of perimembranous ventricular septal defects using the Amplatzer membranous VSD occluder: immediate and midterm results of an

international registry. Catheter Cardiovasc Interv 2006;68(4):620–8.

82. Hijazi ZM, Hakim F, Al-Fadley F, et al. Transcatheter closure of single muscular ventricular septal defects using the Amplatzer muscular VSD occluder: initial results and technical considerations. Catheter Cardiovasc Interv 2000;49(2):167–72.

83. Tzikas A, Ibrahim R, Velasco-Sanchez D, et al. Transcatheter closure of perimembranous ventricular septal defect with the Amplatzer membranous VSD occluder 2: initial world experience and one-year follow-up. Catheter Cardiovasc Interv 2013. [Epub ahead of print].

84. Coggin CJ, Parker KR, Keith JD. Natural history of isolated patent ductus arteriosus and the effect of surgical correction: twenty years' experience at The Hospital for Sick Children, Toronto. Can Med Assoc J 1970;102(7):718–20.

85. Campbell M. Natural history of persistent ductus arteriosus. Br Heart J 1968;30(1):4–13.

86. Campbell M. Patent ductus arteriosus; some notes on prognosis and on pulmonary hypertension. Br Heart J 1955;17(4):511–33.

87. Portsmann W, Wierny L, Warnke H. Closure of persistent ductus arteriosus without thoracotomy. Ger Med Mon 1967;12(6):259–61.

88. Rashkind WJ, Mullins CE, Hellenbrand WE, et al. Nonsurgical closure of patent ductus arteriosus: clinical application of the Rashkind PDA occluder system. Circulation 1987;75(3):583–92.

89. Cambier PA, Kirby WC, Wortham DC, et al. Percutaneous closure of the small (less than 2.5 mm) patent ductus arteriosus using coil embolization. Am J Cardiol 1992;69(8):815–6.

90. Podnar T, Masura J. Percutaneous closure of patent ductus arteriosus using special screwing detachable coils. Cathet Cardiovasc Diagn 1997; 41(4):386–91.

91. Masura J, Gavora P, Podnar T. Transcatheter occlusion of patent ductus arteriosus using a new angled Amplatzer duct occluder: initial clinical experience. Catheter Cardiovasc Interv 2003;58(2):261–7.

92. Pass RH, Hijazi Z, Hsu DT, et al. Multicenter USA Amplatzer patent ductus arteriosus occlusion device trial: initial and one-year results. J Am Coll Cardiol 2004;44(3):513–9.

93. Sanatani S, Potts JE, Ryan A, et al. Coil occlusion of the patent ductus arteriosus: lessons learned. Cardiovasc Intervent Radiol 2000;23(2):87–90.

94. Celermajer DS, Sholler GF, Hughes CF, et al. Persistent ductus arteriosus in adults. A review of surgical experience with 25 patients. Med J Aust 1991;155(4):233–6.

95. Liddy S, Oslizlok P, Walsh KP. Comparison of the results of transcatheter closure of patent ductus arteriosus with newer Amplatzer devices. Catheter Cardiovasc Interv 2013;82(2):253–9.

96. Rao P. Summary and comparison of patent ductus arteriosus closure methods. Philadelphia: Lippincott Williams &Wilkins; 2003.

97. Izzo JL Jr, Gradman AH. Mechanisms and management of hypertensive heart disease: from left ventricular hypertrophy to heart failure. Med Clin North Am 2004;88(5):1257–71.

98. Campbell M. Natural history of coarctation of the aorta. Br Heart J 1970;32:633–40.

99. Lock JE, Bass JL, Amplatz K, et al. Balloon dilation angioplasty of aortic coarctations in infants and children. Circulation 1983;68:109–16.

100. Kan JS, White RI Jr, Mitchell SE, et al. Treatment of restenosis of coarctation by percutaneous transluminal angioplasty. Circulation 1983;68:1087–94.

101. Ebeid MR, Prieto LR, Latson LA. Use of balloon-expandable stents for coarctation of the aorta: initial results and intermediate-term follow-up. J Am Coll Cardiol 1997;30(7):1847–52.

102. Patnaik AN, Srinivas B, Rao DS. Endovascular stenting for native coarctation in older children and adolescents using adult self-expanding (nitinol) iliac stents. Indian Heart J 2009;61(4):353–7.

103. Tyagi S, Singh S, Mukhopadhyay S, et al. Self- and balloon-expandable stent implantation for severe native coarctation of aorta in adults. Am Heart J 2003;146(5):920–8.

104. Sadiq M, Malick NH, Qureshi SA. Simultaneous treatment of native coarctation of the aorta combined with patent ductus arteriosus using a covered stent. Catheter Cardiovasc Interv 2003; 59(3):387–90.

105. Ewert P, Abdul-Khaliq H, Peters B, et al. Transcatheter therapy of long extreme subatretic aortic coarctations with covered stents. Catheter Cardiovasc Interv 2004;63(2):236–9.

106. Fawzy ME, Fathala A, Osman A, et al. Twenty-two years of follow-up results of balloon angioplasty for discreet native coarctation of the aorta in adolescents and adults. Am Heart J 2008;156(5): 910–7.

107. Walhout RJ, Suttorp MJ, Mackaij GJ, et al. Long-term outcome after balloon angioplasty of coarctation of the aorta in adolescents and adults: is aneurysm formation an issue? Catheter Cardiovasc Interv 2009;73(4):549–56.

108. Paddon AJ, Nicholson AA, Ettles DF, et al. Long-term follow-up of percutaneous balloon angioplasty in adult aortic coarctation. Cardiovasc Intervent Radiol 2000;23(5):364–7.

109. Fawzy ME, Awad M, Hassan W, et al. Long-term outcome (up to 15 years) of balloon angioplasty of discrete native coarctation of the aorta in adolescents and adults. J Am Coll Cardiol 2004;43(6): 1062–7.

110. Forbes TJ, Garekar S, Amin Z, et al. Procedural results and acute complications in stenting native

and recurrent coarctation of the aorta in patients over 4 years of age: a multi-institutional study. Catheter Cardiovasc Interv 2007;70(2):276–85.

111. Fawzy ME, Sivanandam V, Pieters F, et al. Long-term effects of balloon angioplasty on systemic hypertension in adolescent and adult patients with coarctation of the aorta. Eur Heart J 1999;20(11): 827–32.

112. Lam YY, Kaya MG, Li W, et al. Effect of endovascular stenting of aortic coarctation on biventricular function in adults. Heart 2007;93(11):1441–7.

113. Hassan W, Awad M, Fawzy ME, et al. Long-term effects of balloon angioplasty on left ventricular hypertrophy in adolescent and adult patients with native coarctation of the aorta. Up to 18 years follow-up results. Catheter Cardiovasc Interv 2007;70(6):881–6.

114. Eicken A, Pensl U, Sebening W, et al. The fate of systemic blood pressure in patients after effectively stented coarctation. Eur Heart J 2006;27(9):1100–5.

115. Roifman I, Therrien J, Ionescu-Ittu R, et al. Coarctation of the aorta and coronary artery disease: fact or fiction? Circulation 2012;126(1):16–21.

Surgical Device Therapy for Heart Failure in the Adult with Congenital Heart Disease

Venkatachalam Mulukutla, MD[a],*,
Wayne J. Franklin, MD[a],*, Chet R. Villa, MD[b],
David Luís Simón Morales, MD[c]

KEYWORDS

- Adult congenital heart disease • Ventricular assist device • Heart failure • Systemic right ventricle

KEY POINTS

- Individuals with congenital heart disease (CHD) are at a great risk for heart failure, and the underlying anatomic features are important predictors of heart failure.
- As the adult with CHD (ACHD) population grows older, multiple events, including years of an altered physiology, the neurohormonal cascade, and many still unknown, culminate in ventricular failure.
- As the ACHD population continues to grow in number and complexity, those with systemic right ventricle or single ventricle are at an increased risk of ventricular failure following surgical palliation.
- Ventricular assist devices have been used with success in bridging ACHD patients to heart transplantation or destination therapy.
- As the ACHD population continues to increase and technological advancement continues, surgical devices will play a significant role in the future.

Congenital heart disease (CHD) has an incidence of approximately 8 per 1000 live births. Fifty years ago only 25% of infants with complex CHD survived beyond their first year of life, but today more than 95% will survive to adulthood.[1] Approximately 15% of children born with CHD have potentially life-threatening defects, and many have complex lesions.[2] With the advent of neonatal repair for complex lesions, modern surgical mortality rates are less than 5%.[3] Today there are more than 1 million adults with CHD, outnumbering pediatric patients with CHD.[4] Individuals with adult congenital heart disease (ACHD) are at a great risk for heart failure, and the underlying anatomic features are important predictors of heart failure. As the ACHD population grows older, multiple events, including years of an altered physiology, the neurohormonal cascade, and many still unknown, culminate in ventricular failure. Surgical device therapy is an effective method in supporting patients with heart failure.

INCIDENCE OF HEART FAILURE IN ADULTS WITH CONGENITAL HEART DISEASE

Adults with CHD have a myriad of primary underlying conditions: tetralogy of Fallot, Ebstein anomaly, single right or left ventricles palliated with a Fontan procedure, or systemic right ventricle anatomy resulting from congenitally corrected transposition of the great arteries (CC-TGA) or D-transposition of the great arteries (D-TGA) after atrial switch

[a] Texas Children's Hospital, Pediatric Cardiology, 6621 Fannin Street, Houston, TX 77030, USA; [b] Cincinnati Children's Hospital Medical Center, Pediatric Cardiology, 3333 Burnet Avenue, Cincinnati, OH 45229, USA; [c] Cincinnati Children's Hospital Medical Center, Cardiovascular Surgery, 3333 Burnet Avenue, Cincinnati, OH 45229, USA
* Corresponding authors.
E-mail addresses: vmulukut@bcm.edu; wjf@bcm.edu

Heart Failure Clin 10 (2014) 197–206
http://dx.doi.org/10.1016/j.hfc.2013.09.016
1551-7136/14/$ – see front matter © 2014 Elsevier Inc. All rights reserved.

palliation. In addition, each surgical technique may have varied clinical outcomes depending on the era. The probability of heart failure in ACHD by congenital diagnosis is illustrated in **Fig. 1**.

Patients with D-TGA born before the mid-1990s are likely to have undergone an atrial switch operation (described by Senning in 1959 and Mustard in 1964), leading to a systemic right ventricle. However, in the last 2 decades the arterial switch (first described by Jatene in 1983) has become the preferred surgical operation because it results in a systemic left ventricle. After follow-up of 15 to 18 years, there has been a documented decrease in the systemic right ventricular (RV) function in 32% to 48% of Mustard and Senning patients.[5] Today, most patients with D-TGA undergo the arterial switch, and many are just now entering their second decade of life.

In CC-TGA the right ventricle is the systemic ventricle, and many patients first present with clinical heart failure in adulthood. The anatomic variations are varied and can include pulmonic stenosis, ventricular septal defect, or tricuspid valve abnormalities. Systemic atrioventricular valve regurgitation may be a harbinger of heart failure, owing to worsening ventricular failure and RV volume overload. Two percent of patients per year can develop complete heart block. Presbitero and colleagues[6] reported that 24% of the patients in the fifth decade of life had heart failure, increasing to 77% by the sixth decade of life. In study by Piran and colleagues,[7] incidence of heart failure in patients with D-TGA subsequent to Mustard procedure was 22%, and 32% in patients with CC-TGA.

In patients born with a single ventricle, many historically underwent the classic atriopulmonary connection procedure, a modification of the approach described in 1971 for tricuspid atresia by Fontan and Baudet.[8] The Fontan procedure, or total cavopulmonary connection, leaves the single-ventricle patient with abnormal venous circulation whereby the venal caval blood returns to the lung passively, with a subpulmonary ventricle. Today the Fontan operation has evolved to being a lateral tunnel through the right atrium, or an extracardiac conduit that connects directly to the branch pulmonary arteries. It is often the last surgical palliation in children born with a functional single ventricle. These patients can do well and survive into adulthood, but long-term follow up past the fifth or sixth decade is not known. In one study, 40% of patients who were palliated via a Fontan procedure developed systolic heart failure.[7]

Tetralogy of Fallot (TOF) is the most common cyanotic heart disease, for which Lillehei performed the first intracardiac repair in 1954. This procedure consisted of repair of a ventricular septal defect and resection of the infundibular region of the RV outflow tract.[9] Today the repair minimizes ventricular incision and infundibular resection, and incorporates a transannular patch. The surgical intervention ultimately leads to distortion of pulmonary valve apparatus and pulmonary regurgitation, which is well tolerated for many years but has an effect on the RV size and function.[3] Norozi and colleagues[10] reported on 94 patients with TOF, of whom 44 had heart failure defined by a brain natriuretic peptide (BNP) level of greater than 100 pg/mL and a maximal oxygen uptake (Vo₂max) of less than 25 m/kg/min, although most were asymptomatic or minimally symptomatic, of New York Heart Association (NYHA) functional class I or II. Complications of progressive RV dilation include right heart failure with decreased exercise tolerance, atrial and ventricular arrhythmias, and sudden cardiac death. The lifetime incidence of sudden cardiac death is 8.8% in postoperative TOF patients in adulthood.[1] Pulmonary valve replacement is considered the treatment of choice, and timing is still debated, with mitigating factors including exercise intolerance, ventricular arrhythmias, and/or RV dysfunction or dilation (RV end-diastolic volume >150 mL/m²).

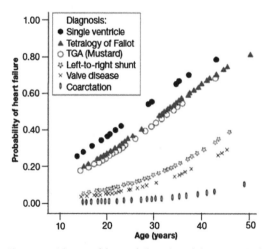

Fig. 1. Incidence of heart failure in adult congenital heart disease. TGA, transposition of the great arteries. (*From* Norozi K, Wessel A, Alpers V, et al. Incidence and risk distribution of heart failure in adolescents and adults with congenital heart disease after cardiac surgery. Am J Cardiol 2006;97(8):1238–43; with permission.)

NEUROHORMONAL ACTIVATION

Neurohormonal activation is an important factor in adults with heart failure. Data have shown that the degree of neurohormonal activation in adults with heart failure is correlated with functional capacity, left ventricular (LV) dysfunction, and mortality.

Study of heart failure in the ACHD population has shown similar findings. Bolger and colleagues[11] showed an elevation in atrial natriuretic peptide (ANP), BNP, endothelin-1 (ET-1), and norepinephrine in the ACHD population with heart failure, as demonstrated in **Fig. 2**, and these correlate with NYHA class, ventricular function, and mortality.

PHARMACOLOGIC TREATMENT

Treatment of adults with congestive heart failure attributable to acquired heart disease has been shown in large randomized controlled trials to be effective in improving mortality. In one of the landmark studies involving angiotensin-converting enzyme (ACE) inhibition, CONSENSUS, patients with NYHA functional class III or IV heart failure and an LV ejection fraction of less than 35% were prescribed enalapril. Patients taking enalapril had a 12-month relative mortality reduction of 31% and a 10-year averaged mortality reduction of 30%.[12] In a meta-analysis involving patients with LV ejection fraction of from less than 35% to 45%, all of whom were NYHA class II to IV, β-blockers decreased mortality by approximately 12% in 1 year and saved 3.8 lives in the first year

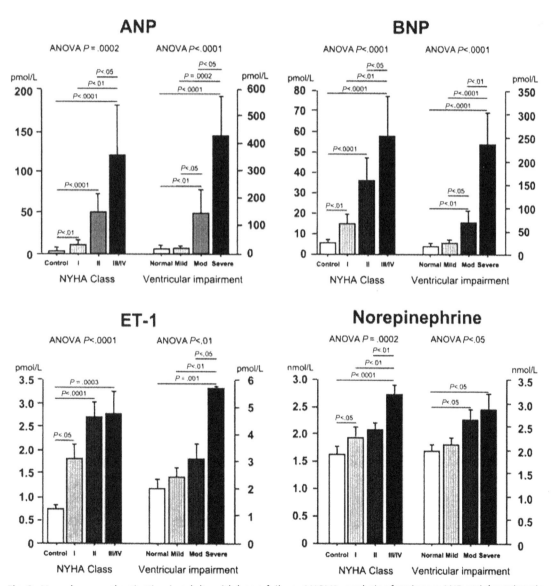

Fig. 2. Neurohormonal activation in adults with heart failure. ANOVA, analysis of variance; ANP, atrial natriuretic peptide; BNP, brain natriuretic peptide; ET-1, endothelin-1; NYHA, New York Heart Association. (*From* Bolger AP, Shama R, Li W, et al. Neurohormonal activation and the chronic heart failure syndrome in adults with congenital heart disease. Circulation 2001;106(1):92–9; with permission.)

per 100 patients treated.[13] The RALES trial proved the benefit of an aldosterone agonist, spironolactone, in NYHA class III or IV heart failure.

In the ACHD population, the data on the benefit of ACE inhibitors, β-blockers, and spironolactone are sparse. Most of the adult literature is pertinent to patients with ischemic heart disease and older patients, and the adult congenital population is much younger on average, has nonischemic cardiomyopathy, or a single ventricle.

Similarly, relatively few studies exist for heart failure in pediatrics. Shaddy and colleagues[14] reported, in a randomized control trial of carvedilol for children with heart failure, that there was no significant improvement in outcomes of clinical heart failure in children and adolescents with systolic heart failure. The study included both systemic right and left ventricles, and suggested that ventricular morphology might be an important factor in determining the effect of this medication. In the ACHD population, the authors often prescribe standard heart failure treatment with the hope that it may be effective. It is clear that despite treatment, many patients will develop heart failure.

Complicating pharmacologic therapy is the high incidence of sick sinus syndrome and other conduction abnormalities in ACHD patients (especially for D-TGA after Senning or Mustard operation, single-ventricle patients after Fontan completion, and complete heart block CC-TGA). Janousek and colleagues[15] reported that in 359 patients after Mustard or Senning operation, there was a prevalence of sinus node dysfunction of 51% at 2 years and 64% at 10 years postoperatively. Incidence of second-degree or third-degree block was 3.2%. In CC-TGA, the risk of heart block is 1% to 2% per year. Use of β-blockers in such a patient population requires close monitoring; the possibility of supraventricular tachyarrhythmia as a result can also be a concern.

DEVICE THERAPY

Many adults with complex CHD have had surgeries that are not curative but palliative. In most cases, the literature includes anecdotal evidence and case reports of device therapy used in the ACHD population.

Balloon Pump

The intra-aortic balloon pump (IABP) is a form of mechanical support that is placed via femoral arterial access in the descending aorta. The balloon expands during diastole to improve coronary perfusion and deflates during systole to improve forward flow, owing to lower systolic afterload. In the recent IABP-Shock II trial, there was no

significant reduction in 30-day mortality in patients with cardiogenic shock following acute myocardial infarction.[16] There are few reports of IABP use in CHD. IABP has been used in the immediate postoperative period following completion of Fontan in 5 series with a total of 21 patients, with survival ranging from 0% to 100%.[16] In one case report, a balloon pump was used in a 20-year-old patient with acute cardiogenic shock following a dual-chamber epicardial lead placement for sinus node dysfunction. The balloon pump was placed in lieu of extracorporeal membrane oxygenation (ECMO) and was weaned off in 72 hours.[17] Thus in specific situations, IABP may be effective for brief periods or before bridging to further support.

Impella (Abiomed)

The Impella device (Abiomed, Danvers, MA) is a minimally invasive catheter-based assist device designed to directly unload the left ventricle and expel blood in the ascending aorta. At present there are two models, one that can pump 2.5 liters per minute and a second that can pump 5 liters per minute. In adults, the Impella 2.5 has been used in high-risk percutaneous coronary interventions and in patients with cardiogenic shock.[18] In the setting of CHD, there is little reported use. The use of an Impella 2.5 and 5.0 was investigated in a mock circulatory system for a failing Fontan. In this model, the left-sided microaxial pumps were not well suited for cavopulmonary support because of severe recirculation.[19]

TandemHeart Percutaneous Ventricular Assist Device

The TandemHeart (Cardiac Assist, Inc, Pittsburgh, PA) is a temporary cardiac assist device, with an external continuous-flow centrifugal pump placed percutaneously (peripheral ventricular assist device [VAD]). One inflow cannula is inserted across the intra-atrial septum into the left atrium, and the pump withdraws blood and propels it into another cannula in the femoral artery. The pump can deliver flow up to 5 liters per minute and may support patients for up 2 weeks. In the literature to date there are no case reports of its use in the ACHD population.

Berlin Heart EXCOR (Pediatric Ventricular Assist Device)

Children with heart failure have limited options for mechanical circulatory support. Fraser and colleagues[20] reported a statistically significant difference in mortality of children with heart failure when comparing the Berlin Heart device with ECMO. The EXCOR (Berlin Heart GmbH, Berlin,

Germany) pediatric VAD is a pneumatically driven pulsatile-flow mechanical circulatory support designed for children. As the progress in developing pediatric devices has been challenging because of size constraints, many options do not exist for these smaller patients.[20] As a result, pediatric patients with CHD have been mainly placed on the Berlin Heart as a bridge to transplantation. Complications can include bleeding, stroke, and infection.

Left Ventricular Assist Devices

According to the Interagency Registry for Mechanically Assisted Circulatory Support (INTERMACS) database, which was established in 2006, there have been more than 6000 adults with heart failure who have been given a left ventricular assist device (LVAD).[21] Patients have received the mechanical circulatory device as a bridge to transplant, a bridge to recovery, or a destination therapy. An LVAD has two cannulas, an inflow cannula usually placed in the left ventricle and an outflow cannula placed in the ascending aorta. There are two categories of LVADs, a pulsatile pump or a continuous-flow pump.[22] The continuous-flow devices use a centrifugal or axial flow pump and have a central rotor containing magnets. Electric current passes through the coils applying force to the magnets, which in turn cause the rotors to spin and the blood to be moved forward.

In a randomized trial comparing devices, 134 patients underwent continuous flow and 66 patients pulsatile flow, and at 2 years there was a statistically significant difference in survival rates, at 58% (continuous flow) versus 24% (pulsatile flow). There were also statistically significant differences favoring continuous-flow devices regarding infection risk, renal and respiratory failure, and the need for pump replacement.[23]

The continuous-flow devices are smaller and have proved to be more durable than their pulsatile counterparts.[24] Today many devices exist, including the HeartMate I/II/III, Debakey MicroMed VAD, Jarvik 2000, and Berlin Heart EXCOR, among others. In most cases, the literature includes anecdotal evidence and case reports of device therapy used in the ACHD population (**Tables 1** and **2**).

Use of LVADs in ACHD
Systemic right ventricles (CC-TGA and D-TGA) In CC-TGA, the morphologic right ventricle is the systemic ventricle, and in D-TGA the morphologic right ventricle is the systemic ventricle after the Mustard or Senning operation. The first case report of LVAD use in D-TGA after a Mustard operation was in 1999.[25] In 2 patients (1 CC-TGA and 1 D-TGA status post Senning) reported by Stewart and colleagues,[26] both had LVAD implantation and both were placed intraperitoneally because of anatomic considerations. The operations resulted in midline abdominal wound dehiscence as a result of tension from placing the LVAD in a more medial position.[26]

With the advent of smaller axial flow assist devices the difficulties of wound dehiscence decreased, but the positioning of the VAD flow cannulas continues to be a challenge. In 2010, Joyce and colleagues[27] reported placing 2 HeartMate II devices in 2 patients (35 and 33 years old old) with D-TGA, and a DeBakey VAD (MicroMed) in a

---

Table 1
Short-term mechanical circulatory support systems available in the United States

Device (Manufacturer)	Position	Pump Type	Minimum Patient Size	Anticoagulation Strategy	Flow Rate (L/min)
ECMO (multiple manufacturers)	Extracorporeal	Centrifugal or roller pump	No minimum	Heparin	Variable
RotaFlow (Maquet)	Extracorporeal	Centrifugal	No minimum	Heparin	<10
PediMag (Thoratec)	Extracorporeal	Centrifugal	<20 kg	Heparin	<1.5
Tandem Heart pVAD (Cardiac Assist)	Extracorporeal or atrial transseptal	Centrifugal	>1.3 m²	Heparin	<5
Impella 2.5, 5.0 (Abiomed)	Transaortic valve	Axial	>1.3 m²ᵃ	Heparin	<2.5; <5
IABP (Maquet)	Intra-aortic	Counterpulsation	>1.3 m²	None	<1.5
AB5000 (Abiomed)	Extracorporeal	Displacement	>1.3 m²	Heparin	<6
CentriMag (Thoratec)	Extracorporeal	Centrifugal	>20 kg	Heparin	<10

ᵃ In addition, the manufacturer recommends left ventricular long-axis dimension of 7–11 cm.

Table 2
Mid-term and long-term mechanical circulatory support systems available in the United States

Device (Manufacturer)	Position	Pump Type	Minimum Patient Size	Long-Term Anticoagulation Strategy	Flow Rate (L/min)
EXCOR (Berlin Heart)	Extracorporeal	Pulsatile	>3 kg	Warfarin and ASA/ dipyridamole	Variable[a]
PVAD/IVAD (Thoratec)	Extracorporeal/ preperitoneal pocket	Pulsatile	>0.7 m²	Warfarin and ASA/ dipyridamole/ pentoxifylline	<7
Duraheart (Terumo Heart)	Preperitoneal pocket	Continuous	>1.1 m²	Warfarin and ASA	<8
SynCardia TAH (CardioWest)	Extracorporeal	Pulsatile	>1.7 m²[b]	Warfarin and ASA/ dipyridamole/ pentoxifylline	<9.5
Heartware HVAD (Heartware)	Pericardial	Continuous	>1.2 m²	Warfarin and ASA	<10
HeartMate II (Thoratec)	Preperitoneal pocket	Continuous	>1.3 m²	Warfarin and ASA/ dipyridamole	<10
Jarvik 2000 (Jarvik Heart)	Left ventricle	Continuous	>1.2 m²	Warfarin and ASA/ dipyridamole	<7

Abbreviation: ASA, aspirin (acetylsalicylic acid).
[a] Dependent on pump size (available sizes 10, 25, 30, 50, 60 mL).
[b] Also requires >10 cm between the sternum and the 10th vertebral body measured by computed tomography imaging.

25-year old with CC-TGA. A problem was encountered when placing the cannula anteriorly, which created obstruction by the moderator band in the right ventricle; when moved to a placement more posterior to the moderator band, a dramatic improvement was noticed in the rate of blood flow.[28] Concerns of tricuspid regurgitation were well tolerated in these patients. Of these 3 cases, 1 patient underwent successful transplantation and 2 were awaiting a donor.[27] Agusala and colleagues[28] reported a case of a Jarvik 2000 VAD in a 41-year-old patient with D-TGA status post Mustard who had a failing systemic right ventricle. The patient initially did well, but later developed multiorgan dysfunction complicated by infection, pancreatitis, coagulopathy, and bleeding, and died on postoperative day 47.

The largest case series was reported by Shah and colleagues,[29] in which 6 patients (3 with CC-TGA and 3 with D-TGA) underwent placement of a VAD, comprising 3 HeartMate II, 1 Jarvik 2000, 1 HeartMate SVE, and 1 HeartWare HVAD. The average age of implantation was 41 years, and there were 2 patients with single-ventricle physiology. Five patients survived to discharge and 1 patient who had previous Mustard operation died 27 days after surgery. One patient underwent successful transplantation, and several patients were listed for destination therapy. The longest

implanted VAD was in a patient with D-TGA status post Mustard who had been on device support for 988 days as destination therapy.

Fontan Since the inception of the Fontan operation for tricuspid atresia, the operation has evolved to palliate a large number of patients born with a single ventricle. Many of these patients who have reached adulthood have failing "Fontan circulation" secondary to chronically elevated central venous pressure or failure of a single systemic right or left ventricle. In the setting of an atriopulmonary Fontan, many patients have been converted to lateral tunnel or extracardiac Fontan, and have undergone an atrial Maze procedure (Fontan conversion). In one case report reported by Newcomb and colleagues,[30] a patient underwent a Fontan conversion, and remained in a low cardiac output with increasing ionotropic support including IABP without improvement. The patient was implanted with a Thoratec VAD 10 days after the operation and underwent successful orthotopic heart transplantation 5 months later.

In January 2003, a 14-year-old boy who had tricuspid atresia who had undergone Fontan procedure at 4 years presented with dyspnea and cyanosis, and was found to have thrombus in the hypoplastic right ventricle. He underwent creation of an extracardiac conduit, but was unable to be weaned from bypass. He was implanted with a HeartMate implantable pneumatic (IP) left ventricular assist system (LVAS), as illustrated in **Fig. 3**, and was supported for 5 weeks before undergoing successful heart transplantation.[31]

In the case series by Shah and colleagues,[29] two patients with Fontan physiology and NYHA functional class IV underwent successful LVAD implantation (HeartMate II). One patient had dextrocardia, hypoplastic right ventricle, pulmonary valve stenosis, atrial and ventricular septal defect, partial anomalous pulmonary venous return, and interrupted inferior vena cava, and had undergone a previous Potts and central shunt and, ultimately, a Fontan completion. The technical difficulties of implantation of an LVAD in a patient with dextrocardia on the left versus levocardia on the right are illustrated in **Fig. 4**. The second patient had D-TGA, a ventricular septal defect and pulmonary

valve stenosis, and a hypoplastic right ventricle, and had undergone a previous Waterston-Cooley shunt followed by Fontan completion. Both patients underwent VAD as destination therapy; one patient passed away after 261 days and the other was living at 493 days.[29]

Griffiths and colleagues[32] reported on 34 patients with failing Fontan circulation who were evaluated for heart transplantation. Eighteen had impaired ventricular function and 16 had preserved ventricular function, and 20 of the patients underwent heart transplantation. Of note, patients with preserved ventricular function had a higher mortality independent of whether they underwent transplantation. This consideration is important when evaluating patients with failing Fontan physiology and preserved ventricular function because they would not benefit from a VAD, whose failure may be due to any of numerous conditions such

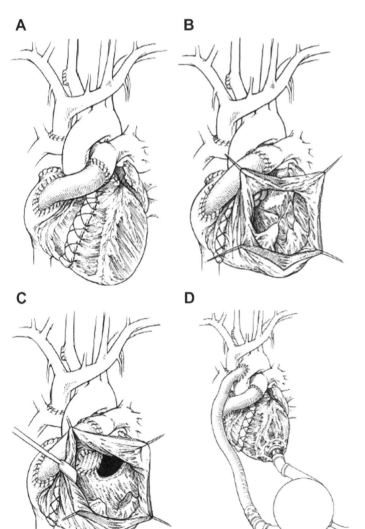

A
B
C
D

Fig. 3. The HeartMate IP LVAS shown in tricuspid atresia and Fontan. (*A*) The modified Fontan procedure. (*B*) The nonfunctional right ventricle as seen through the ventricular cavity. (*C*) After complete mitral valve excision, a pouch is constructed from the remaining viable myocardium and the left atrium, to serve as a reservoir for the inlet cannula. (*D*) The completed implantation of the left ventricular assist device. (*From* Frazier O, Gregoric I, Messner G. Total circulatory support with an LVAD in an adolescent with a previous Fontan procedure. Tex Heart Inst J 2005;32(3):402–4; with permission. Copyright 2006 by the Texas Heart Institute, Houston.)

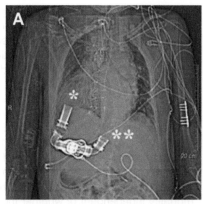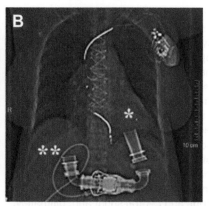

Fig. 4. Implantation of a left ventricular assist device in Fontan with dextrocardia. (*A*) Radiographic image shows the "mirror-image" orientation of a HeartMate II ventricular assist device implanted over the right abdomen in a patient with dextrocardia (Patient 2). Note that the inlet cannula (*asterisk*) is to the right of the outflow cannula (*double asterisk*). (*B*) Radiographic image shows the "normal" orientation of a HeartMate II ventricular assist device, with the inlet cannula to the left of the outflow cannula. (*From* Shah N, Lam W, Rodriguez F, et al. Clinical outcomes after ventricular assist device implantation in adults with complex congenital heart disease. J Heart Lung Transplant 2013;32(6):615–20; with permission.)

as ascites, pleural effusions, protein-losing enteropathy, plastic bronchitis, tachyarrhythmia, and Fontan pathway obstruction.

Right Ventricular Assist Devices

Implantation of an LVAD complicated by RV failure has a poor prognosis, and has led to placement of an additional right ventricular assist device (RVAD) in select patients. Ochiai and colleagues[33] reviewed 245 patients who underwent LVAD placement, only 9% of whom required RVAD insertion after LVAD placement. Clinical predictors included female gender and nonischemic etiology. In the ACHD population, a single VAD has been placed in the failing systemic single ventricle or systemic right ventricle.

In patients with TOF or Ebstein anomaly, patients have 2 ventricles; as well as a systemic left ventricle they may have a dysfunctional subpulmonary right ventricle, leading to right heart failure. In the literature there have been no case reports of placement of an RVAD. In TOF, surgical or percutaneous replacement of the pulmonary valve is the most common approach, and in Ebstein anomaly with severe RV failure, consideration can be given to repair or replacement of the tricuspid valve using one of several surgical approaches.

ANTITHROMBOTIC THERAPY STRATEGY

Anticoagulation in patients with an LVAD is critical, and there are many different institutional protocols on the optimal strategy. There is a substantial alteration in the prothrombotic profile, and these abnormalities often reverse with removal of the device. Rossi and colleagues[34] reviewed 17 institutional practices of axial-flow LVADs and recommended an optimal strategy of 100 mg/d of aspirin with a targeted international normalized ratio (INR) of 2.5 on warfarin that would inhibit 70% of platelets. Boyle and colleagues[35] reviewed 331 outpatients with the HeartMate II who were treated with 81 mg aspirin and warfarin. In total, there were 10 thrombotic events and 58 hemorrhagic events with a median INR of 2.1 at discharge and 1.9 at 6 months. Because of the low thromboembolic rate, an optimal INR of 1.5 to 2.5 was recommended. An increase in bleeding with an INR greater than 2.5 was seen, and 33% of the hemorrhagic strokes occurred with an INR higher than 3.0. There was a 40% increase in ischemic stroke with an INR less than 1.5.[35]

SUMMARY

As the ACHD population continues to grow in number and complexity, those with systemic right ventricle or single ventricle are at an increased risk of ventricular failure resulting from surgical palliation. VADs have been used with success in bridging ACHD patients to heart transplantation or destination therapy. As the ACHD population continues to increase in the future and technological advancement continues, surgical devices will continue to play a significant role.

REFERENCES

1. Warnes CA, Williams RG, Bashore TM, et al. ACC/ AHA 2008 guidelines for the management of adults with congenital heart disease: a report of the

American College of Cardiology/American Heart Association Task Force on Practice Guidelines. J Am Coll Cardiol 2008;52:e143–263.

2. Wren C, Reinhardt Z, Khawaja K. Twenty year trends in diagnosis of life threatening neonatal cardiovascular malformations. Arch Dis Child Fetal Neonatal Ed 2008;93:F33–5.

3. Warnes C. The adult with congenital heart disease: born to be bad? J Am Coll Cardiol 2005;46(1):1–8.

4. Shaddy R, Webb G. Applying heart failure guidelines to adult congenital heart disease patients. Expert Rev Cardiovasc Ther 2008;6(2):165–74.

5. Puley G, Siu S, Connely M, et al. Arrhythmia and survival in patients >18 years of age after the Mustard procedure for complete transposition of the great arteries. Am J Cardiol 1999;83(7):1080–4.

6. Presbitero P, Somerville J, Rabajoli F, et al. Corrected transposition of the great arteries without associated defects in adult patients: clinical profile and follow up. Br Heart J 1995;74:57–9.

7. Piran S, Veldtman G, Siu S, et al. Heart failure and ventricular dysfunction in patients with single or systemic right ventricles. Circulation 2002;105(10): 1189–94.

8. Fontan F, Baudet E. Surgical repair of tricuspid atresia. Thorax 1971;26:240–8.

9. Lillehei C, Varco R, Cohen M, et al. The first open heart corrections of tetralogy of Fallot. A 26 to 31 year follow-up of 106 patients. Ann Surg 1986;204: 490–502.

10. Norozi K, Wessel A, Alpers V, et al. Incidence and risk distribution of heart failure in adolescents and adults with congenital heart disease after cardiac surgery. Am J Cardiol 2006;97(8):1238–43.

11. Bolger AP, Shama R, Li W, et al. Neurohormonal activation and the chronic heart failure syndrome in adults with congenital heart disease. Circulation 2001;106(1):92–9.

12. Effects of enalapril on mortality in severe congestive heart failure. Results of the Cooperative North Scandinavian Enalapril Survival Study (CONSENSUS). The CONSENSUS Trial Study Group. N Engl J Med 1987;316(23):1429.

13. Brophy JM, Joseph L, Rouleau JL. Beta-blockers in congestive heart failure. A Bayesian meta-analysis. Ann Intern Med 2001;134(7):550.

14. Shaddy RE, Boucek MM, Hsu DT, et al. Carvedilol for children and adolescents with heart failure: a randomized controlled trial. JAMA 2007;298(10): 1171–9.

15. Janousek J, Paul T, Luhmer I, et al. Atrial baffle procedures for complete transposition of the great arteries: natural course of sinus node dysfunction and risk factors for dysrhythmias and sudden death. Z Kardiol 1994;83(12):933–8.

16. Thiele H, Schuler G, Neumann FJ, et al. Intraaortic balloon support for myocardial infarction with cardiogenic shock. N Engl J Med 2012;367(14): 1287–96.

17. Moran A, Blume E, Quinn R. Intra-aortic balloon pump use in the failing Fontan circulation. Congenit Heart Dis 2008;3:60–2.

18. Lauten A, Engstrom AE, Jung C, et al. Percutaneous left-ventricular support with the Impella-2.5-assist device in acute cardiogenic shock: results of the Impella-EUROSHOCK-registry. Circ Heart Fail 2013; 6(1):23–30.

19. Haggerty CM, Fynn-Thompson F, McElhinney DB, et al. Experimental and numeric investigation of Impella pumps as cavopulmonary assistance for a failing Fontan. Thorac Cardiovasc Surg 2012; 144(3):563–9.

20. Fraser CD Jr, Jaquiss RD, Rosenthal DN, et al. Prospective trial of a pediatric ventricular assist device. N Engl J Med 2012;367(6):532–41.

21. Rodriguez L, Suarez E. Ventricular assist devices therapy: new technology, new hope? Methodist Debakey Cardiovasc J 2013;9(1):32–7.

22. Slaughter MS, Rogers JG, Frazier OH, et al. Advanced heart failure treated with continuous-flow left ventricular assist device. N Engl J Med 2009; 361:2241–51.

23. Slaughter MS, Pagani FD, Rogers JG, et al. Clinical management of continuous-flow left ventricular assist devices in advanced heart failure. J Heart Lung Transplant 2010;29(4):S1–39.

24. Schulman AR, Martens TP, Christos PJ, et al. Comparisons of infection complications between continuous flow and pulsatile flow left ventricular assist devices. J Thorac Cardiovasc Surg 2007;133(3):841–2.

25. Wiklund L, Svensson S, Berggren H. Implantation of a left ventricular assist device, back-to-front, in an adolescent with a failing mustard procedure. J Thorac Cardiovasc Surg 1999;118:755–6.

26. Stewart AS, Gorman RC, Pocchetino A, et al. Left ventricular assist device for right side assistance in patients with transposition. Ann Thorac Surg 2002; 74:912–4.

27. Joyce DL, Crow SS, John R, et al. Mechanical circulatory support in patients with heart failure secondary to transposition of the great arteries. J Heart Lung Transplant 2010;29(11):1302–5.

28. Agusala K, Bogaev R, Franklin W. Ventricular assist device placement in an adult with D-transposition of the great arteries with prior Mustard operation. Congenit Heart Dis 2010;5(6):635–7.

29. Shah N, Lam W, Rodriguez F, et al. Clinical outcomes after ventricular assist device implantation in adults with complex congenital heart disease. J Heart Lung Transplant 2013;32(6):615–20.

30. Newcomb AE, Negri JC, Brizard CP, et al. Successful left ventricular assist device bridge to transplantation after failure of a Fontan revision. J Heart Lung Transplant 2006;25(3):365–7.

31. Frazier O, Gregoric I, Messner G. Total circulatory support with an LVAD in an adolescent with a previous Fontan procedure. Tex Heart Inst J 2005;32(3): 402–4.

32. Griffiths E, Kaza A, Wyler von Ballmoos M, et al. Evaluating failing Fontans for heart transplantation: predictors of mortality. Ann Thorac Surg 2009; 88(2):558–64.

33. Ochiai Y, McCarthy P, Smedira N, et al. Predictors of severe right ventricular failure after implantable left ventricular assist device insertion: analysis of 245 patients. Circulation 2002;106(12 Suppl 1): I198–202.

34. Rossi M, Serraino G, Jiritano F, et al. What is the optimal anticoagulation in patients with a left ventricular assist device? Interact Cardiovasc Thorac Surg 2012;15:733–40.

35. Boyle AJ, Russell SD, Teuteberg JJ, et al. Low thromboembolism and pump thrombosis with the HeartMate II left ventricular assist device: analysis of outpatient anti-coagulation. J Heart Lung Transplant 2009;28:881–7.

Heart Transplantation in Adults with Congenital Heart Disease

Garrick C. Stewart, MD[a],*, John E. Mayer Jr, MD[b]

KEYWORDS

- Heart transplantation • Heart defects • Congenital • Heart failure • Patient selection

KEY POINTS

- Heart transplantation has become an increasingly common and effective therapy for adults with end-stage congenital heart disease (CHD) because of advances in patient selection and surgical technique.
- Indications for transplantation in CHD are largely similar to those for other forms of heart failure given the absence of specific guideline-based listing criteria.
- Pretransplant assessment of CHD patients emphasizes careful evaluation of cardiac anatomy, pulmonary vascular disease, allosensitization, hepatic dysfunction, and neuropsychiatric status.
- Cardiac transplant for CHD should be performed by surgeons experienced in congenital heart surgery given the complexities of CHD anatomy and the frequent need for adjunctive vascular reconstruction.
- Patients with a failed Fontan circulation have a higher posttransplant mortality than those with other CHD due to risk of infection, bleeding, and posttransplant right heart failure.

INTRODUCTION

Advances in medical and surgical inventions have led to remarkable improvements in the survival and quality of life of patients with CHD. The population of adults living with CHD is estimated to be increasing 5% per year and more than 85% of individuals born with CHD survive into adulthood.[1,2] Myocardial dysfunction in CHD can arise from prevailing hemodynamic insults from residual or uncorrected lesions or from previous palliative procedures that are now failing.[3] The burden of heart failure in patients with complex CHD will continue to increase as survivors of complex neonatal palliation from the 1980s and 1990s survive into adulthood. As a consequence, more adult CHD patients suffering from heart failure will merit consideration for cardiac transplantation as treatment of end-stage disease (**Box 1**).[4]

Historically, many transplant programs have been reluctant to offer transplantation to adults with CHD due to excess surgical risk related to multiple prior operations, recipient sensitization, and poor outcomes. Once deemed unacceptably risky or even ineffective, transplantation has become an increasingly common and effective therapy for adults with end-stage CHD because of advances in patient selection and surgical technique. Patients with CHD now account for 3% of adult heart transplants and more than 40% of heart-lung transplants in the United States.[5,6] Although an early hazard after transplantation for CHD remains, the intermediate-term and long-term survival rates for patients after transplant are similar to those transplanted for other causes of failure.[7,8] The continued improvement in outcomes after transplantation hinges on careful consideration of each patient's unique

Disclosures: The authors have no disclosures relevant to the content in this article.
[a] Division of Cardiovascular Medicine, Center for Advanced Heart Disease, Brigham and Women's Hospital, 75 Francis Street, Boston, MA 02115, USA; [b] Cardiovascular Surgery, Boston Children's Hospital, 300 Longwood Avenue, Boston, MA 02115, USA
* Corresponding author.
E-mail address: gcstewart@partners.org

Heart Failure Clin 10 (2014) 207–218
http://dx.doi.org/10.1016/j.hfc.2013.09.007
1551-7136/14/$ – see front matter © 2014 Elsevier Inc. All rights reserved.

Box 1
Common forms of congenital heart disease leading to transplant in adulthood

Single-ventricle physiology

Fontan circulation

Congenitally corrected transposition of the great arteries

D-transposition after Mustard or Senning operation in which the systemic ventricle is the morphologic right ventricle

Tetralogy of Fallot with early-era surgery, long-standing shunt, or severe pulmonic regurgitation

Unoperated atrioventricular septal defects

Eisenmenger syndrome

---

anatomy and physiology. This review focuses on adults with CHD who have advanced heart failure and highlights the indications for transplant listing, elements of the transplant evaluation, operative considerations, and posttransplant outcomes.

INDICATIONS FOR TRANSPLANT

Although specific criteria for transplant in adults with CHD do not exist, indications for transplant are similar to those for non-CHD patients.[9,10] The most common reason for transplant is unremitting moderate-to-severe heart failure symptoms consistent with New York Heart Association (NYHA) class III-IV functional capacity despite optimal, guideline-based medical and device therapies (**Box 2**).[11,12] After the development of heart failure symptoms, palliative or corrective surgery for CHD is usually preferable to transplant listing. The possibility for surgical remediation should be reviewed by a congenital heart surgeon prior to transplant listing. Transplant is also appropriate in patients who are dependent on either continuous intravenous inotropes or a mechanical support device, because each of these treatments suggests a level of illness associated with a high mortality. Less commonly used indications for transplant include refractory ventricular tachycardia or angina not amenable to other therapies.

Exercise intolerance carries important prognostic significance in heart failure stemming from CHD.[13] Self-reported exercise tolerance in CHD is poorly correlated with objective measures of exercise capacity, so standardized testing is required.[14] Cardiopulmonary exercise testing (CPET) has become the single most important test for assessing appropriateness of transplant listing for all causes of end-stage heart failure. Transplant should never be based solely on CPET results; rather, CPET data should be thoughtfully integrated into the assessment of disease severity.[9] A maximal exercise test as assessed by a respiratory exchange ratio (RER) greater than 1.05 is required to determine if functional limitation is due to heart disease.[15] A reduced peak oxygen uptake is associated with a high mortality from heart failure and is the traditional CPET metric used for transplant listing.[16] Reduced peak oxygen uptake has been shown to predict hospital admission and death in CHD. It is not known whether the same threshold for listing should be used in CHD or if the thresholds are independent of the underlying congenital defect.[17]

In younger patients and in women, the peak oxygen uptake, which is indexed to body weight, can be misleading, so a less than 50% predicted uptake for age and gender can be used as an alternative transplant listing measure. For those patients who fail to reach maximal exercise (RER <1.05), the ventilation equivalent of carbon dioxide slope can be used to gauge cardiac limitations, with higher numbers reflecting more severe heart failure. This can be less useful in some forms of

---

Box 2
Indications for heart transplantation in adults with congenital heart disease

NYHA class III/IV symptoms from structural heart disease not amenable to correction or palliation

Cardiogenic shock requiring inotropes or an MCS device

Reduced functional capacity on CPET with maximal effort

- Peak oxygen uptake $\leq$12 mL/kg/min (or $\leq$14 mL/kg/min if intolerant to β-blockers)
- Peak oxygen uptake <50% predicted
- If submaximal effort (RER <1.05) a ventilation equivalent of carbon dioxide slope >35

Intractable life-threatening arrhythmias refractory to medical, ablative and device therapies

Intractable angina refractory to medical therapy or revascularization

Adapted from Mehra MR, Kobashigawa J, Starling R, et al. Listing criteria for heart transplantation: International Society for Heart and Lung Transplantation guidelines for the care of cardiac transplant candidates–2006. J Heart Lung Transplant 2006;25:1024; and Kinkhabwala MP, Mancini D. Patient selection for cardiac transplant in 2012. Expert Rev Cardiovasc Ther 2013;11:182.

CHD in which this ratio is universally elevated, for example, in the setting of right-to-left intracardiac shunting. In circumstances where there is ambiguity among the criteria for transplant listing, the heart failure survival score can be used to risk stratify transplant candidates, although it has not been validated in the adult CHD population.[18,19]

Identification of early end-organ dysfunction can be an important clue to a declining circulatory status. It is imperative that transplant listing occurs prior to multiple organ system dysfunction, given the long expected waitlist times for transplantation.[11] Several specific markers of adverse heart failure prognosis in CHD are worth highlighting. The development of renal failure and anemia are important markers of increased mortality in CHD.[20] Persistent hyponatremia is also an indicator of adverse prognosis in patients with heart failure and CHD, independent of hemodynamic status.[21,22] Other markers of increased mortality in heart failure include repeated heart failure hospitalizations, intolerance to angiotensin-converting enzyme inhibitors or β-adrenergic blockers, recurrent implantable defibrillator shocks, and high or increasing diuretic requirements.[23–27] Awareness of myriad signposts marking downward disease trajectory can trigger referral for heart transplantation while salvage of the failing circulation is still possible.

TRANSPLANT EVALUATION

Given the scarcity of donor organs, transplant listing is restricted to patients most likely to realize the greatest benefit from a cardiac allograft. The pretransplantation evaluation requires a multidisciplinary approach to assess the cardiopulmonary, renal, infectious, neurologic, and psychosocial substrate of the patient. Cardiac catheterization as well as imaging with MRI or CT can delineate the unique anatomic features of each CHD patient to aid surgical planning. Contraindications for transplantation in CHD emphasize the cumulative burden of extracardiac comorbidities (**Table 1**).[9,28] Transplant for CHD is contraindicated if there are multiple severe congenital abnormalities. Relative contraindications specific to the CHD population include heterotaxy syndromes, particularly when there are complex venous drainage anomalies, extensive systemic artery to pulmonary collateral vessels, immune deficiency related to specific genetic syndromes, or asplenia in the case of right atrial isomerism. Multiple prior sternotomies are not a contraindication to transplantation.[29]

Several specific considerations during the transplant evaluation are of particular relevance to the CHD population.[30] These include assessment of pulmonary hypertension, allosensitization, hepatic function, and neuropsychiatric status. Given these complexities, the American College of Cardiology/American Heart Association Guidelines for the Management of Adults with CHD make a class I recommendation that patients with CHD and heart failure who may require transplant should be evaluated and managed in a tertiary care center with medical and surgical expertise in the management of both CHD and heart transplantation.[28]

Pulmonary Hypertension

Right ventricular failure is a common cause of morbidity and mortality after cardiac transplantation, accounting for approximately 20% of early deaths.[31] Patients with CHD are particularly prone to developing pulmonary hypertension due to longstanding left-to-right shunting, pulmonary

---

Table 1
Contraindications to cardiac transplantation for congenital heart disease

Absolute Contraindications	Relative Contraindications
• Multiple organ system failure • Active malignancy • Cognitive and/or behavioral deficits that interfere with compliance • Severe metabolic disease • Active hepatitis C infection • Multiple other severe congenital abnormalities	• Diabetes with end-organ dysfunction • Elevated PVR • Irreversible chronic kidney disease • Severe cerebrovascular or peripheral vascular disease not amenable to revascularization • Obesity • Active tobacco or substance abuse • Positive serology for human immunodeficiency virus • Immune deficiencies related to specific genetic syndromes • Heterotaxy syndromes • Extensive collateral vessels • Asplenia in the case of right atrial isomerism

Data from Refs.[9,28,29]

arterial (PA) abnormalities, and systemic ventricular failure. Invasive hemodynamic assessment is required to diagnose pulmonary hypertension, which has been associated with posttransplant right heart failure.[32] The presence of PA hypertension (defined as PA systolic pressure >60 mm Hg) is a relative contraindication to transplantation when the pulmonary vascular resistance (PVR) is greater than 5 Wood units, the indexed PVR is greater than 6, or the transpulmonary gradient exceeds 16 mm Hg to 20 mm Hg.[9] Precise cutoff values may vary from center to center.

Vasodilator challenges may be performed during a right heart catheterization to assess for reversibility in the PVR elevations once pulmonary capillary wedge pressure has been optimized. Commonly used vasodilators include prostacyclines, nitric oxide, and nitroprusside. A fall of at least 20% in mean PA pressure and restoration of PVR below 2.5 Wood units without a decrease in cardiac index is reassuring. If medical therapy over days or weeks fails to reduce wedge pressure less than 25 mm Hg and the PA systolic pressure to less than 60 mm Hg, the reversibility of elevated PVR cannot be determined.[9] Often, the only way to fully unload the systemic ventricle is by inotrope infusion and/or mechanical circulatory support (MCS) in order to determine if the PVR is reversible. Even reversible pretransplant pulmonary hypertension predicts a higher risk of mortality after cardiac transplantation, although it is not a strict contraindication to isolated heart transplant.[33] If "fixed" pulmonary hypertension present, the risk of right heart failure after isolated heart transplant is too high and dual heart-lung transplantation must be considered.

The PVR evaluation is particularly challenging in the complex CHD population, many of whom have single-ventricle physiology or residual intracardiac shunting. For example, patients with a failing Fontan circulation can have pulmonary vascular abnormalities, in situ thrombosis and thromboembolism related to low pulmonary blood flow, differential right and left lung blood flow, and multiple sources of pulmonary blood flow (eg, residual antegrade flow across an oversewn pulmonary valve or venovenous collateral). It is not known whether or not the same PVR cutoffs used to guide listing eligibility are valid in the CHD population or what levels of PVR might preclude successful transplantation.[8]

Allosensitization

Many adult CHD patients have undergone multiple prior surgeries with exposure to blood products and homograft materials that increase the risk of allosensitization. Fresh cryopreserved allografts are often used for the reconstruction of atretic, hypoplastic, or stenotic structures during congenital heart surgery. Antibodies to HLA have been shown to persist late after CHD surgery that uses allograft material, such as single-ventricle palliation.[34,35] Late sensitization is also observed in patients undergoing childhood CHD surgery without allograft material and is likely related to blood product exposure. Both class I and class II anti-HLA antibodies can persist for a decade or more after CHD surgery. Other causes of increased sensitization include pregnancy and the use of MCS as a bridge to transplant.[36] High levels of preformed circulating lymphocytotoxic antibodies increase the risk of hyperacute, acute, and chronic rejection after transplantation.

Time constraints for donor organ allocation and organ scarcity preclude full HLA matching in heart transplantation. Panel-reactive antibody tests and solid-state, single-bead assays are used to identify the presence of HLA antibodies, estimate the risk of rejection with a given donor, and guide the need for prospective crossmatching. Patients undergoing transplant for CHD are more likely to have elevations in panel-reactive antibodies than adults with other diagnoses.[37] In practice, most centers avoid transplant in the case of high or moderate concentrations of donor-specific HLA antibodies. Strategies to increase the donor pool for sensitized patients, such as desensitization with intravenous immunoglobulin and plasmapheresis, or the use of virtual crossmatching, are now widely used.[38] Even so, the prevalence of such presensitized patients among the CHD population translates into longer waiting times for transplantation and increased risk of death while on the waiting list and may contribute to poor graft and overall survival after transplant.[39]

Hepatic Function

Underlying cirrhosis and portal hypertension are associated with poor prognosis after heart transplantation. Recognition of hepatic dysfunction in adult CHD patients may warrant more intensification of heart failure treatment to decongest the systemic venous circulation and correct abnormal liver function parameters, such as elevation in transaminases or total bilirubin. Signs of hepatic dysfunction may also prompt earlier consideration for transplant evaluation before cardiac cirrhosis develops.[40] There has been increasing interest in the use of the Model for End-Stage Liver Disease (MELD) score to predict postcardiac transplant outcomes.[41] Chronic cardiac hepatopathy and elevations in the MELD score can frequently resolve after transplantation, so the score cannot be used in isolation to guide transplant eligibility.[41,42]

Traditional methods for estimating hepatic dysfunction and surgical risk, such as the MELD score or Child-Turcotte-Pugh class, may also be inadequate in the CHD population where liver synthetic dysfunction may lead to atypical pattern of biochemical abnormalities.[43,44] Patients with biochemical, clinical, or radiographic evidence of advanced liver disease should be evaluated thoroughly for cirrhosis. This evaluation often involves liver biopsy to identify and stage bridging fibrosis, with the recognition that many patients with chronic hepatic congestion from right heart failure have some degree of fibrosis even in the absence of cirrhosis.[45] Given the higher risk of irreversible hepatic injury in patients with a failing Fontan circulation despite often normal liver synthetic function, many such patients undergo concomitant evaluation by a liver transplant team for possible heart-liver cotransplantation.[46,47]

Neuropsychiatric Status and Social Supports

The psychological strain on individuals and their families or other social supports during a transplant listing of indeterminate length cannot be minimized. Once a matching donor organ is found, adherence to the complex medical regimen after heart transplantation requires a robust psychological foundation. As a consequence, the neurologic status and development of patients with CHD is pertinent to the transplant evaluation. The neuropsychiatric status of all potential transplant candidates requires expert adjudication by mental health professionals working in collaboration with the heart transplant team.

Neurodevelopmental delay has been linked to some forms of CHD and may place adult CHD patients at risk for posttransplant complications linked to medication nonadherence unless a supportive social milieu is confirmed.[48] Adults with CHD approaching transplant may also carry the burden of childhood or adolescent behavioral and psychosocial issues related to chronic illness, prolonged hospitalization, or other adjustment disorders. Common neurologic complications of CHD include stroke and brain abscess.[49,50] Many CHD patients are further exposed to the attendant neurologic complications of repeated corrective or palliative cardiac surgeries during their use, including those arising from cardiac bypass and hypothermic circulatory arrest.[51] Once cleared for transplant listing, the mental health status of CHD patients with neurocognitive vulnerabilities requires careful monitoring and support through the waitlist period and after successful transplant surgery.

TRANSPLANT WAITING LIST

Approximately 3% of patients on the adult transplant waiting list have CHD as their primary indication for transplant. Approximately 90% of patients with CHD are listed at an adult transplant program, with the balance listed at pediatric transplant programs.[8] Adults with CHD have a longer waitlist time than non-CHD patients. This disparity persists despite a greater percentage of time in the highest waitlist priority (status 1A or 1B) among CHD patients. Reasons for longer waitlist times may include concerns over sensitization or the need for extra tissue for cardiac allograft implantation, which excludes many donors simultaneously giving lungs because the added vasculature required can interfere with lung procurement. In addition, there may be a desire among transplant programs to wait for the ideal donor given the younger age of listed CHD patients.

CHD patients have elevated waitlist mortality despite being younger and possessing fewer comorbidities compared with others listed for transplant. In addition, some experts have challenged traditional transplant indications in CHD populations because common triggers, such as reduced oxygen uptake on cardiopulmonary testing, may prompt transplant listing too late in the disease process for CHD candidates.[8] For example, CHD patients are likely to have a lower body mass index at transplantation, suggesting a greater degree of neurohumoral activation consistent with consequent cardiac cachexia, which has been consistently linked to poor outcomes.[8]

The high waitlist mortality for CHD may also be linked to the less frequent use of MCS devices as a means of bridging to transplantation (see article by Mulukutla and colleagues, elsewhere in this issue).[8] CHD patients are less likely to have MCS at listing or transplantation compared with non-CHD patients.[52] Furthermore, the use of MCS in CHD is not associated with improved rates of survival to transplant in contrast to patients with cardiomyopathies.[8] The few reports of MCS in adults with complex CHD have suggested that they fare worse than those with cardiomyopathy.[53] Residual shunting, unfavorable ventricular anatomy, multiple prior sternotomies, and a complex systemic arterial to PA collateral circulation may further dissuade implant of left ventricular assist devices.[54] Patients with complex CHD and single-ventricle physiologies have limited options for advanced MCS, with contemporary devices designed for adults with cardiomyopathies.[55] Patients with a failing Fontan circulatory can have circulatory failure despite preserved ventricular systolic function, precluding an indication for single-ventricle MCS.[56] Because many patients with complex CHD cannot receive or would not benefit from isolated systemic ventricular assist devices, a total artificial heart may be required. There is an urgent need to improve MCS bridging options for adult CHD patients awaiting transplant.

TRANSPLANT OPERATION

Several unique features of the CHD population make transplantation technically challenging and add to the duration and complexity of transplant surgery. CHD patients often come to transplant having had previous cardiac surgery for staged repairs or palliative procedures. Between 23% and 84% of patients undergoing transplant for CHD have a history of prior surgery for CHD repair or palliation.[57] These operations can distort anatomy and leave patients with dense adhesions that must be carefully dissected at the time of transplant. In addition to adhesions, end-stage CHD patients often have a distended right heart, further complicating resternotomy. Alternative cannulation sites are often required to establish cardiopulmonary bypass. Dissection in cyanotic patients is further complicated by the development dense networks of collaterals that may bleed profusely if disrupted. The risk of bleeding is further increased by the coagulopathy seen in cyanotic patients with a high hematocrit.[58] Systemic to pulmonary collaterals in the posterior mediastinum result in increased pulmonary venous return, which can compromise exposure during surgery. Patients with hepatic dysfunction, as in the failing Fontan circulation, may also be predisposed to coagulopathy.

Traditionally, orthotopic heart transplantation has been conducted with either biatrial or bicaval anastomoses, with the latter the most popular technique worldwide. Modifications to these classic surgical techniques are required in 60% to 75% of patients undergoing transplantation for CHD due to unusual anatomy or distortions caused by prior surgeries.[59] Despite the complexities and improvisations required during congenital heart surgery, only a few anatomic sites are of paramount interest. These include the sites of anastomosis between the donor and recipient—the points of systemic and pulmonary venous return along with the two great vessels (**Table 2**).[60]

Table 2
Relevant morphologic considerations for transplant surgery in congenital heart disease

Anatomic Site	Possible Anomalies
Pulmonary venous return	• Total or partial anomalous pulmonary venous return • Severe stenosis, hypoplasia, or atresia of pulmonary veins[a]
Systemic venous return	• Left superior vena cava with or without bridging innominate vein • Interrupted inferior vena cava with azygous continuation • Absence of right superior vena cava
Atria	• Situs ambiguous (right and left atrial isomerism or single large atrium) • Situs inversus (mirror-image atrial arrangement) • Distortion due to previous surgery (eg, Mustard, Senning, or Fontan procedure)
Pulmonary artery	• Hypoplasia or atresia of main pulmonary artery and/or main branches • Distortion from previous surgery (eg, Blalock-Taussig shunt, Glenn, or Fontan) • Severe hypoplasia or absence of extrapulmonary branches of pulmonary arteries[a]
Ascending aorta and aortic arch	• Aortic hypoplasia, interruption or coarctation (most often previously repaired) • Distortion from previous surgery (eg, arch repair, Damus-Kaye-Stansel procedure, truncus arteriosus repair, or arterial switch operation) • Abnormal spatial relationship to pulmonary artery (eg, transposition of the great arteries, double-outlet ventricle) • Right-sided aortic arch

[a] Requires heart-lung transplantation.

Adapted from Hosseinpour AR, Gonzalez-Calle A, Adsuar-Gomez A, et al. Surgical technique for heart transplantation: a strategy for congenital heart disease. Eur J Cardiothorac Surg 2013;44(4):598–604; with permission.

Anomalies at each anastomotic site must be addressed at the time of transplantation.

Reconstruction of anastomotic sites is often required. Such reconstruction is usually done with living tissue from the donor or recipient rather than prosthetic material in order to minimize the risk of bleeding and infection. This requires careful planning and close collaboration between the donor and recipient surgical teams so that as much tissue can be harvested as possible, including extra length of the superior vena cava and innominate vein along with great vessels and pericardium.[61] The need for additional donor tissue for allograft implantation in CHD patients has raised concerns that prolonged waitlist times may be inevitable given the resultant exclusion of donors simultaneously donating lungs. These myriad surgical complexities mean that CHD patients are much more likely to have prolonged allograft ischemic times (>4 h) compared with non-CHD transplant recipients, whether or not it is a reoperation.[8]

OUTCOMES AFTER HEART TRANSPLANT

Outcomes after heart transplantation for cardiomyopathy have steadily improved, yet survival rates after transplant for CHD have remained the same.[8] The increasing complexity of CHD presenting for transplant may be masking the overall trend toward better survival.[62] Within the first 30 days after transplant, patients are at risk for perioperative complications largely due to comorbidities present prior to transplant as well as complex surgical anatomy.[5] Between 1 month and 1 year, the greatest hazard in transplant comes from rejection, which necessitates aggressive early immune suppression, thereby exposing patients to risk of infection. After 1 year, primary risk of death comes from malignancy, coronary allograft vasculopathy, noncytomegalovirus infection, and renal failure.[5]

Pretransplant heart disease etiology has a major effect on posttransplant survival. In data from the United Network for Organ Sharing (UNOS), risk of death within 30 days is significantly higher in patients with CHD whether or not reoperation is required (18.9% vs 9.6% reoperation; 16.6% vs 6.3% nonreoperation).[8] In the International Society for Heart and Lung Transplantation Registry, patients with nonischemic cardiomyopathy have 86% 1-year survival after transplant, compared to 81% in ischemic cardiomyopathy and 79% in CHD.[5] These data reinforce the importance of thoughtful pretransplant evaluation, careful surgical planning, and operation by experienced surgeons at high-volume CHD/transplant centers (**Box 3**). A recent single-center report suggests that in the

> **Box 3**
> **Select risk factors for mortality after transplant for congenital heart disease**
>
> Previous Fontan operation
>
> PVR >4 Wood units
>
> Prolonged ischemic time (>4 h)
>
> Prior Glenn operation
>
> Cytomegalovirus mismatch
>
> Low body mass index
>
> *Data from* Patel ND, Weiss ES, Allen JG, et al. Heart transplantation for adults with congenital heart disease: analysis of the United network for organ sharing database. Ann Thorac Surg 2009;88:819; and Lamour JM, Kanter KR, Naftel DC, et al. The effect of age, diagnosis, and previous surgery in children and adults undergoing heart transplantation for congenital heart disease. J Am Coll Cardiol 2009;54:163.

modern era, using careful donor and recipient selection, CHD patients have excellent early and midterm survival rates after transplant that rival those for other etiologies of end-stage heart failure.[7]

Patients with CHD undergoing transplant are more likely to die of primary graft failure, multiple organ system failure, stroke, and renal failure compared with their non-CHD counterparts.[63] In the early postoperative period, CHD patients are also at a higher risk of reoperation and dialysis.[37] The presence of CHD alone may not confer an increased of dying from acute or chronic rejection despite a higher prevalence of allosensitization.[37] Yet an analysis of the UNOS data set suggests there is a lower frequency of induction immunosuppression and chronic corticosteroid maintenance among CHD patients, factors associated with improved survival in other adult transplant recipients.[64]

Beyond the first year, patients with CHD actually have a lower risk of long-term mortality than those with ischemic cardiomyopathy. This striking difference in early and late hazard is a signature feature of transplant in adults with CHD. The relative youth and paucity of extracardiac comorbidities in the CHD patients undergoing transplant seem protective in the long run. By 10 years after transplant, CHD patients have a slight survival advantage compared with the non-CHD population.[8,37,61]

Fontan Transplants

An increasing number of single-ventricle palliation procedures have been performed in the past 30 years, contributing to a growing prevalence of patients presenting for transplant with Fontan circuits and late Fontan failure.[56,65] Fontan physiology has been linked to a striking 8-fold adjusted relative risk of early death after transplant.[63] One-year survival in Fontan patients is 71% compared with 83% in the non-Fontan CHD population.[63] These less favorable outcomes may be related to technical challenges of multiple earlier palliative procedures and individual anatomic differences. In addition, Fontan patients are more likely to have protein-losing enteropathy, with resulting cachexia, edema, and lymphopenia, making them more vulnerable to infection.[66] Anomalies within the pulmonary vascular and/or dual blood supplies may make assessment of PVR difficult. Just because the Fontan circuit allows passive flow from the systemic venous system through the pulmonary bed does not necessarily mean PVR is low enough to tolerate transplant.[67] Lastly, the presence of aortopulmnoary collaterals in some Fontan patients coupled with coagulopathy from hepatic congestion increases the risk of postoperative bleeding.[43] Patients with Fontan physiology exemplify the remarkable heterogeneity in peritransplant management and outcomes within the CHD population.

HEART-LUNG TRANSPLANT

Combined heart-lung transplantation remains the only option for many patients with previous repaired CHD associated with significant pulmonary vascular obstructive disease. CHD is the most common indication for dual heart-lung transplantation, accounting for approximately 36% of cases between 1982 and 2011.[6] Common indications for combined transplant include single-ventricle physiology with pulmonary vascular disease or primary systemic ventricular failure with irreversible secondary pulmonary hypertension. Survival after heart-lung transplant is significantly less than after isolated heart transplant.[57] Actuarial survival at 10 years after heart-lung transplant is only 20%. A pretransplant diagnosis of Eisenmenger syndrome has the best overall survival among all indications for heart-lung transplantation.[6] In select patients with simple CHD and pulmonary vascular disease, lung transplantation coupled with surgical repair of the primary intracardiac lesion has been proposed as a mechanism to optimize donor allocation.[68]

RETRANSPLANTATION

Retransplantation accounts for only 3.5% of heart transplants.[5] A recent analysis from UNOS revealed that adult CHD patients are retransplanted more often than other recipients (4.7% vs 3.4%).[64] Adults with CHD receiving a heart transplant are younger than the non-CHD population, so may be eligible for retransplantation should they suffer late graft failure, most commonly due to allograft coronary disease. Survival after retransplant is worse than after primary transplant, with the risk of death approximately 70% higher compared with de novo transplant.[69] A higher rate of comorbidities, such as chronic kidney disease, among cardiac retransplant recipients contributes to decreased survival.[70] Specific factors linked to decrease retransplant survival include early retransplantation, high-grade rejection in the first transplant, older recipient age, and posttransplant malignancy.[71] The responsibility for individual transplant patients must be carefully balanced against the obligation to fairly allocate scarce donor organs.[72] Retransplantation is reserved for a highly select group of elective recipients with coronary vasculopathy or graft failure who have few comorbid conditions.

ETHICAL CONSIDERATIONS

Improving outcomes with medical therapy for heart failure coupled with a shortage of donor organs generates an imperative to restrict transplantation to those most disabled by heart failure and who are also most likely to derive maximum longevity. The utilitarian principle of providing the greatest good to the greatest number of heart failure patients underpins the rationing of scarce donor organs. In previous eras, the less favorable short-term and long-term outcomes of transplant recipients for CHD raised the ethical dilemma of allocating an organ to a recipient actuarially less likely to derive benefit compared with those with an ischemic or nonischemic cardiomyopathy. This creates a tension between the societal good of allocating organs to the best candidates versus the duty to care for an individual patient and respect for autonomy.[73]

Although the CHD population is expanding, CHD is likely to remain an uncommon indication for transplant for the foreseeable future. Transplantation often remains the only viable option to support the circulation of patients with complex CHD anatomy or residual shunting. MCS platforms, which in theory have an unlimited supply, do not confer the same benefits in the CHD, because most were designed to support the failing left ventricle and not for complex CHD anatomy.[52] Given the long waitlist time for transplant in CHD and the early hazard after surgery, one strategy to uncouple the higher-risk CHD population from the traditional waiting list is to use alternative donor lists. Such lists match high-risk recipients to older donor or more marginal donor hearts.[74] Despite expanding the donor pool, alternative transplant lists are not the answer to address the disparity in early outcomes and such lists remain available at only a few high-volume centers. Indiscriminate use of alternative donor lists could erode the progress seen in CHD outcomes and raises some concerns about equity in solid organ allocation yet may be the last remaining chance for high-risk transplant candidates.

The ethical landscape for adult CHD transplant has changed in recent years thanks to improving short-term and long-term outcomes. The percentage of CHD patients listed for transplant has remained stable even as the adult CHD population continues to expand. This suggests that the selection criteria for listing adults with CHD have become more stringent, perhaps with an emphasis on earlier-stage disease before critical end-organ dysfunction. Increased awareness of the special features of the CHD during the prelisting evaluation may have played some role. Thoughtful surgical planning and donor selection can produce outcomes in highly selected CHD patients that are on par with non-CHD patients. The contemporary pool of CHD transplant candidates is likely to realize the utility of transplantation, making the allocation of a donor organ to a CHD recipient more ethically defensible than in previous eras.

ACKNOWLEDGMENTS

Dr Stewart would like to thank the Kenneth L. Baughman Clinician Scholar Program in Cardiovascular Medicine at Brigham and Women's Hospital for its ongoing support.

REFERENCES

1. Brickner ME, Hillis LD, Lange RA. Congenital heart disease in adults. Second of two parts. N Engl J Med 2000;342:334–42.
2. Warnes CA, Liberthson R, Danielson GK, et al. Task force 1: the changing profile of congenital heart disease in adult life. J Am Coll Cardiol 2001;37: 1170–5.
3. Perloff JK, Warnes CA. Challenges posed by adults with repaired congenital heart disease. Circulation 2001;103:2637–43.
4. Opotowsky AR, Siddiqi OK, Webb GD. Trends in hospitalizations for adults with congenital heart disease in the U.S. J Am Coll Cardiol 2009;54:460–7.
5. Stehlik J, Edwards LB, Kucheryavaya AY, et al. The Registry of the International Society for Heart and Lung Transplantation: 29th official adult heart transplant report–2012. J Heart Lung Transplant 2012; 31:1052–64.
6. Christie JD, Edwards LB, Kucheryavaya AY, et al. The Registry of the International Society for Heart and Lung Transplantation: 29th adult lung and heart-lung transplant report-2012. J Heart Lung Transplant 2012;31:1073–86.
7. Bhama JK, Shulman J, Bermudez CA, et al. Heart transplantation for adults with congenital heart disease: results in the modern era. J Heart Lung Transplant 2013;32:499–504.
8. Davies RR, Russo MJ, Yang J, et al. Listing and transplanting adults with congenital heart disease. Circulation 2011;123:759–67.
9. Mehra MR, Kobashigawa J, Starling R, et al. Listing criteria for heart transplantation: International Society for Heart and Lung Transplantation guidelines for the care of cardiac transplant candidates–2006. J Heart Lung Transplant 2006;25:1024–42.
10. Kittleson MM, Kobashigawa JA. Management of advanced heart failure: the role of heart transplantation. Circulation 2011;123:1569–74.
11. Mancini D, Lietz K. Selection of cardiac transplantation candidates in 2010. Circulation 2010;122: 173–83.
12. Kinkhabwala MP, Mancini D. Patient selection for cardiac transplant in 2012. Expert Rev Cardiovasc Ther 2013;11:179–91.
13. Diller GP, Dimopoulos K, Okonko D, et al. Exercise intolerance in adult congenital heart disease: comparative severity, correlates, and prognostic implication. Circulation 2005;112:828–35.
14. Ehlert N, Hess J, Hager A. Shifts in exercise capacity are not reported adequately in patients with congenital heart disease. Congenit Heart Dis 2012;7:448–54.
15. Balady GJ, Arena R, Sietsema K, et al. Clinician's Guide to cardiopulmonary exercise testing in adults: a scientific statement from the American Heart Association. Circulation 2010;122:191–225.
16. Mancini DM, Eisen H, Kussmaul W, et al. Value of peak exercise oxygen consumption for optimal timing of cardiac transplantation in ambulatory patients with heart failure. Circulation 1991;83: 778–86.
17. Fernandes SM, Alexander ME, Graham DA, et al. Exercise testing identifies patients at increased risk for morbidity and mortality following Fontan surgery. Congenit Heart Dis 2011;6:294–303.
18. Aaronson KD, Schwartz JS, Chen TM, et al. Development and prospective validation of a clinical index to predict survival in ambulatory patients referred for cardiac transplant evaluation. Circulation 1997;95:2660–7.
19. Goda A, Lund LH, Mancini D. The Heart Failure Survival Score outperforms the peak oxygen consumption for heart transplantation selection in the era of device therapy. J Heart Lung Transplant 2011;30:315–25.
20. Dimopoulos K, Diller GP, Koltsida E, et al. Prevalence, predictors, and prognostic value of renal

dysfunction in adults with congenital heart disease. Circulation 2008;117:2320–8.

21. Gheorghiade M, Rossi JS, Cotts W, et al. Characterization and prognostic value of persistent hyponatremia in patients with severe heart failure in the ESCAPE Trial. Arch Intern Med 2007;167:1998–2005.

22. Dimopoulos K, Diller GP, Petraco R, et al. Hyponatraemia: a strong predictor of mortality in adults with congenital heart disease. Eur Heart J 2010;31:595–601.

23. Setoguchi S, Stevenson LW, Schneeweiss S. Repeated hospitalizations predict mortality in the community population with heart failure. Am Heart J 2007;154:260–6.

24. Kittleson M, Hurwitz S, Shah MR, et al. Development of circulatory-renal limitations to angiotensin-converting enzyme inhibitors identifies patients with severe heart failure and early mortality. J Am Coll Cardiol 2003;41:2029–35.

25. Fonarow GC, Abraham WT, Albert NM, et al. Influence of beta-blocker continuation or withdrawal on outcomes in patients hospitalized with heart failure: findings from the OPTIMIZE-HF program. J Am Coll Cardiol 2008;52:190–9.

26. Neuberg GW, Miller AB, O'Connor CM, et al. Diuretic resistance predicts mortality in patients with advanced heart failure. Am Heart J 2002;144:31–8.

27. Poole JE, Johnson GW, Hellkamp AS, et al. Prognostic importance of defibrillator shocks in patients with heart failure. N Engl J Med 2008;359:1009–17.

28. Warnes CA, Williams RG, Bashore TM, et al. ACC/AHA 2008 guidelines for the management of adults with congenital heart disease: a report of the American College of Cardiology/American Heart Association Task Force on Practice Guidelines (Writing Committee to Develop Guidelines on the Management of Adults With Congenital Heart Disease). Developed in Collaboration With the American Society of Echocardiography, Heart Rhythm Society, International Society for Adult Congenital Heart Disease, Society for Cardiovascular Angiography and Interventions, and Society of Thoracic Surgeons. J Am Coll Cardiol 2008;52:e143–263.

29. Attenhofer Jost CH, Schmidt D, Huebler M, et al. Heart transplantation in congenital heart disease: in whom to consider and when? J Transplant 2013;2013:376027.

30. Sian Pincott E, Burch M. Indications for heart transplantation in congenital heart disease. Curr Cardiol Rev 2011;7:51–8.

31. Stobierska-Dzierzek B, Awad H, Michler RE. The evolving management of acute right-sided heart failure in cardiac transplant recipients. J Am Coll Cardiol 2001;38:923–31.

32. Costard-Jackle A, Fowler MB. Influence of preoperative pulmonary artery pressure on mortality after heart transplantation: testing of potential reversibility of pulmonary hypertension with nitroprusside is useful in defining a high risk group. J Am Coll Cardiol 1992;19:48–54.

33. Butler J, Stankewicz MA, Wu J, et al. Pre-transplant reversible pulmonary hypertension predicts higher risk for mortality after cardiac transplantation. J Heart Lung Transplant 2005;24:170–7.

34. Breinholt JP 3rd, Hawkins JA, Lambert LM, et al. A prospective analysis of the simmunogenicity of cryopreserved nonvalved allografts used in pediatric heart surgery. Circulation 2000;102:III179–82.

35. O'Connor MJ, Lind C, Tang X, et al. Persistence of anti-human leukocyte antibodies in congenital heart disease late after surgery using allografts and whole blood. J Heart Lung Transplant 2013;32:390–7.

36. Pagani FD, Dyke DB, Wright S, et al. Development of anti-major histocompatibility complex class I or II antibodies following left ventricular assist device implantation: effects on subsequent allograft rejection and survival. J Heart Lung Transplant 2001;20:646–53.

37. Patel ND, Weiss ES, Allen JG, et al. Heart transplantation for adults with congenital heart disease: analysis of the United network for organ sharing database. Ann Thorac Surg 2009;88:814–21 [discussion: 821–2].

38. Kobashigawa J, Mehra M, West L, et al. Report from a consensus conference on the sensitized patient awaiting heart transplantation. J Heart Lung Transplant 2009;28:213–25.

39. Rossano JW, Morales DL, Zafar F, et al. Impact of antibodies against human leukocyte antigens on long-term outcome in pediatric heart transplant patients: an analysis of the United Network for Organ Sharing database. J Thorac Cardiovasc Surg 2010;140:694–9, 699.e1–2.

40. Kim MS, Kato TS, Farr M, et al. Hepatic dysfunction in ambulatory patients with heart failure: application of the MELD scoring system for outcome prediction. J Am Coll Cardiol 2013;61:2253–61.

41. Chokshi A, Cheema FH, Schaefle KJ, et al. Hepatic dysfunction and survival after orthotopic heart transplantation: application of the MELD scoring system for outcome prediction. J Heart Lung Transplant 2012;31:591–600.

42. Dichtl W, Vogel W, Dunst KM, et al. Cardiac hepatopathy before and after heart transplantation. Transpl Int 2005;18:697–702.

43. Kiesewetter CH, Sheron N, Vettukattill JJ, et al. Hepatic changes in the failing Fontan circulation. Heart 2007;93:579–84.

44. van Nieuwenhuizen RC, Peters M, Lubbers LJ, et al. Abnormalities in liver function and

coagulation profile following the Fontan procedure. Heart 1999;82:40–6.

45. Samsky MD, Patel CB, Dewald TA, et al. Cardiohepatic interactions in heart failure: an overview and clinical implications. J Am Coll Cardiol 2013;61: 2397–405.

46. Baek JS, Bae EJ, Ko JS, et al. Late hepatic complications after Fontan operation; non-invasive markers of hepatic fibrosis and risk factors. Heart 2010;96:1750–5.

47. Cannon RM, Hughes MG, Jones CM, et al. A review of the United States experience with combined heart-liver transplantation. Transpl Int 2012; 25:1223–8.

48. Marino BS, Lipkin PH, Newburger JW, et al. Neurodevelopmental outcomes in children with congenital heart disease: evaluation and management: a scientific statement from the American Heart Association. Circulation 2012;126:1143–72.

49. Ammash N, Warnes CA. Cerebrovascular events in adult patients with cyanotic congenital heart disease. J Am Coll Cardiol 1996;28:768–72.

50. Rodan L, McCrindle BW, Manlhiot C, et al. Stroke recurrence in children with congenital heart disease. Ann Neurol 2012;72:103–11.

51. Miatton M, De Wolf D, Francois K, et al. Neurocognitive consequences of surgically corrected congenital heart defects: a review. Neuropsychol Rev 2006;16:65–85.

52. Rossano JW, Kaufman BD, Rame JE. Ethical considerations related to the use of mechanical support in congenital heart disease. World J Pediatr Congenit Heart Surg 2013;4:70–4.

53. Shah NR, Lam WW, Rodriguez FH 3rd, et al. Clinical outcomes after ventricular assist device implantation in adults with complex congenital heart disease. J Heart Lung Transplant 2013;32: 615–20.

54. Clark JB, Pauliks LB, Myers JL, et al. Mechanical circulatory support for end-stage heart failure in repaired and palliated congenital heart disease. Curr Cardiol Rev 2011;7:102–9.

55. Miller LW, Pagani FD, Russell SD, et al. Use of a continuous-flow device in patients awaiting heart transplantation. N Engl J Med 2007;357: 885–96.

56. Simpson KE, Cibulka N, Lee CK, et al. Failed Fontan heart transplant candidates with preserved vs impaired ventricular ejection: 2 distinct patient populations. J Heart Lung Transplant 2012;31: 545–7.

57. Goerler H, Simon A, Gohrbandt B, et al. Heart-lung and lung transplantation in grown-up congenital heart disease: long-term single centre experience. Eur J Cardiothorac Surg 2007;32:926–31.

58. Jensen AS, Johansson PI, Idorn L, et al. The haematocrit - an important factor causing impaired haemostasis in patients with cyanotic congenital heart disease. Int J Cardiol 2013; 167(4):1317–21.

59. Hasan A, Au J, Hamilton JR, et al. Orthotopic heart transplantation for congenital heart disease. Technical considerations. Eur J Cardiothorac Surg 1993;7:65–70.

60. Hosseinpour AR, Gonzalez-Calle A, Adsuar-Gomez A, et al. Surgical technique for heart transplantation: a strategy for congenital heart disease. Eur J Cardiothorac Surg 2013;44(4): 598–604.

61. Hosseinpour AR, Cullen S, Tsang VT. Transplantation for adults with congenital heart disease. Eur J Cardiothorac Surg 2006;30:508–14.

62. Chen JM, Davies RR, Mital SR, et al. Trends and outcomes in transplantation for complex congenital heart disease: 1984 to 2004. Ann Thorac Surg 2004;78:1352–61 [discussion: 1352–61].

63. Lamour JM, Kanter KR, Naftel DC, et al. The effect of age, diagnosis, and previous surgery in children and adults undergoing heart transplantation for congenital heart disease. J Am Coll Cardiol 2009; 54:160–5.

64. Karamlou T, Hirsch J, Welke K, et al. A United Network for Organ Sharing analysis of heart transplantation in adults with congenital heart disease: outcomes and factors associated with mortality and retransplantation. J Thorac Cardiovasc Surg 2010;140:161–8.

65. Khairy P, Fernandes SM, Mayer JE Jr, et al. Long-term survival, modes of death, and predictors of mortality in patients with Fontan surgery. Circulation 2008;117:85–92.

66. Bernstein D, Naftel D, Chin C, et al. Outcome of listing for cardiac transplantation for failed Fontan: a multi-institutional study. Circulation 2006;114: 273–80.

67. Mitchell MB, Campbell DN, Boucek MM. Heart transplantation for the failing Fontan circulation. Semin Thorac Cardiovasc Surg Pediatr Card Surg Annu 2004;7:56–64.

68. Pigula FA, Gandhi SK, Ristich J, et al. Cardiopulmonary transplantation for congenital heart disease in the adult. J Heart Lung Transplant 2001; 20:297–303.

69. Shuhaiber JH, Kim JB, Hur K, et al. Comparison of survival in primary and repeat heart transplantation from 1987 through 2004 in the United States. Ann Thorac Surg 2007;83:2135–41.

70. Tsao L, Uriel N, Leitz K, et al. Higher rate of comorbidities after cardiac retransplantation contributes to decreased survival. J Heart Lung Transplant 2009;28:1072–4.

71. Goerler H, Simon A, Gohrbandt B, et al. Cardiac re-transplantation: is it justified in times of critical donor organ shortage? Long-term single-center experience. Eur J Cardiothorac Surg 2008;34: 1185–90.

72. Kaufman BD, Jessup M. Adult and pediatric perspectives on heart retransplant. World J Pediatr Congenit Heart Surg 2013;4:75–9.

73. Gries CJ, White DB, Truog RD, et al. An official American Thoracic Society/International Society for Heart and Lung Transplantation/Society of Critical Care Medicine/Association of Organ and Procurement Organizations/United Network of Organ Sharing Statement: ethical and policy considerations in organ donation after circulatory determination of death. Am J Respir Crit Care Med 2013; 188:103–9.

74. Alexander JW, Zola JC. Expanding the donor pool: use of marginal donors for solid organ transplantation. Clin Transplant 1996;10:1–19.

Heart Failure in Congenital Heart Disease
A Confluence of Acquired and Congenital

Akl C. Fahed, MD[a,b], Amy E. Roberts, MD[c],
Seema Mital, MD[d], Neal K. Lakdawala, MD[e,f],*

KEYWORDS

- Heart failure • Congenital heart disease • Genomics • Adult

KEY POINTS

- Heart failure (HF) is a major cause of morbidity and mortality in adults with congenital heart disease (ACHD) and the current approach for its treatment is rarely evidence based.
- Rare monogenic causes of congenital heart disease (CHD) and HF include Noonan syndrome, Williams-Beuren syndrome, and 22q11 syndrome.
- Overlapping molecular pathways between CHD and HF exist, and their interrogation will create a better understanding of the development of HF in CHD.
- HF in ACHD is most commonly a result of a confluence between inherited complex genetic factors and acquired stressors caused by the defect.
- Current technologies such as next-generation sequencing and iPS will contribute to the understanding of this confluence and lead to novel therapeutics.

INTRODUCTION

Congenital heart disease (CHD) encompasses all malformations of the heart that occur in utero and exist at birth and is estimated to affect at least 8.1 per 1000 live births.[1] The prevalence of complex and hemodynamically significant lesions, which result in early deaths if not addressed via surgical or percutaneous methods, is 2.3 per 1000 infants.[2] The past 3 decades have witnessed marked progress in pediatric cardiology and cardiac surgery, allowing patients to survive to adulthood. As a result, the adult population with CHD (ACHD) outnumbers the pediatric population with

CHD in the United States.[2,3] An analysis of 71,686 patients with CHD between 1987 and 2005 revealed that infant CHD mortality has decreased dramatically, but with a shifting mortality burden toward adulthood.[4] Heart failure (HF) is the major problem in ACHD, because nearly one-quarter of patients develop heart failure at 30 years.[5] The events inciting HF in patients with ACHD are different than in other forms of HF; however, there are limited data available to guide their management. Consensus guidelines for diagnosis and treatment of HF are often used for patients with ACHD with HF because adequate controlled data are lacking for this subpopulation.[6]

The authors have no conflicts of interest to disclose.
^a Department of Genetics, Harvard Medical School, 77 Avenue Louis Pasteur, Boston, MA 02115, USA;
^b Department of Medicine, Massachusetts General Hospital, 55 Fruit Street, Boston, MA 02114, USA;
^c Division of Genetics, Department of Cardiology, Boston Children's Hospital, 300 Longwood Avenue, Boston, MA 02115, USA; ^d Division of Cardiology, Department of Pediatrics, Hospital for Sick Children, University of Toronto, 555 University Avenue, Toronto, ON M5G 1X8, Canada; ^e Division of Cardiovascular Medicine, Brigham and Women's Hospital, 75 Francis Street, Boston, MA 02115, USA; ^f Division of Cardiology, VA Boston Health Care, Harvard Medical School, 1400 VFW Parkway, Boston, MA, USA
* Corresponding author. Division of Cardiovascular Medicine, Brigham and Women's Hospital, 75 Francis Street, Boston, MA 02115.
E-mail address: nlakdawala@partners.org

Heart Failure Clin 10 (2014) 219–227
http://dx.doi.org/10.1016/j.hfc.2013.09.017
1551-7136/14/$ – see front matter Published by Elsevier Inc.

Advances in cardiac genetics have paralleled improvements in the treatment of CHD. Over the past 2 decades, 50% to 70% of the genetic causes of inherited cardiomyopathies were established through increasingly powerful methods of DNA analysis. Discovery of the genetics of nonsyndromic CHD lags behind the inherited cardiomyopathies. Sequencing initially identified mutations in transcription factor genes involved in heart development in familial cases, and most sporadic CHD has remained unexplained. This is likely because of the complexity of the underlying genetic causes; multiple mutations may increase the risk of CHD, in an additive fashion, or manifest in the presence of environmental factors and result in cardiac malformation. Current research emphasizes the important role of gene-environment interactions and epigenetics in CHD.

As the molecular signatures of CHD and HF are characterized with the use of available technology, it is increasingly appreciated that at least some disease pathways are shared. Determining the molecular basis of HF in ACHD will play a crucial role in developing treatment strategies for this growing population. This article summarizes the limited current knowledge of the genetics of HF in ACHD, and discusses how innovative therapies may be discovered for this population.

ROUTES TO HF IN PATIENTS WITH CHD

The progression to HF in patients with CHD involves proven and hypothesized mechanisms, which we classify into 3 routes (**Figs. 1** and **2**). The first route is purely acquired and mechanical, with no genetic element, and includes incomplete or palliative correction of a lesion leading to a chronic state of hemodynamic stress and subsequent heart failure.[6] The probability of heart failure in CHD lesions such as tetralogy of Fallot (TOF), and transposition of the great arteries (TGA) can be as high as 80% at 50 years of age, whereas it is around 20% to 30% for isolated valvular disease or defects that result in left-to-right shunt.[6] Additional myocardial insults can complicate surgery, including injury to the myocardium, coronary arteries, and conduction system.[6] Postsurgical conduction disease may require permanent ventricular pacing, which can lead to progressive contractile dysfunction.[6] Because these insults often occur in the first years of life, the effects of altered hemodynamics or tissue injury accumulate over the years, resulting in early development of HF.

Although the increased prevalence of HF in ACHD is primarily a result of a volume or pressure overload, whereby the starting point is an abnormal heart, an independent genetic component is also present. This second route (depicted in **Fig. 1**) delineates a purely genetic component that causes both cardiac malformation and a cardiomyopathy that result in HF, unrelated to hemodynamic stress. Many of the pathways involved in cardiac development in utero are also involved in myocardial structure and stability. Therefore, certain molecular perturbations can cause both a cardiac defect at birth and a cardiomyopathy that can present later in life, often in childhood. As described in greater detail later, Noonan syndrome (NS) is the second most frequent syndromic form of CHD and can

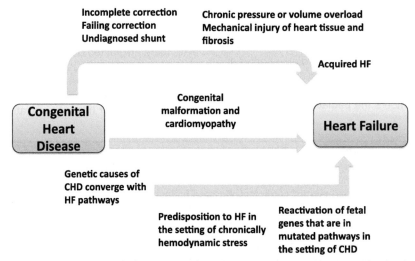

Fig. 1. The hypothesized mechanisms linking CHD with HF. We propose 3 putative routes that lead to HF in ACHD: rare monogenic entities that cause both CHD and HF (*middle arrow*); severe CHD lesions in which acquired hemodynamic effects of CHD or surgery result in HF (*top arrow*); and, most commonly, a combined effect of complex genetics in overlapping pathways and acquired stressors caused by the lesion (*bottom arrow*).

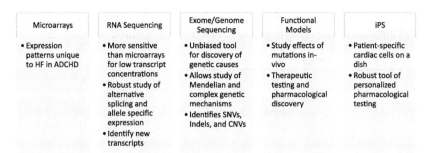

Microarrays	RNA Sequencing	Exome/Genome Sequencing	Functional Models	iPS
• Expression patterns unique to HF in ADCHD	• More sensitive than microarrays for low transcript concentrations • Robust study of alternative splicing and allele specific expression • Identify new transcripts	• Unbiased tool for discovery of genetic causes • Allows study of Mendelian and complex genetic mechanisms • Identifies SNVs, Indels, and CNVs	• Study effects of mutations in-vivo • Therapeutic testing and pharmacological discovery	• Patient-specific cardiac cells on a dish • Robust tool of personalized pharmacological testing

Fig. 2. Current genomic technologies and proposed mechanisms of contribution to the understanding of HF in ACHD. iPS, induced pluripotent stem cells. ACHD, adults with congenital heart disease; CNV, copy number variation; SNV, single nucleotide variants.

cause both CHD and cardiomyopathy. Another example of congenital cardiomyopathy is left ventricular noncompaction (LVNC), a heterogeneous disorder that often results in HF. LVNC has been associated with CHD including atrial and ventricular septal defects, Ebstein anomaly, and outflow tract lesions, and is caused by genes such as *MYH7* and the transcription factor *NKX2-5*, among others.[7-10]

In a Dutch registry of 10,808 patients with CHD followed for 21 years (median), the incidence of HF admissions was 1.2 per 1000 patient years and median age at first HF admission was 46.7 years. This incidence of HF admissions in patients with ACHD is more than 10 times what is reported in an age-matched cohort without CHD (0.1 per 1000 person years).[11] The true prevalence of HF is thought to be higher because not all HF events in patients with CHD resulted in hospital admission. Low-prevalence CHD lesions such as TGA and TOF that result in HF via markedly abnormal hemodynamics do not solely account for the epidemic of HF in CHD. Moreover, gene mutations that cause both cardiomyopathy and CHD are rare. Therefore, it is unlikely that these two routes alone explain the high incidence of HF in CHD, which suggests additional mechanisms through which patients with CHD can develop HF. This mechanism is the third route shown in **Fig. 1**, which is a combination of congenital genetic risk and acquired hemodynamic stressors. There is significant overlap in the molecular pathways that result in CHD during development and those that are responsible for the integrity of the postnatal myocardium. This overlap suggests that molecular perturbations that result in abnormal cardiac development can increase the risk for HF in adulthood, especially in the presence of chronically perturbed hemodynamics. HF also involves the reactivation of many fetal genes. The reactivation of a mutated pathway is expected to exacerbate the progression to HF in the setting of CHD. With the current era of high-throughput

DNA, RNA, protein, and metabolic analysis, this hypothesis can be studied using a systems biology approach to investigate the development of HF in patients with CHD, particularly those with mild phenotypes whose progression to HF might not be justified by the degree of volume or pressure overload caused by the lesion.

MONOGENIC CAUSES OF HF IN CARDIOMYOPATHY AND CHD

The genetic basis of hypertrophic cardiomyopathy (HCM) was first described in 1990.[12,13] Following this discovery, the principal genetic causes of hypertrophic, dilated, and arrhythmogenic cardiomyopathies have been identified. Depending on phenotype, a disease-causing mutation can be found in 30% to 70% of patients. Culprit genes encode structural proteins such as those that form the sarcomere, cellular cytoskeleton, or ion channels (**Table 1**).[14] Genetic testing for inherited cardiomyopathies is clinically available and improves the efficiency of family screening, enabling early diagnosis and timely clinical management in at-risk individuals.[15]

As an alternative, the clinical application of CHD genetics remains limited. Monogenic causes of CHD are estimated to account for only 5% to 10% of disease, usually related to loss-of-function mutations in transcription factor genes and other signaling molecules that disturb molecular pathways during cardiac development (see **Table 1**).[16] Monogenic causes have predominantly been identified in syndromic cases in which CHD occurs with noncardiac congenital malformations.[16] In only a minority of presentations is genetic testing available and useful. Genetic testing is available for most syndromic cases. To name few examples, Holt-Oram syndrome, which causes CHD and upper limb malformations, is caused by mutations in *TBX5* and *SALL4* genes.[16] Alagille syndrome, causing CHD along with liver disease, is caused by mutations in the *JAG1* or *NOTCH2* genes.[16]

Table 1
Comparison of differences and similarities between CHD and cardiomyopathy

	CHD	Cardiomyopathy
Differences		
Phenotype	Wide spectrum of cardiac malformations including the valves, septa, and great vessels	Dilation or hypertrophy of the myocardium ± disease of the conduction system; results in HF or SCD
Expression	Present at birth (by definition)	Typical disease onset is in adolescence or adulthood, but can express at any age
Genetics	LOF mutations in transcription factor genes and other signaling molecules that disturb molecular pathways during cardiac development	Mutations in structural genes involving proteins of the sarcomere, cellular cytoskeleton, or ion channels
Population attributable risk of genetic causes (%)	5–10	50–70
Clinical genetic testing	Not recommended except in rare syndromic cases	Recommended in most familial cases
Similarities		
Phenotype	Several syndromes with CHD and congenital CMP; co-occurrence of LVNC with CHD	
Expression	Congenital cardiomyopathies occurring in the setting of CHD	
Genetics	Multiple shared pathways between heart development and myocardial disease; few genes that cause both CHD and congenital CMP; multiple genes that cause CHD have altered expression in the setting of HF	

Abbreviations: CMP, cardiomyopathy; LOF, loss of function; SCD, sudden cardiac death.

Among the nonsyndromic genes, *GATA4* and *Nkx2-5* are two well-established genes in familial CHD,[16] and are also available for clinical genetic testing. The genetic cause of nonsyndromic CHD is less well understood, and clinical genetic testing is not routinely advised for such patients.[17,18] However, there are several genetically characterized syndromes in which CHD and HF are common morbidities, including NS, Williams-Beuren syndrome (WBS), and 22.q11.2 deletion syndrome.

NS, in which HCM is the second most common cardiac manifestation, is a representative example. NS results from abnormal RAS-MAPK signaling, which normally regulates cellular proliferation, differentiation, and survival.[19] Mutations in different components of the RAS-MAPK pathway have been described, including *PTPN11, KRAS, SOS1, NRAS, RAF1, SHOC2*, and *CBL*[19,20]; which typically result in constitutive activation.[19] The 20% of patients with NS who develop HCM present with a wide phenotypic spectrum, with approximately 25% dying of HF in the first year of life.[19] The CHD manifestations of NS are pulmonary stenosis, present in more than 50% of cases, and secundum atrial septal defect in 6% to 10%. Other

less common malformations include ventricular septal defect, atrioventricular canal, aortic stenosis, and coarctation.[19] Common extracardiac manifestations of NS include short stature and facial dysmorphism.[20] Adults with NS have cardiac complications of the syndrome that frequently result in HF, whether caused by the cardiomyopathy, the associated valvular disease, or both.[21] The limited natural history data in NS suggest that cardiovascular complications are a major cause of mortality.[22] NS with multiple lentigenes (formerly known as LEOPARD [lentigines, electrocardiogram abnormalities, ocular hypertelorism, pulmonic stenosis, abnormalities of genitalia, retardation of growth, and deafness] syndrome) is similar to NS, is caused by loss of function mutations in the *PTPN11* gene, and has a high frequency (>70%) of associated HCM.[23] Additional manifestations of this rare syndrome include multiple lentigines and sensorineural deafness.[24]

WBS is caused by a microdeletion on chromosome 7q11.23, a region that includes 26 to 28 genes.[25] The syndrome is characterized in most cases by supravalvular aortic stenosis (SVAS), mental retardation, and distinctive facial features.[25]

Loss of 1 allele of the *ELN* gene, which encodes elastin and resides on the 7q11.23 locus, causes familial SVAS without the other manifestations of WBS.[25] Severe SVAS in children leads to cardiac hypertrophy and HF unless corrected surgically. Adults with SVAS have high risk of cardiovascular complications; of 113 patients with median 6-year follow-up, 7.3% developed new-onset HF.[26]

The 22q11.2 microdeletion syndrome (also known as DiGeorge or velocardiofacial syndrome) has a diverse phenotypic spectrum. Common manifestations include ventricular outflow tract defects, facial dysmorphism, hypocalcemia, and immunodeficiency.[21] The syndrome is caused by a 1.5-Mb to 3-Mb hemizygous deletion on chromosome 22q11.2 and most clinical manifestations, especially the cardiac malformations, are explained by the loss of 1 allele of the *TBX1* gene.[21] The most common outflow tract defects seen in the syndrome are TOF, type B interrupted aortic arch (IAA), and truncus arteriosus (TA). Microdeletion in the same region may cause isolated CHD without obvious extracardiac syndromic manifestations.[21] Complications of these malformations in adulthood are common and include recoarctation of an IAA that was previously surgically reconstructed, residual or acquired obstruction of the left ventricular outflow tract, or arrhythmias that arise after repair of TOF.[21] Genetic testing for 22q11.2 deletion is readily available and recommended for CHD lesions typical of the 22q11.2 syndrome, including aortic arch abnormalities.[27] Genetic diagnosis may have clinical implications, because in patients with isolated TOF and 22q11.2 deletion there is evidence for an increased prevalence of aortic root dilatation.[28]

Several other genes have been associated with familial forms of nonsyndromic CHD. Evidence is most robust for loss of function (LOF) mutations in *GATA4*, *TBX5*, and *NKX2-5*, which are transcription factors expressed in the developing heart,[16] although other transcription factors and signaling molecules have been implicated. The transcripts of these three genes form a complex that regulates downstream targets involved in the regulation of cardiac development. LOF mutations in these genes can be a result of nonsense or frameshift mutations that cause a truncated protein or can be caused by copy number variation (CNV), which result in loss or gain of a copy of a gene. For example, at least 10% of TOF are caused by de novo CNVs.[29] In addition to identifying the role of CNVs in CHD, the advent of exome sequencing is starting to yield a better understanding of novel molecular causes of CHD. A recent study showed that de novo LOF mutations in histone-modifying genes contribute to 10% of severe CHD,

highlighting a unique role for epigenetic mechanisms involved in the molecular pathophysiology of CHD.[18] Identification of CHD as part of a genetic syndrome would allow prediction of not only cardiac but also extracardiac outcomes as well as interventions to modify them (eg, aggressive monitoring and treatment of hypertension and of coronary artery lesions in WBS that may contribute to cardiac hypertrophy and dysfunction). This development may help personalize the care of the adult patient with CHD at risk for HF.

OVERLAPPING PATHWAYS IN CHD AND HF GENETICS

Although the genetics of CHD and HF in humans has been studied separately, with the few directly shared disease genes described to date, there is significant evidence from model organisms and in vitro studies that similar molecular pathways are involved (**Table 2**). Several genes involved in embryonic cardiac development continue to be expressed in the adult heart, in which they play a role in maintaining cardiomyocyte survival and integrity. *GATA4* and *GATA6* are transcription factor genes that are mutated in familial cases of CHD.[16] In addition to their role in cardiac development, they are potent activators of cardiac promoters such as atrial natriuretic factor and B-type natriuretic peptide in the adult heart.[30] They also regulate the transcription of cardiac sarcomere genes, namely alpha-myosin and beta-myosin heavy chain.[30] Moreover, *GATA4* is

---

Table 2
Canonical pathways from IPA analysis of CHD candidate genes that have major roles in HF

Pathway	Candidate Genes in CHD
Wnt/β-catenin signaling	SOX2, GJA1, CREBBP
HIF1α signaling	CREBBP, HRAS, NAA10
Cardiac hypertrophy signaling	NKX2-5, ADCY2, SOS1, CREBBP, HRAS, GATA4
Noonan pathway	SOS1, PTPN11
BMP signaling pathway	NKX2-5, SOS1, CREBBP, HRAS, PITX2
TGF-β signaling	NKX2-5, SOS1, CREBBP, HRAS, PITX2
JAK/Stat signaling	PTPN11, SOS1, HRAS
RAR activation	NSD1, ADCY2, CREBBP, PML, CITED2
PPARα/RXRα activation	ADCY2, SOS1, CREBBP, HRAS, MED12

Abbreviations: BMP, bone morphogenetic protein; TGF, transforming growth factor.

a survival factor for adult cardiomyocytes because it also regulates the antiapoptotic gene BCL-X.[31] Myocyte apoptosis is a major element in the pathophysiology of HF, and genetic or pharmacologic enhancement of GATA4 can prevent cardiomyocyte toxicity and drug-induced cardiotoxicity, such as with doxorubicin treatment, in which GATA4 depletion is an early event.[31] These data suggest that GATA4 is a potential target in HF treatment, and that patients with CHD with LOF mutations in their GATA4 or GATA6 genes might have increased apoptosis of their cardiomyocytes predisposing them to HF in the setting of other insults such as volume overload caused by CHD. GATA4 also plays a role in calcium-calcineurin signaling responsible for cardiac hypertrophy and HF.[32] Calcineurin dephosphorylates nuclear factor of activated T cells (NFATC), which results in its translocation to the nucleus, where it binds GATA4 and activates transcription of a hypertrophic gene program.[32] NFATC transcription factor is essential for valve formation in mice,[33] and mutations in NFATC1 have been associated with CHD in humans.[34,35] Recent murine data also suggest an important role for NFATC transcription factors in the cardiomyocyte response to stress.[36] Calcineurin also activates calmodulin-dependent protein kinase and results in phosphorylation of histone deacetylase (HDAC), a nuclear protein causing its dissociation from the transcription factor myocyte enhancer factor 2 (MEF2) and its externalization from the nucleus.[32] MEF2 transcription factors are the second effectors of calcineurin signaling, and also play critical roles in both cardiac development and normal postnatal myocardial survival.[37] This calcium-dependent signaling pathway constitutes an excellent potential target in HF and/or cardiac hypertrophy.[32]

Epigenetics, particularly the role of molecules such as HDAC that are responsible for DNA methylation and histone modifications, represents another shared pathway in CHD and HF. The importance of increased DNA methylation of genes in cardiomyopathy hearts compared with controls has been described,[38,39] and a large exome sequencing project recently identified that de novo truncating mutations in similar histone-modifying genes is seen in ~10% of sporadic CHD.[18] HF progression involves a pattern of gene expression including reexpression of fetal genes involved in cardiac development, increased expression of genes encoding extracellular matrix proteins, altered calcium signaling, and histone modification.[40] These processes involve genes that can be mutated in the setting of CHD. Therefore, preexisting defects in these pathways can potentially worsen the progression to HF in patients with CHD. Addressing this hypothesis is a methodological challenge that has only recently become possible with the advent of technologies such as next-generation sequencing. Although this article does not explore all potential overlapping molecular pathways in HF and CHD, the examples of epigenetics, transcription factors, and calcium-dependent signaling that are discussed serve as putative examples. Using IPA (Ingenuity Systems, www.ingenuity.com), a software toolkit to model and analyze complex biologic systems, we performed a rapid analysis of canonical pathways on a set of 146 literature-curated genes known to be involved in CHD in humans or in animal models. This analysis yielded multiple pathways that are known to be involved in HF (see **Table 2**). Genes involved in hypoxia-inducible factor (HIF) 1-alpha signaling are activated in cardiac hypertrophy,[41] whereas their downregulation is associated with the development of TGA in mice.[42] Other signaling pathways such as Wnt/β-catenin, transforming growth factor-β, and JAK/Stat are similarly involved in HF and, at the same time, harbor CHD candidate genes. In understanding the genomics of HF there have been many milestones, but most of the work has been focused on identifying the molecular signature of ischemic and nonischemic cardiomyopathies and trying to target the ensuing HF.[43,44] Patients with CHD with HF constitute a smaller niche that has not been interrogated. Studies of gene expression profiles through RNA sequencing of human hearts with CHD and HF and corresponding controls will be valuable to the understanding of the unique molecular causes of HF in patients with CHD.

THE FUTURE OF PERSONALIZED TREATMENT OF HF IN ACHD

Current treatment of HF in ACHD involves therapies that limit neurohumoral activation and are based on extrapolation from adults with HF unrelated to CHD. Although using beta-adrenergic blockers, aldosterone antagonism, and angiotensin inhibition has intuitive appeal, there are limited data to support the use of these drugs in the ACHD population with HF. Emerging data challenge the notion that conventional HF therapies can be extrapolated to patients with ACHD with HF. For example, a recent trial of valsartan in patients with a systemic right ventricle failed to show any beneficial effect on the primary end point of right ventricular ejection fraction, and most secondary end points.[45] This trial suggests that the ACHD population might have unique genetic and acquired factors that make medications used in common causes of HF ineffective. Pharmacogenomic studies have established that single-nucleotide polymorphisms (SNPs) in adrenergic receptors could modify the response to β-blockers.[46] In patients with CHD, SNPs in HF pathways targeted by pharmacotherapy can potentially result in resistance to drug therapy. Such studies are needed for patients with CHD to have better tailored therapies. In one successful example, polymorphisms in the renin-angiotensisn-aldosterone system genes were used to identify a subgroup of high-risk patients with single ventricles that did not show reverse remodeling after staged surgery.[47] This high-risk subset may benefit from earlier volume-unloading surgery before injury becomes irreversible. A study in surgically repaired patients with TOF identified variations in HIF1-alpha genes that were associated with right ventricle dilatation and dysfunction during follow-up likely related to maladaptive response to hypoxia and hemodynamic load.[48] It raised the possibility that earlier repair of TOF may limit hypoxic injury of the myocardium and promote better long-term adaptation. These studies show the power of genomics in guiding clinical decisions, including surgical decisions. These studies need to be done in adult patients with CHD to determine whether the effect of genetic variations on adverse ventricular remodeling persists into adulthood.

Another promising aspect of how genomics can help tailor therapy in HF in ACHD is targeted therapy for particular pathways known to be involved in the progression to heart failure. Although it is early to discuss therapeutics because most of the complex genetic aspects of HF in CHD remain incompletely understood, there has been at least one example with inhibition of the pathways that leads to HCM in NS, in which a clinical trial using a MEK1 inhibitor is underway (www.clinicaltrials.gov NCT01556568). Once other pathways are clearly defined, similar targeted therapy for the prevention of HF in other forms of ACHD may follow. Progress toward this goal has been enabled by high-throughput sequencing technologies and the availability of patient-specific induced pluripotent stem cells (iPS) from patients with cardiomyopathies in which drug-specific cardiotoxicity was shown at the single-cell level.[49] These cells could be used for rapid screening of cardioactive drugs with the patient's genetic background, an approach being assessed in primary cardiomyopathy.[50,51]

SUMMARY

HF is a major cause of morbidity and mortality in ACHD and the current approach for its treatment is rarely evidence based. Rare monogenic causes of CHD and HF include NS, WBS, and 22q11 syndrome. Overlapping molecular pathways between CHD and HF exist, and their interrogation will lead to a better understanding of the development of HF in CHD. HF in ACHD is most commonly a result of a confluence between inherited complex genetic factors and acquired stressors caused by the defect. Current technologies such as next-generation sequencing and iPS will contribute to the understanding of this confluence and lead to novel therapeutics.

REFERENCES

1. Montana E, Khoury MJ, Cragan JD, et al. Trends and outcomes after prenatal diagnosis of congenital cardiac malformations by fetal echocardiography in a well defined birth population, Atlanta, Georgia, 1990-1994. J Am Coll Cardiol 1996;28(7):1805–9.
2. Webb CL, Jenkins KJ, Karpawich PP, et al. Collaborative care for adults with congenital heart disease. Circulation 2002;105(19):2318–23.
3. Greutmann M, Tobler D. Changing epidemiology and mortality in adult congenital heart disease: looking into the future. Future Cardiol 2012;8(2):171–7.
4. Khairy P, Ionescu-Ittu R, Mackie AS, et al. Changing mortality in congenital heart disease. J Am Coll Cardiol 2010;56(14):1149–57.
5. Norozi K, Wessel A, Alpers V, et al. Incidence and risk distribution of heart failure in adolescents and adults with congenital heart disease after cardiac surgery. Am J Cardiol 2006;97(8):1238–43.
6. Parekh DR. A review of heart failure in adults with congenital heart disease. Methodist Debakey Cardiovasc J 2011;7(2):26–32.
7. Cavusoglu Y, Ata N, Timuralp B, et al. Noncompaction of the ventricular myocardium: report of two cases with bicuspid aortic valve demonstrating poor prognosis and with prominent right ventricular involvement. Echocardiography 2003;20(4):379–83.
8. Ichida F, Tsubata S, Bowles KR, et al. Novel gene mutations in patients with left ventricular noncompaction or Barth syndrome. Circulation 2001; 103(9):1256–63.
9. Puley G, Siu S, Connelly M, et al. Arrhythmia and survival in patients >18 years of age after the Mustard procedure for complete transposition of the great arteries. Am J Cardiol 1999;83(7):1080–4.
10. Wessels MW, De Graaf BM, Cohen-Overbeek TE, et al. A new syndrome with noncompaction cardiomyopathy, bradycardia, pulmonary stenosis, atrial septal defect and heterotaxy with suggestive linkage to chromosome 6p. Hum Genet 2008;122(6):595–603.
11. Zomer AC, Vaartjes I, van der Velde ET, et al. Heart failure admissions in adults with congenital heart disease; risk factors and prognosis. Int J Cardiol 2013;168:2487–93.

12. Jarcho JA, McKenna W, Pare JA, et al. Mapping a gene for familial hypertrophic cardiomyopathy to chromosome 14q1. N Engl J Med 1989;321(20): 1372–8.

13. Geisterfer-Lowrance AA, Kass S, Tanigawa G, et al. A molecular basis for familial hypertrophic cardiomyopathy: a beta cardiac myosin heavy chain gene missense mutation. Cell 1990;62(5): 999–1006.

14. Teekakirikul P, Kelly MA, Rehm HL, et al. Inherited cardiomyopathies: molecular genetics and clinical genetic testing in the postgenomic era. J Mol Diagn 2013;15(2):158–70.

15. Ingles J, McGaughran J, Scuffham PA, et al. A cost-effectiveness model of genetic testing for the evaluation of families with hypertrophic cardiomyopathy. Heart 2012;98(8):625–30.

16. Fahed AC, Gelb BD, Seidman JG, et al. Genetics of congenital heart disease: the glass half empty. Circ Res 2013;112(4):707–20.

17. Gelb B, Brueckner M, Chung W, et al. The Congenital Heart Disease Genetic Network Study: rationale, design, and early results. Circ Res 2013; 112(4):698–706.

18. Zaidi S, Choi M, Wakimoto H, et al. De novo mutations in histone-modifying genes in congenital heart disease. Nature 2013;498(7453):220–3.

19. Roberts AE, Allanson JE, Tartaglia M, et al. Noonan syndrome. Lancet 2013;381(9863):333–42.

20. Tartaglia M, Kalidas K, Shaw A, et al. PTPN11 mutations in Noonan syndrome: molecular spectrum, genotype-phenotype correlation, and phenotypic heterogeneity. Am J Hum Genet 2002;70(6): 1555–63.

21. Lin AE, Basson CT, Goldmuntz E, et al. Adults with genetic syndromes and cardiovascular abnormalities: clinical history and management. Genet Med 2008;10(7):469–94.

22. Shaw AC, Kalidas K, Crosby AH, et al. The natural history of Noonan syndrome: a long-term follow-up study. Arch Dis Child 2007;92(2):128–32.

23. Carcavilla A, Santome JL, Pinto I, et al. LEOPARD syndrome: a variant of Noonan syndrome strongly associated with hypertrophic cardiomyopathy. Rev Esp Cardiol 2013;66(5):350–6.

24. Gorlin RJ, Anderson RC, Blaw M. Multiple lentigenes syndrome. Am J Dis Child 1969;117(6): 652–62.

25. Pober BR. Williams-Beuren syndrome. N Engl J Med 2010;362(3):239–52.

26. Greutmann M, Tobler D, Sharma NC, et al. Cardiac outcomes in adults with supravalvar aortic stenosis. Eur Heart J 2012;33(19):2442–50.

27. Peyvandi S, Lupo PJ, Garbarini J, et al. 22q11.2 deletions in patients with conotruncal defects: data from 1,610 consecutive cases. Pediatr Cardiol 2013;34:1687–94.

28. John AS, Rychik J, Khan M, et al. 22q11.2 deletion syndrome as a risk factor for aortic root dilation in tetralogy of Fallot. Cardiol Young 2013;1–8. [E-pub ahead of print].

29. Greenway SC, Pereira AC, Lin JC, et al. De novo copy number variants identify new genes and loci in isolated sporadic tetralogy of Fallot. Nat Genet 2009;41(8):931–5.

30. Charron F, Paradis P, Bronchain O, et al. Cooperative interaction between GATA-4 and GATA-6 regulates myocardial gene expression. Mol Cell Biol 1999;19(6):4355–65.

31. Aries A, Paradis P, Lefebvre C, et al. Essential role of GATA-4 in cell survival and drug-induced cardiotoxicity. Proc Natl Acad Sci U S A 2004;101(18): 6975–80.

32. Epstein JA, Rader DJ, Parmacek MS. Perspective: cardiovascular disease in the postgenomic era—lessons learned and challenges ahead. Endocrinology 2002;143(6):2045–50.

33. de la Pompa JL, Timmerman LA, Takimoto H, et al. Role of the NF-ATc transcription factor in morphogenesis of cardiac valves and septum. Nature 1998;392(6672):182–6.

34. Abdul-Sater Z, Yehya A, Beresian J, et al. Two heterozygous mutations in NFATC1 in a patient with tricuspid atresia. PLoS One 2012;7(11): e49532.

35. Yehya A, Souki R, Bitar F, et al. Differential duplication of an intronic region in the NFATC1 gene in patients with congenital heart disease. Genome 2006; 49(9):1092–8.

36. Azzam R, Hariri F, El-Hachem N, et al. Regulation of de novo ceramide synthesis: the role of dihydroceramide desaturase and transcriptional factors NFATC and Hand2 in the hypoxic mouse heart. DNA Cell Biol 2013;32(6):310–9.

37. Planavila A, Dominguez E, Navarro M, et al. Dilated cardiomyopathy and mitochondrial dysfunction in Sirt1-deficient mice: a role for Sirt1-Mef2 in adult heart. J Mol Cell Cardiol 2012;53(4):521–31.

38. Movassagh M, Choy MK, Goddard M, et al. Differential DNA methylation correlates with differential expression of angiogenic factors in human heart failure. PloS One 2010;5(1):e8564.

39. Haberland M, Montgomery RL, Olson EN. The many roles of histone deacetylases in development and physiology: implications for disease and therapy. Nat Rev Genet 2009;10(1):32–42.

40. Creemers EE, Wilde AA, Pinto YM. Heart failure: advances through genomics. Nat Rev Genet 2011;12(5):357–62.

41. Krishnan J, Suter M, Windak R, et al. Activation of a HIF1alpha-PPARgamma axis underlies the integration of glycolytic and lipid anabolic pathways in pathologic cardiac hypertrophy. Cell Metab 2009; 9(6):512–24.

42. Amati F, Diano L, Campagnolo L, et al. Hif1alpha down-regulation is associated with transposition of great arteries in mice treated with a retinoic acid antagonist. BMC Genomics 2010;11:497.

43. Piran S, Liu P, Morales A, et al. Where genome meets phenome: rationale for integrating genetic and protein biomarkers in the diagnosis and management of dilated cardiomyopathy and heart failure. J Am Coll Cardiol 2012;60(4):283–9.

44. Lin D, Hollander Z, Meredith A, et al. Molecular signatures of end-stage heart failure. J Card Fail 2011; 17(10):867–74.

45. van der Bom T, Winter MM, Bouma BJ, et al. Effect of valsartan on systemic right ventricular function: a double-blind, randomized, placebo-controlled pilot trial. Circulation 2013;127(3):322–30.

46. Dorn GW 2nd. Adrenergic signaling polymorphisms and their impact on cardiovascular disease. Physiol Rev 2010;90(3):1013–62.

47. Mital S, Chung WK, Colan SD, et al. Renin-angiotensin-aldosterone genotype influences ventricular remodeling in infants with single ventricle. Circulation 2011;123(21):2353–62.

48. Jeewa A, Manickaraj AK, Mertens L, et al. Genetic determinants of right-ventricular remodeling after tetralogy of Fallot repair. Pediatr Res 2012;72(4): 407–13.

49. Mordwinkin NM, Burridge PW, Wu JC. A review of human pluripotent stem cell-derived cardiomyocytes for high-throughput drug discovery, cardiotoxicity screening, and publication standards. J Cardiovasc Transl Res 2013;6(1):22–30.

50. Lan F, Lee AS, Liang P, et al. Abnormal calcium handling properties underlie familial hypertrophic cardiomyopathy pathology in patient-specific induced pluripotent stem cells. Cell Stem Cell 2013;12(1): 101–13.

51. Liang P, Lan F, Lee AS, et al. Drug screening using a library of human induced pluripotent stem cell-derived cardiomyocytes reveals disease-specific patterns of cardiotoxicity. Circulation 2013; 127(16):1677–91.

Index

Note: Page numbers of article titles are in **boldface** type.

Heart Failure Clin 10 (2014) 229–232
http://dx.doi.org/10.1016/S1551-7136(13)00136-0
1551-7136/14/$ – see front matter © 2014 Elsevier Inc. All rights reserved.

heartfailure.theclinics.com

Printed and bound by CPI Group (UK) Ltd, Croydon, CR0 4YY

03/10/2024

01040378-0004